PARKINSON'S DISEASE

THE LIFE CYCLE OF THE DOPAMINE NEURON

ANNALS OF THE NEW YORK ACADEMY OF SCIENCES

Volume 991

PARKINSON'S DISEASE

THE LIFE CYCLE OF THE DOPAMINE NEURON

*Edited by Howard J. Federoff, Robert E. Burke,
Stanley Fahn, and Gary Fiskum*

The New York Academy of Sciences
New York, New York
2003

Library of Congress Cataloging-in-Publication Data

Parkinson's disease: the life cycle of the dopamine neuron / edited by Howard J. Federoff . . . [et al.].
    p. ; cm. -- (Annals of the New York Academy of Sciences ; v. 991)
"This volume is the result of a conference entitled Parkinson's disease: the life cycle of the dopamine neuron, sponsored by the New York Academy of Sciences held on September 18-20, 2002 in Princeton, New Jersey"--Contents p.
Includes bibliographical references and index.
    ISBN 1-57331-448-X (cloth : alk. paper) -- ISBN 1-57331-449-8 (paper : alk. paper)
    1. Parkinson's disease--Pathophysiology--Congresses. 2. Parkinson's disease--Molecular aspects--Congresses. 3. Dopaminergic neurons--Congresses. 4. Dopaminergic mechanisms--Congresses.
    [DNLM: 1. Parkinson's Disease--Congresses. 2. Dopamine--biosynthesis--Congresses. WL 359 P25176 2003] I. Federoff, Howard. II. Series.
    Q11.N5 vol. 991
    [RC382]
    500 s--dc21
    [616.8/33

                                                                            2003009584

GYAT / PCP
Printed in the United States of America
ISBN 1-57331-448-X (cloth)
ISBN 1-57331-449-8 (paper)
ISSN 0077-8923

ANNALS OF THE NEW YORK ACADEMY OF SCIENCES

Volume 991
June 2003

PARKINSON'S DISEASE

THE LIFE CYCLE OF THE DOPAMINE NEURON

Editors
HOWARD J. FEDEROFF, ROBERT E. BURKE, STANLEY FAHN,
AND GARY FISKUM

Conference Organizers
HOWARD J. FEDEROFF, ROBERT E. BURKE, STANLEY FAHN,
GARY FISKUM, AND OLE ISACSON

This volume is the result of a conference entitled **Parkinson's Disease: The Life Cycle of the Dopamine Neuron**, which was sponsored by the New York Academy of Sciences and held September 18–20 in Princeton, New Jersey.

CONTENTS

Preface. *By* HOWARD J. FEDEROFF. ix

Part I. Clinical Syndrome

Description of Parkinson's Disease as a Clinical Syndrome.
By STANLEY FAHN 1

Physiology and Pathophysiology of Parkinson's Disease. *By* CLEMENT
HAMANI AND ANDRES M. LOZANO 15

PET Studies on the Function of Dopamine in Health and Parkinson's Disease.
By DAVID J. BROOKS 22

Part II. Development

Midbrain Dopaminergic Neurons: Determination of Their Developmental
Fate by Transcription Factors. *By* HORST H. SIMON, LAVINIA BHATT,
DANIEL GHERBASSI, PAOLA SGADÓ, AND LAVINIA ALBERÍ 36

Transcriptional Control of Dopamine Neuron Development. *By* ÅSA WALLÉN
AND THOMAS PERLMANN 48

Transcription Factors in the Development of Midbrain Dopamine Neurons. *By* J. PETER H. BURBACH, SIMONE SMITS, AND MARTEN P. SMIDT 61

Postnatal Developmental Programmed Cell Death in Dopamine Neurons. *By* ROBERT E. BURKE 69

Part III. From Molecules to Organism: The Molecules

The Cast of Molecular Characters in Parkinson's Disease: Felons, Conspirators, and Suspects. *By* KAH LEONG LIM, VALINA L. DAWSON, AND TED M. DAWSON 80

Oxidative Modifications of α-Synuclein. *By* HARRY ISCHIROPOULOS 93

Parkin and Endoplasmic Reticulum Stress. *By* RYOSUKE TAKAHASHI, YUZURU IMAI, NOBUTAKA HATTORI, AND YOSHIKUNI MIZUNO 101

Parkinson's Disease and Related α-Synucleinopathies Are Brain Amyloidoses. *By* JOHN Q. TROJANOWSKI AND VIRGINIA M-Y. LEE 107

Part IV. From Molecules to Organism: The Cells

Mitochondrial Mechanisms of Neural Cell Death and Neuroprotective Interventions in Parkinson's Disease. *By* GARY FISKUM, ANATOLY STARKOV, BRIAN M. POLSTER, AND CHRISTOS CHINOPOULOS 111

Mitochondria, Oxidative Damage, and Inflammation in Parkinson's Disease. *By* M. FLINT BEAL 120

Apoptosis Inducing Factor and PARP-Mediated Injury in the MPTP Mouse Model of Parkinson's Disease. *By* HONGMIN WANG, MIKA SHIMOJI, SEONG-WOON YU, TED M. DAWSON, AND VALINA L. DAWSON 132

Cellular Models to Study Dopaminergic Injury Responses. *By* TIMOTHY J. COLLIER, KATHY STEECE-COLLIER, SUSAN MCGUIRE, AND CARYL E. SORTWELL 140

Convergent Pathobiologic Model of Parkinson's Disease. *By* KATHLEEN A. MAGUIRE-ZEISS AND HOWARD J. FEDEROFF 152

The Relationship between Lewy Body Disease, Parkinson's Disease, and Alzheimer's Disease. *By* JOHN HARDY 167

Part V. From Molecules to Organism: The Organism

Transgenic Models of α-Synuclein Pathology: Past, Present, and Future. *By* MAKOTO HASHIMOTO, EDWARD ROCKENSTEIN, AND ELIEZER MASLIAH . . 171

The 1-Methyl-4-Phenyl-1,2,3,6-Tetrahydropyridine Mouse Model: A Tool to Explore the Pathogenesis of Parkinson's Disease. *By* SERGE PRZEDBORSKI AND MIQUEL VILA 189

Pathophysiology of Parkinson's Disease: The MPTP Primate Model of the Human Disorder. *By* THOMAS WICHMANN AND MAHLON R. DELONG. . . 199

The Role of Glial Reaction and Inflammation in Parkinson's Disease. *By* E. C. HIRSCH, T. BREIDERT, E. ROUSSELET, S. HUNOT, A. HARTMANN, AND P. P. MICHEL 214

Part VI. Convergence of Cell Genesis and Cell Transfer

Induction of Adult Neurogenesis: Molecular Manipulation of Neural Precursors *in Situ. By* PAOLA ARLOTTA, SANJAY S. MAGAVI, AND JEFFREY D. MACKLIS 229

Molecular Mechanisms of Neuronal Cell Death. *By* KIM A. HEIDENREICH 237

Redox State as a Central Modulator of Precursor Cell Function. *By* MARK NOBLE, JOEL SMITH, JENNIFER POWER, AND MARGOT MAYER-PRÖSCHEL 251

COX-2 and Neurodegeneration in Parkinson's Disease. *By* P. TEISMANN, M. VILA, D.-K. CHOI, K. TIEU, D. C. WU, V. JACKSON-LEWIS, AND S. PRZEDBORSKI 272

Part VII. Poster Papers

Striatopallidal Changes in a Preclinical Rat Model of Parkinson's Disease. *By* A. E. GRISSELL, T. M. BUCHANAN, AND M. A. ARIANO 278

Neurotoxicity-Induced Changes in Striatal Dopamine Receptor Function. *By* ANNA-LIISA BROWNELL, IRIS Y. CHEN, XUKUI WANG, MEIXIANG YU, AND BRUCE G. JENKINS 281

The Developmental Time Course of Glial Cell Line–Derived Neurotrophic Factor (GDNF) and GDNF Receptor α-1 mRNA Expression in the Striatum and Substantia Nigra. *By* JINWHAN CHO, NIKOLAI G. KHOLODILOV, AND ROBERT E. BURKE 284

Subcellular Compartmentalization of P-ERKs in the Lewy Body Disease Substantia Nigra. *By* CHARLEEN T. CHU AND JIAN-HUI ZHU 288

Altered Striatal Neuronal Morphology Is Associated with Astrogliosis in a Chronic Mouse Model of Parkinson's Disease. *By* A. G. DERVAN, S. TOTTERDELL, Y.-S. LAU, AND G. E. MEREDITH 291

Is the Initial Insult in Parkinson's Disease and Dementia with Lewy Bodies a Neuritic Dystrophy? *By* JOHN E. DUDA, BENOIT I. GIASSON, VIRGINIA M-Y. LEE, AND JOHN Q. TROJANOWSKI 295

Neuroplasticity in the MPTP-Lesioned Mouse and Nonhuman Primate. *By* MICHAEL W. JAKOWEC, BETH FISHER, KERRY NIXON, ELIZABETH HOGG, CHARLES MESHUL, SAMUEL BREMMER, TOM MCNEILL, AND GISELLE M. PETZINGER 298

An Experimental Infection by Filterable Forms of *Nocardia asteroides* and Late-Onset Movement Disorder in Mice. *By* S. KOHBATA AND C. KADOYA 302

A Characterization of Dopaminergic Neurodegeneration in Organotypic Cultures. *By* GERALDINE J. KRESS AND IAN J. REYNOLDS 304

Developmental Cell Death and Oxidative Stress: Lessons from Nigral Dopamine Neurons. *By* LAURENT GROC, TANGELLA JACKSON HUNTER, HAO JIANG, LAURENT BEZIN, AND ROBERT A. LEVINE 307

Identification of a Novel Gene Linked to Parkin via a Bidirectional Promoter. *By* PAUL J. LOCKHART, ANDREW B. WEST, CASEY A. O'FARRELL, AND MATTHEW J. FARRER 311

Gene Expression Analysis of the MPTP-Lesioned Substantia Nigra in Mice. *By* R. M. MILLER, C. CASACELI, L. CHEN, AND H. J. FEDEROFF 315

Neuroimaging and Proteomic Tracking of Neurodegeneration in MPTP-Treated Mice. *By* HOWARD E. GENDELMAN, CHRISTOPHER J. DESTACHE, MARINA L. ZELIVYANSKAYA, JAY A. NELSON, MICHAEL D. BOSKA, TONI M. BISKUP, MICHAEL K. MCCARTHY, KIMBERLY A. CARLSON, CRAIG NEMECHEK, ERIC J. BENNER, AND R. LEE MOSLEY 319

PCBs and Dopamine Function: Neurological Effects of Polychlorinated Biphenyls: Does Occupational Exposure Alter Dopamine-Mediated Function? *By* RICHARD F. SEEGAL 322

A Murine Model of ALS-PDC with Behavioral and Neuropathological Features of Parkinsonism. *By* J. D. SCHULZ, J. M. B. WILSON, AND C. A. SHAW 326

Neuroprotective Ganglioside Derivatives. *By* K. CONN, S. DOHERTY, P. EISENHAUER, R. FINE, J. WELLS, AND M. D. ULLMAN 330

Redox- and Metalloregulated RNA Bioaptamer Targets of Proteins Associated with Parkinson's and Other Neurodegenerative Diseases: Factors of Relevance in the Life Cycle of Cells. *By* JOSEF H. WISSLER 333

Dopaminergic Stimulatory Polypeptides from Immortalized Striatal Cells. *By* ALFRED HELLER, MARTIN GROSS, SUZANNE HESSEFORT, NANCY BUBULA, AND LISA WON 339

Glutathione and Ascorbate: Their Role in Protein Glutathione Mixed Disulfide Formation during Oxidative Stress and Potential Relevance to Parkinson's Disease. *By* GAIL D. ZEEVALK, LAURA P. BERNARD, AND JULIE EHRHART 342

Dopaminergic Neurons in Human Striatum and Neurogenesis in Adult Monkey Striatum. *By* MARTINE COSSETTE, ANDRÉANNE BÉDARD, AND ANDRÉ PARENT 346

Secreted Factors from Primary Midbrain Glia Regulate Nurr1 Activity. *By* Y. LUO AND H. J. FEDEROFF 350

Development of Nurr1 Stable Cell Lines for the Identification of Downstream Targets. *By* YU LUO, LEIGH A. HENRICKSEN, KATHLEEN A. MAGUIRE-ZEISS, AND HOWARD J. FEDEROFF 354

* * *

Index of Contributors 359

The conference on which these proceedings are based was made possible by an educational grant from the U.S. Army Medical Research and Materiel Command.

Preface

Parkinson's disease and its motor manifestations result predominantly from a loss of midbrain dopamine neurons. Although other neuronal populations are also affected in the disease, we conceptualized this meeting and volume around the theme of the life cycle of the dopamine neuron. By bringing together neurologists, neuro-surgeons, developmental biologists, neuropathologists, fly geneticists, systems and other neuroscientists, and molecular biologists, we hoped for an extensive inter-disciplinary exchange of ideas to occur. By all accounts this did happen: the level of discussion throughout the meeting ranged over the entire spectrum of scientific approaches and levels of inquiry.

This meeting would not have occurred without the thoughtful suggestions of Col. Karl Friedl, Ph.D., and Stephen Grate, Ph.D. As important, the support provided by Col. Friedl and the Department of Defense was essential to achieving the proper set-ting, balance of participants, and sponsorship by the prestigious New York Academy of Sciences. The inspiration for the meeting arose from the highly interactive and prescient Organizing Committee. The New York Academy of Sciences' Dr. Rashid Shaikh, Renée Wilkerson-Brown, and other staff members provided critical guid-ance and operations assistance that made the meeting successful. The completion of the proceedings would not have been possible without the stewardship of the New York Academy of Sciences' Richard Stiefel. On behalf of the Organizing Committee I am extremely thankful to all who contributed to making Parkinson's Disease: The Life Cycle of the Dopamine Neuron a most enjoyable and stimulating conference and, it is hoped, a useful book.

HOWARD J. FEDEROFF, M.D., PH.D.
Professor of Neurology
University of Rochester School of Medicine

Description of Parkinson's Disease as a Clinical Syndrome

STANLEY FAHN

Department of Neurology, Columbia University College of Physicians & Surgeons, New York, New York 10032, USA

ABSTRACT: Parkinsonism is a clinical syndrome comprising combinations of motor problems—namely, bradykinesia, resting tremor, rigidity, flexed posture, "freezing," and loss of postural reflexes. Parkinson's disease (PD) is the major cause of parkinsonism. PD is a slowly progressive parkinsonian syndrome that begins insidiously and usually affects one side of the body before spreading to involve the other side. Pathology shows loss of neuromelanin-containing monoamine neurons, particularly dopamine (DA) neurons in the substantia nigra pars compacta. A pathologic hallmark is the presence of cytoplasmic eosinophilic inclusions (Lewy bodies) in monoamine neurons. The loss of DA content in the nigrostriatal neurons accounts for many of the motor symptoms, which can be ameliorated by DA replacement therapy—that is, levodopa. Most cases are sporadic, of unknown etiology; but rare cases of monogenic mutations (10 genes at present count) show that there are multiple causes for the neuronal degeneration. The pathogenesis of PD remains unknown. Clinical fluctuations and dyskinesias are frequent complications of levodopa therapy; these, as well as some motor features of PD, improve by resetting the abnormal brain physiology towards normal by surgical therapy. Nonmotor symptoms (depression, lack of motivation, passivity, and dementia) are common. As the disease progresses, even motor symptoms become intractable to therapy. No proven means of slowing progression have yet been found.

KEYWORDS: Parkinson's disease; parkinsonism; Lewy body; dopamine; levodopa

HISTORICAL INTRODUCTION

Clinical Description

By amazing coincidence, James Parkinson published a monograph describing the entity subsequently bearing his name in the same year, 1817, that the New York Academy of Sciences was founded.[1] He described six individuals with the clinical features. One was followed in detail over a long period of time; the other five consisted of brief descriptions, including two whom he had met walking in the street and another whom he had observed at a distance. Such distant observations without a medical examination demonstrates how readily distinguishable the condition is

Address for correspondence: Dr. Stanley Fahn, Neurological Institute, 710 West 168th Street, New York, NY 10032. Voice: 212-305-5295; fax: 212-305-3530.
fahn@neuro.columbia.edu

Ann. N.Y. Acad. Sci. 991: 1–14 (2003). © 2003 New York Academy of Sciences.

merely from the patients' appearance of flexed posture, resting tremor, and shuffling gait. Parkinson's opening description has the key essentials: "Involuntary tremulous motion, with lessened muscular power, in parts not in action and even when supported; with a propensity to bend the trunk forward, and to pass from a walking to a running pace: the senses and intellects being uninjured." Despite the small number of patients examined, Parkinson provided a detailed description of the symptoms and also discussed the progressive worsening of the disorder, which he called the *shaking palsy* and by the Latin term *paralysis agitans*.

In his monograph, Parkinson reviewed the different kinds of tremors previously reported and specifically cited the tremor in his "An Essay on the Shaking Palsy" as occurring when the body part is at rest and not during an active voluntary movement. Seventy years later Charcot emphasized that tremor need not be present in the disorder and argued against the term *paralysis agitans*; he suggested, instead, that the name of the disorder be *Parkinson's disease* (see Goetz, 1987[2] for English translation).

The terms *paralysis* and *palsy* in *paralysis agitans* and *shaking palsy* are also inappropriate. There is no true paralysis. Today, the "lessened muscular power" mentioned by Parkinson is recognized to be a slowness of movement that is called *akinesia, hypokinesia,* or *bradykinesia*, all three terms often being used interchangeably. These terms represent a paucity of movement in the absence of weakness or paralysis.

Recognition and development of the term *akinesia* came about slowly. Charcot, in his Tuesday Lessons of 1888, related slowness to rigidity and specifically excluded weakness as a cause (see Ref. 2). Gowers in 1893[3] described Parkinson's disease as consisting of tremor, weakness, rigidity, flexed posture, and short steps, with slowness due in part to rigidity. Oppenheim in 1911[4] mentioned that impairment and retardation of active movements might occur in the absence of rigidity. He did not relate it to weakness. Wechsler in the 1932 edition of his textbook[5] commented on the special difficulty of initiation of movement as a feature of slowness. Wilson in his large neurology opus of 1940[6] used the terms *akinesia, akinesis,* and *hypokinesia*. Under these terms, he related the masked facies, the unblinking eyes, the poverty of movement, and the patient sitting immobile. Schwab, England, and Peterson devoted an entire paper in 1959[7] to the subject of akinesia, which by this time was firmly established as the "lessened muscular power" mentioned by Parkinson. Within the definition of *akinesia*, these authors mentioned fatigue, decrementing amplitude of movements, difficulty shifting to other contraction patterns, apathy, inability to complete actions, difficulty initiating an act, and the ability to reach normal movement briefly under sudden motivation. Furthermore, they described the difficulty for a patient with Parkinson's disease to execute two motor events simultaneously, all under the rubric of *akinesia*.

Pathology of Parkinson's Disease

It was many years after Parkinson's original description before the basal ganglia were recognized by Meynert in 1871[8] as being involved in disorders of abnormal movements. And it was not until 1895 that the substantia nigra was suggested to be affected in Parkinson's disease. Brissaud (1895)[9] suggested this on the basis of a report by Blocq and Marinesco (1893)[10] of a tuberculoma in that site that was associated with hemiparkinsonian tremor. These authors were careful to point out that the pyramidal tract and the brachium conjuctivum above and below the level of the lesion contained no degenerating fibers. The importance of the substantia nigra was emphasized by Tretiakoff in 1919,[11] who studied the substantia nigra in nine cases of Parkinson's disease, one case of hemiparkinsonism, and three cases of postencephalitic parkinsonism, finding lesions in this nucleus in all cases. With the hemiparkinsonian case Tretiakoff found a lesion in the nigra on the opposite side, concluding that the nucleus served the motor activity on the contralateral side of the body. The substantia nigra, so named because of its normal content of neuromelanin pigment, was noted to show depigmentation, loss of nerve cells, and gliosis. These findings remain the histopathologic features of the disease. In his study, Tretiakoff also confirmed the earlier observation of Lewy (1914),[12] who had discovered the presence of cytoplasmic inclusions in Parkinson's disease, now widely recognized as the major pathologic hallmark of the disorder and referred to as *Lewy bodies*.

Foix and Nicolesco made a detailed study of the pathology of Parkinson's disease in 1925[13] and found that the most constant and severe lesions are in the substantia nigra. Since then many workers, including Hassler (1938)[14] and Greenfield and Bosanquet (1953),[15] have confirmed these findings and added other observations, including involvement of other brain stem nuclei such as the locus ceruleus.

Biochemistry of Parkinson's Disease

Prior to 1957, the parkinsonian syndrome in animals and humans induced by reserpine was thought to be due to a depletion of brain serotonin. But in that year Carlsson and colleagues[16] discovered that L-dopa reversed the reserpine-induced parkinsonian state in rabbits; while the precursor of serotonin, L-5-hydroxytryptophan, did not. L-dopa is the precursor to dopamine and norepinephrine, and at that time it was thought that dopamine did not have an independent function but served solely as a precursor of norepinephrine. In 1958, after he developed a method for its chemical assay, Carlsson determined that dopamine was present in brain.[17] By the following year the regional distribution of dopamine was mapped out in brain in both animals[18] and humans.[19] In 1959, at the International Catecholamine Symposium, Carlsson suggested that Parkinson's disease was related to brain dopamine.[20] In 1960, Ehringer and Hornykiewicz, using Carlsson's methodology, measured dopamine and norepinephrine in humans with basal ganglia disorders and discovered a neostriatal dopamine deficiency in parkinsonism.[21] Thus began the modern era of understanding parkinsonism and the role of dopamine in brain. Carlsson's contributions eventually led to his being awarded the Nobel Prize in Physiology and Medicine in 2000.

DISTINGUISHING BETWEEN PARKINSON'S DISEASE AND PARKINSONISM

The syndrome of parkinsonism must be understood before understanding what is Parkinson's disease. Today, the term *parkinsonism* is defined by any combination of six specific motoric features: tremor at rest, bradykinesia, rigidity, loss of postural reflexes, flexed posture (FIG. 1), and the freezing phenomenon (where the feet are

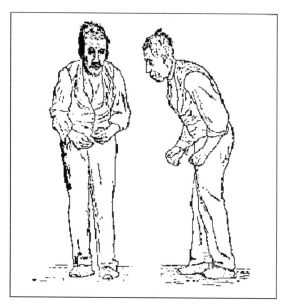

FIGURE 1. Drawing of a patient with Parkinson disease demonstrating the flexed posture typically seen in this disorder. (Modified from Gowers, 1893, p. 639.[3])

transiently "glued to the ground")[22] (TABLE 1). Not all six of these cardinal features need be present, but at least two should be before the diagnosis of parkinsonism is made, with at least one of them being tremor at rest or bradykinesia. Parkinsonism is classified into four categories (TABLE 2). PD or primary parkinsonism will be the principal focus of this volume. It is the category that is most commonly encountered by the general clinician; it is also the category on which much research has been carried out and the one we know the most about. The great majority of cases of primary parkinsonism are sporadic, but in the last few years several gene mutations have been discovered to cause PD (TABLE 3). Whether primary parkinsonism is genetic or idiopathic in etiology, the common denominator is that it is not caused by known insults to the brain (the main feature of secondary parkinsonism) and is not associated with other motoric neurologic features (the main feature of Parkinson-plus syndromes). The uncovering of genetic causes of primary parkinsonism has shed light on probable pathogenetic mechanisms that may be a factor in even the more common idiopathic cases of PD. It may even turn out that many of the idiopathic cases will be linked to gene mutations, this discovery is yet to be made. Although the term *idiopathic PD* has been applied to primary parkinsonism, the fact that there are now known genetic causes encourages us to adopt instead the term *primary parkinsonism*, for the former term implies that the etiology is unknown.

Three of the most helpful clues that one is likely to be dealing with PD rather than another category of parkinsonism are: (1) an asymmetrical onset of symptoms (PD often begins on one side of the body); (2) the presence of rest tremor (although rest tremor may be absent in patients with PD, it is almost always absent in Parkinson-

TABLE 1. Six cardinal clinical features of parkinsonism

Tremor at rest	Flexed posture of neck, trunk, and limbs
Rigidity	Loss of postural reflexes
Bradykinesia/hypokinesia/akinesia	Freezing phenomenon

TABLE 2. Classification of the parkinsonian states

Primary parkinsonism (Parkinson's disease)
  Sporadic
  Known genetic etiology (see Table 3)
Secondary parkinsonism (environmental etiology
  Drugs
    Dopamine receptor blockers (most commonly antipsychotic medications)
    Dopamine storage depletors (reserpine, tetrabenazine)
  Postencephalitic
  Toxins: Mn,CO, MPTP, cyanide
  Vascular
  Brain tumors
  Head trauma
  Normal-pressure hydrocephalus
Parkinsonism-plus syndromes
  Progressive supranuclear palsy
  Multiple system atrophy
  Cortical-basal ganglionic degeneration
  Parkinson-dementia-ALS complex of Guam
  Progressive pallidal atrophy
  Diffuse Lewy body disease (DLBD)
Heredodegenerative disorders
  Alzheimer's disease
  Wilson's disease
  Huntington's disease
  Frontotemporal dementia (tau mutation on chromosome 17q21)
  X-linked dystonia-parkinsonism (in Filipino men; known as lubag)

plus syndromes); and (3) substantial clinical response to adequate levodopa therapy (usually, Parkinson-plus syndromes do not respond to levodopa therapy). In this chapter, we will concentrate on PD and not the other categories of parkinsonism. One common misdiagnosis as PD is the presence of tremor due to the entity known as *essential tremor*, which can even be unilateral, although it more commonly is bilateral. Helpful in the diagnosis is that the tremor due to PD is a rest tremor (tremor appears with the affected body part is at rest), whereas the tremor due to essential tremor is not present at rest, but appears with holding the arms in front of the body and increases in amplitude with activity of the arm, such as with handwriting or performing the finger-to-nose maneuver.

TABLE 3. Genetic forms of primary parkinsonism

Name of gene	Protein	Chromosome
Autosomal dominant transmission		
PARK1	α-synculein	4q21-q22
PARK3	?	2p13
PARK4	Iowa pedigree: PD/ET	4p15
PARK5	ubiquitin C terminal hydrolase-L1 (UCH-L1)	4p14
PARK8	?	12p11.2-q13.1
Dopa-responsive dystonia	GTP cyclohydrolase 1	14q22.1-q22.2
Autosomal recessive transmission		
PARK2	parkin (ubiquitin ligase)	6q25.2-q27
PARK6	?	1p35-p36
PARK7	DJ-1	1p36
PARK9	?	1p36
PARK10	?	1p32
Tyrosine hydroxylase deficiencey		11p11.5

CLINICAL FEATURES AND EPIDEMIOLOGY OF PARKINSON'S DISEASE

The symptoms of PD begin insidiously and gradually worsen. Rest tremor, because it is so obvious, is often the first symptom recognized by the patient. But the illness sometimes begins with bradykinesia; and in some patients, tremor may never develop. Bradykinesia manifests as slowness, such as slower and smaller handwriting, decreased arm swing and leg stride when walking, decreased facial expression, and decreased amplitude of voice. Rest tremor can be intermittent at the beginning, being present only in stressful situations; eventually it tends to be present most of the time and worsens in amplitude with stress or excitement. There is a steady worsening of symptoms over time; if untreated, the symptoms lead to disability with severe immobility and falling. The early symptoms and signs of PD—rest tremor, bradykinesia, and rigidity—are related to progressive loss of nigrostriatal dopamine. These signs and symptoms result from striatal dopamine deficiency and are usually correctable by levodopa and dopamine agonists. As PD progresses over time, symptoms that do not respond to levodopa develop, such as flexed posture, the freezing phenomenon, and loss of postural reflexes; these are often referred to as non-dopamine-related features of PD. Moreover, bradykinesia that responded to levodopa in the early stage of PD increases as the disease worsens and no longer fully responds to levodopa. It is particularly these intractable motoric symptoms that lead to the disabilities of increasing immobility and balance difficulties (FIG. 2).

While the motor symptoms of PD dominate the clinical picture—and even define the parkinsonian syndrome—many patients with PD have other complaints that have been classified as *nonmotor* (see TABLE 4). These include fatigue, depression, anxiety, sleep disturbances, constipation, bladder and other autonomic disturbances (sexual, gastrointestinal), and sensory complaints. Sensory symptoms include pain,

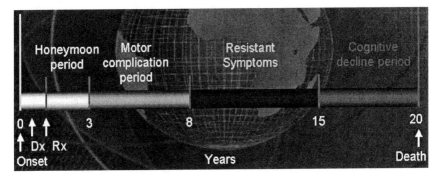

FIGURE 2. Diagram of a typical clinical course of Parkinson's disease despite therapy.

TABLE 4. Nonmotor features of Parkinson's disease

Personality and behavior	Autonomic
depression'	hypotension
fear	bladder problems
anxiety	constipation
passivity	sexual dysfunction
dependence	seborrhea
loss of motivation, apathy	sweating
Cognition and mental	**Sleep problems**
bradyphrenia	sleep fragmentation
"tip of the tongue" phenomenon	REM sleep behavior disorder
dementia	excessive daytime sleepiness
Sensory	altered sleep-wake cycle
pain	**Fatigue**
paresthesiae	
numbness	
burning	
akathisia	
restless legs syndrome	

numbness, tingling, and burning in the affected limbs; these occur in about 40% of patients. Behavioral and mental alterations are common and include changes in mood, decreased motivation and apathy, slowness in thinking (bradyphrenia), and a declining cognition that can progress to dementia. Dementia is most common in those with an older age at onset of PD and can occur in about 40% of such patients; this becomes more disabling than the motoric features of PD (FIG. 2).

The development of dementia in a patient with parkinsonism remains a difficult differential diagnosis. If the patient's parkinsonian features did not respond to levodopa, the diagnosis is likely to be Alzheimer disease, which can occasionally present with features of parkinsonism. If the presenting parkinsonism responded to levodopa and the patient developed dementia over time, the diagnosis could be either

PD or diffuse Lewy body disease (DLBD) (also called dementia with Lewy bodies). If hallucinations occur with or without levodopa therapy, DLBD is the most likely diagnosis. DLBD is a condition where Lewy bodies are present in the cerebral cortex as well as in the brain stem nuclei. The heredodegenerative disease known as *frontotemporal dementia* is an autosomal dominant disorder due to mutations in the tau gene on chromosome 17; the full syndrome presents with dementia, loss of inhibition, parkinsonism, and sometimes muscle wasting.

Although PD can develop at any age, it begins most commonly in older adults, with a peak age at onset at around 60 years. The likelihood of developing PD increases with age, with a lifetime risk of about 2%.[23] A positive family history doubles the risk of developing PD to about 4%. Twin studies indicate that PD with an onset under the age of 50 years is more likely to have a genetic relationship than PD with a later age at onset.[24] Males have higher prevalence and incidence rates than females. Patients with PD can live 20 or more years, depending on the age at onset. The mortality rate is about 1.6 times that of normal individuals of the same age.[25] Death in PD is usually due to some concurrent unrelated illness or due to the effects of decreased mobility, aspiration, or increased falling with subsequent physical injury. At the present time, approximately 850,000 individuals in the U.S. have PD, with the number expected to grow as the population ages.

There are no practical diagnostic laboratory tests for PD, and the diagnosis rests on the clinical features and on excluding other causes of parkinsonism. The research tool of fluorodopa (FDOPA) positron emission tomography (PET) measures levodopa uptake into dopamine nerve terminals, and this shows a decline of about 8% per year of the striatal uptake. A similar result is seen using ligands for the dopamine transporter, either by PET or by single-photon emission computed tomography (SPECT); these ligands also label the dopamine nerve terminals. All these neuroimaging techniques reveal decreased dopaminergic nerve terminals in the striatum in both PD and the Parkinson-plus syndromes and do not distinguish between them. A substantial response to levodopa is most helpful in the differential diagnosis, indicating presynaptic dopamine deficiency with intact postsynaptic dopamine receptors, features typical of PD.

Some adults may develop a more benign form of PD, in which the symptoms respond to very-low-dosage levodopa, and the disease does not worsen severely with time. This form is usually due to the autosomal dominant disorder known as doparesponsive dystonia, which typically begins in childhood as a dystonia. But when it starts in adult life, it can present with parkinsonism. There is no neuronal degeneration. The pathogenesis is due to a biochemical deficiency involving dopamine synthesis. The gene defect is for an enzyme (GTP cyclohydrolase I) required to synthesize the cofactor for tyrosine hydroxylase activity, the crucial rate-limiting first step in the synthesis of dopamine and norepinephrine. Infantile parkinsonism is due to the autosomal recessive deficiency of tyrosine hydroxylase, another cause of a biochemical dopamine deficiency disorder.

PATHOLOGY, BIOCHEMISTRY AND PHYSIOLOGY OF PARKINSON'S DISEASE

PD and the Parkinson-plus syndromes have in common a degeneration of substantia nigra pars compacta dopaminergic neurons, with a resulting deficiency of striatal

TABLE 5. Dopamine concentration in striatum is associated with severity of bradykinesia

Severety of bradykinesia	Caudate nucleus	Putamen
Mild	0.58 (13)	0.44 (12)
Marked	0.44 (9)	0.05 (9)
Normal controls	2.65 (28)	3.44 (28)

NOTE: Date from Bernheimer *et al.*[26] Results are means in μg/g fresh tissue. Numbers in parentheses are the number of cases studied.

dopamine due to loss of the nigrostriatal neurons. Accompanying this neuronal loss is an increase in glial cells in the nigra and a loss of the neuromelanin normally contained in the dopaminergic neurons. In PD, intracytoplasmic eosinophilic inclusions, called Lewy bodies, are usually present in many of the surviving neurons. It is recognized today that not all patients with PD have Lewy bodies; those with the homozygous mutation in the PARK2 gene—mainly young-onset PD patients—have nigral neuronal degeneration without Lewy bodies. Lewy bodies contain many proteins, including the fibrillar form of α-synuclein, discovered because PARK1's mutations involve the gene for this protein. There are no Lewy bodies in the Parkinson-plus syndromes.

With the progressive loss of the nigrostriatal dopaminergic neurons, there is a corresponding decrease of dopamine content in both the nigra and the striatum, which, as mentioned above, accounts particularly for the bradykinesia and rigidity in PD. There are compensatory changes, such as supersensitivity of dopamine receptors, so that symptoms of PD are first encountered only when there is about an 80% reduction of dopamine concentration in the putamen (or a loss of 60% of nigral dopaminergic neurons).[26] With further loss of dopamine concentration, parkinsonian bradykinesia becomes more severe (TABLE 5). The progressive loss of the dopaminergic nigrostriatal pathway can be detected *in vivo* using PET and SPECT scanning; these show a continuing reduction of FDOPA and dopamine transporter ligand binding in the striatum.[27–31]

The consequence of nigrostriatal loss is an altered physiology downstream from the striatum. The striatum contains D1 and D2 receptors. The current thinking is that dopamine is excitatory at the D1 receptor and inhibitory at the D2 receptor. Deficiency of dopamine at these receptors results in alteration at the downstream nuclei: excessive activity of the subthalamic nucleus and globus pallidus interna, and increased inhibition in the thalamus and cerebral cortex.[32–34] These altered physiological patterns are restored towards normal with treatment by levodopa.

CAUSES AND PATHOGENESIS OF PD AND PARKINSON-PLUS SYNDROMES

Other than known genetic causes of PD (TABLE 3), the etiology of these disorders remains unknown. Three (PARK1, PARK2, and PARK5) of the four identified mutated genes causing PD—involving the proteins α-synuclein, parkin, and ubiquitin C terminal hydrolase-L1—point to an impairment of protein degradation with a buildup of toxic proteins that cannot be degraded via the ubiquitin-proteasomal path-

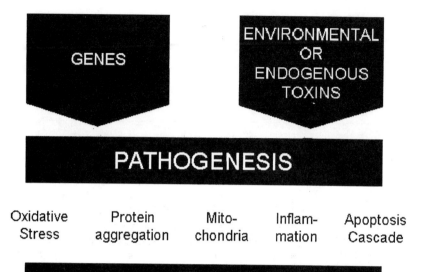

FIGURE 3. Diagram of the concept of the etiology and pathogenesis of Parkinson's disease.

way. The fourth, PARK7—involving a nuclear protein of unknown function—appears also to play a role in protein degradation. These findings have led to the concept that perhaps most, if not all, cases of sporadic PD have an impairment of protein degradation. A current hypothesis is that oxidative stress with the formation of oxyradicals, such as dopamine quinone, can lead to reactions with α-synuclein to form oligomers of α-synuclein (so-called protofibrils), which accumulate because they cannot be degraded by the ubiquitin-proteasomal pathway, leading finally to cell death.[35] Other pathogenetic mechanisms being considered are (1) other effects from oxidative stress, such as the reaction of oxyradicals with nitric oxide to form the highly reactive peroxynitrite radical; (2) impaired mitochondria leading to both reduced ATP production and accumulation of electrons that aggravate oxidative stress, with the final outcome being apoptosis and cell death; and (3) inflammatory changes in the nigra, producing cytokines that augment apoptosis (FIG. 3). These actions lead to an apoptotic cascade that leads to cell death. These concepts on pathogenesis are leading researchers to test agents that affect these potential mechanisms in an attempt to reduce the rate of neurodegeneration in PD.

THERAPY OF PARKINSON'S DISEASE

Neuroprotective Therapy

So far no drug or surgical approach has been shown unequivocally to slow the rate of progression of PD, but if any drug should be proved to delay the progression of the disease process, it should be incorporated in treatment early in the course of the disease. There are some controlled clinical trials that were sufficiently positive to have raised the possibility that the propargylamine agents selegiline and rasagiline and the mitochondrial enhancing agent coenzyme Q_{10} could have some neuroprotective qualities.[36–38] Larger clinical trials with neuroimaging of striatal dopamine nerve terminals would be necessary to provide adequate documentation of neuroprotection.

Symptomatic Therapy

Dopamine replacement therapy is the major medical approach to treating PD, and a variety of dopaminergic agents are available (TABLE 6). The most powerful drug is levodopa. It is usually administered with a peripheral decarboxylase inhibitor to prevent formation of dopamine in the peripheral tissues. In addition to being metabolized by aromatic amino acid decarboxylase, levodopa is also metabolized by catechol-O-methyltransferase (COMT) to form 3-O-methyldopa. The use of a COMT inhibitor with levodopa can extend the plasma half-life of levodopa without increasing its peak plasma concentration and can thereby prolong the duration of action of each dose of levodopa. Although levodopa is the most effective drug to treat the symptoms of PD, about 60% of patients develop troublesome complications of disabling response fluctuations (the "wearing-off" effect) and dyskinesias after five years of levodopa therapy; younger patients (less than 60 years of age) are particularly prone to developing these problems even sooner.

The next most powerful drugs in treating PD symptoms are the dopamine agonists. Several of these are available. Apomorphine may be the most powerful, but it needs to be injected or taken sublingually. The others agonists are effective orally. Pergolide, pramipexole, and ropinirole appear to be equally effective; and all are more powerful than bromocriptine. Cabergoline and lisuride are not available in the U.S. Cabergoline has the longest half-life and therefore may prove ultimately to be most useful. Compared to levodopa, dopamine agonists are more likely to cause hallucinations, confusion, and psychosis, especially in the elderly. Thus, it is safer to use levodopa in patients over the age of 70 years. They are also more likely to cause drowsiness and, after several years of use, can cause leg edema. On the other hand, controlled clinical trials have revealed that dopamine agonist therapy is less likely to produce dyskinesias and the wearing-off phenomenon than levodopa.[39,40] But these trials also showed that levodopa provides greater symptomatic benefit than do dopamine agonists. The neuroimaging component of these studies reveals that striatal dopamine nerve terminals disappear at a faster rate with levodopa treatment than with the agonists. There is uncertainty about how to apply the information gleaned from these studies to the patient; a frank discussion between physician and patient should lead to the appropriate treatment for that individual.

TABLE 6. Dopaminergic agents used in the treatment of Parkinson's disease

Dopamine precursor: levodopa	Dopamine agonists: bromocriptine, pergolide, pramipexole, ropinirole, apomorphine, and cabergoline
Peripheral decarboxylase inhibitors: carbidopa, benserazide	Dopamine releaser: amantadine
Catechol-O-methyltransferase inhibitors: tolcapone, entacapone	MAO type B inhibitor: selegiline, rasagiline

Amantadine has several actions: it has antimuscarinic effects, but more importantly it can activate release of dopamine from nerve terminals, block dopamine uptake into the nerve terminals, and block glutamate receptors. Its dopaminergic actions make it a useful drug to relieve symptoms in about two-thirds of patients, but it can induce livedo reticularis, ankle edema, visual hallucinations, and confusion. Its antiglutamatergic action is useful in reducing the severity of levodopa-induced dyskinesias. The elderly do not tolerate amantadine well because of the adverse mental effects. Monoamine oxidase type B (MAO-B) inhibitors (e.g., selegiline) offer mildly effective symptomatic benefit and are without the hypertensive "cheese effect" seen with MAO-A inhibitors; therefore, they can be used in the presence of levodopa therapy. Although there has been considerable debate about the possible protective benefit of selegiline, recent studies evaluating its long-term use indicate that selegiline is associated with less freezing of gait and with a slower rate of clinical worsening compared to placebo-treated subjects. These benefits appear to be separate from its mild symptomatic effects because all subjects were receiving the symptomatic benefit from concurrent levodopa therapy.[36] Nondopaminergic agents are also useful to treat many PD symptoms, both motoric and nonmotoric; they are beyond the scope of this review.

Surgical Therapy

Surgery for PD is becoming increasingly available as new techniques of electrical stimulation have been developed and a better understanding of basal ganglia physiology has been attained. Stereotaxic deep brain stimulation (DBS) is fast becoming the treatment of choice because ablative lesioning involves greater risk of inducing neurological deficits. With stimulating electrodes, the stimulation can be adjusted, and the electrodes can be removed if necessary. However, DBS is more costly than creating a lesion in the target, and frequent adjustments of the stimulator are usually needed. The location of the stereotaxic target is the other major factor that needs to be individualized for each patient. The thalamus, particularly the ventral intermediate nucleus, appears to be the most successful target for controlling tremor, but this target does not eliminate bradykinesia; so stereotaxic thalamotomy or thalamic DBS is not a preferred choice today. The globus pallidus interna is a more satisfactory target for controlling choreic and dystonic dyskinesias due to levodopa therapy. But the subthalamic nucleus appears to be the best target for controlling bradykinesia. DBS of the subthalamic nucleus, by reducing bradykinesia, allows for a reduction of levodopa dosage, thus reducing the severity of dyskinesias as well. This surgical approach seems the most promising. Surgical procedures for patients with PD are best performed at specialty centers by an experienced team consisting of a neurosurgeon, a neurophysiologist to monitor the target during the operative procedure, and a neurologist to program the stimulators. The patient needs close follow-up to adjust the stimulator settings to their optimum.

REFERENCES

1. PARKINSON, J. 1817. An Essay on the Shaking Palsy. Sherwood, Neely, and Jones. London.
2. GOETZ, C.G. 1987. Charcot, the Clinician: the Tuesday Lessons. Excerpts from Nine Case Presentations on General Neurology Delivered at the Salpetriere Hospital in

1887-88 by Jean-Martin Charcot. Translated with commentary: pp. 123–124. Raven Press. New York.
3. GOWERS, W.R. 1893. A Manual of Diseases of the Nervous System, Vol. II, 2nd edit.: p. 644. Blakiston. Philadelphia.
4. OPPENHEIM, H. 1911. Textbook of Nervous Diseases for Physicians and Students, 5th edit., trans. by H. Bruce: pp. 1301–1302. Otto Schulze. Edinburgh.
5. WECHSLER, I.S. 1932. A Textbook of Clinical Neurology, 2nd edit.: p. 576. W.B. Saunders. Philadelphia.
6. WILSON, S.A.K. 1940. Neurology, vol. II: p. 793. Williams & Wilkins. Baltimore.
7. SCHWAB, R.S., A.C. ENGLAND & E. PETERSON. 1959. Akinesia in Parkinson's disease. Neurology 9: 65–72.
8. MEYNERT, T. 1871. Ueber Beitrage zur differential Diagnose der paralytischen Irrsinns. Wiener Med. Presse 11: 645–647.
9. BRISSAUD, E. 1895. Lecons sur les Maladies Nerveuses. Masson et Cie. Paris.
10. BLOCQ, P. & G. MARINESCO. 1893. Sur un cas de tremblement Parkinsonien hemiplegique, symptomatique d'une tumeur de peduncle cerebral. C. R. Soc. Biol. Paris 5: 105–111.
11. TRETIAKOFF, C. 1919. Contribution a l'etude de l'anatomie pathologique du locus niger de Soemmering avec quelques dedutions relatives a la pathogenie des troubles du tonus musculaire et de la maladie de Parkinson. These de Paris.
12. LEWY, F.H. 1914. Zur pathologischen Anatomie der Paralysis agitans. Dtsch. Z. Nervenheilk 1: 50–55.
13. FOIX, C. & I. NICOLESCO. 1925. Anatomie Cerebrale; Les Noyeux Gris Centraux et la Region Mesencephalo-Sous-Opitique, Suive d'un Appendice sur l'Anatomie Pathologique de la Maladie de Parkinson. Masson et Cie. Paris.
14. HASSLER, R. 1938. Zur Pathologie der Paralysis Agitans und des postenzephalitischen Parkinsonismus. J. Psychol. Neurol. 48: 387–476.
15. GREENFIELD, J.G. & F.D. BOSANQUET. 1953. The brain-stem lesions in parkinsonism. J. Neurol. Neurosurg. Psychiatry 16: 213–226.
16. CARLSSON, A., M. LINDQVIST & T. MAGNUSSON. 1957. 3,4-Dihydroxyphenylalanine and 5-hydroxytryptophan as reserpine antagonists. Nature 180: 1200.
17. CARLSSON, A., M. LINDQVIST, T. MAGNUSSON & B. WALDECK. 1958. On the presence of 3-hydroxytyramine in brain. Science 127: 471.
18. BERTLER, A. & E. ROSENGREN. 1959. Occurrence and distribution of catechol amines in brain. Acta Physiol. Scand. 47: 350–361.
19. SANO, I., T. GAMO, Y. KAKIMOTO, et al. 1959. Distribution of catechol compounds in human brain. Biochim. Biophys. Acta 32: 586–587.
20. CARLSSON, A. 1959. The occurrence, distribution and physiological role of catecholamines in the nervous system. Pharmacol. Rev. 11: 490–493.
21. EHRINGER, H. & O. HORNYKIEWICZ. 1960. Verteilung von Noradrenalin und Dopamin (3-Hydroxytyramin) im Gehirn des Menschen und ihr Verhalten bei Erkrankungen der extrapyramidalen Systems. Klin. Wochenschr. 38: 1236–1239.
22. FAHN, S. & S. PRZEDBORSKI. 2000. Parkinsonism. In Merritt's Neurology, 10th edit. L.P. Rowland, Ed.: 679–693. Lippincott Williams & Wilkins. Philadelphia.
23. ELBAZ, A., J.H. BOWER, D.M. MARAGANORE, et al. 2002. Risk tables for parkinsonism and Parkinson's disease. J. Clin. Epidemiol. 55(1): 25–31.
24. TANNER, C.M., R. OTTMAN, S.M. GOLDMAN, et al. 1999. Parkinson disease in twins— an etiologic study. JAMA 281: 341–346.
25. ELBAZ, A., J.H. BOWER, B.J. PETERSON, et al. 2003. Survival study of Parkinson disease in Olmsted county, Minnesota. Arch. Neurol. 60(1): 91–96.
26. BERNHEIMER, H., W. BIRKMAYER, O. HORNYKIEWICZ, et al. 1973. Brain dopamine and the syndromes of Parkinson and Huntington. J. Neurol. Sci. 20: 415–455.
27. SNOW, B.J., C.S. LEE, M. SCHULZER, et al. 1994. Longitudinal fluorodopa positron emission tomographic studies of the evolution of idiopathic Parkinsonism. Ann. Neurol. 36: 759–764.
28. SEIBYL, J.P., K.L. MAREK, D. QUINLAN, et al. 1995. Decreased single-photon emission computed tomographic [(123)]I beta-CIT striatal uptake correlates with symptom severity in Parkinson's disease. Ann. Neurol. 38: 589–598.

29. EIDELBERG, D., J.R. MOELLER, T. ISIKAWA, et al. 1995. Assessment of disease severity in parkinsonism with fluorine-18- fluorodeoxyglucose and PET. J. Nucl. Med. **36:** 378–383.
30. MORRISH, P.K., G.V. SAWLE & D.J. BROOKS. 1996. An [F-18]dopa-PET and clinical study of the rate of progression in Parkinson's disease. Brain **119:** 585–591.
31. BENAMER, H.T.S., J. PATTERSON, D.J. WYPER, et al. 2000. Correlation of Parkinson's disease severity and duration with I-123- FP-CIT SPECT striatal uptake. Mov. Disord. **15**(4): 692–698.
32. PENNEY, J.B., JR. & A.B. YOUNG. 1986. Striatal inhomogeneities and basal ganglia function. Mov. Disord. **1:** 3–14.
33. MILLER, W.C. & M.R. DELONG. 1988. Parkinsonian symptomatology: an anatomical and physiological analysis. Ann. N.Y. Acad. Sci. **515:** 287–302.
34. MITCHELL, I.J., C.E. CLARKE, S. BOYCE, et al. 1989. Neural mechanisms underlying parkinsonian symptoms based upon regional uptake of 2-deoxyglucose in monkeys exposed to 1-methyl-4-phenyl-1,2,3,6-tetrahydropyridine. Neuroscience **32:** 213–226.
35. CONWAY, K.A., J.C. ROCHET, R.M. BIEGANSKI & P.T.J. LANSBURY. 2001. Kinetic stabilization of the alpha-synuclein protofibril by a dopamine-alpha-synuclein adduct. Science **294:** 1267–1268.
36. SHOULSON, I., D. OAKES, S. FAHN, et al.; PARKINSON STUDY GROUP. 2002. Impact of sustained deprenyl (selegiline) in levodopa-treated Parkinson's disease: a randomized placebo-controlled extension of the deprenyl and tocopherol antioxidative therapy of parkinsonism trial. Ann. Neurol. **51**(5): 604–612.
37. PARKINSON STUDY GROUP. 2002. A controlled trial of rasagiline in early Parkinson disease—the TEMPO study. Arch. Neurol. **59**(12): 1937–1943.
38. SHULTS, C.W., D. OAKES, K. KIEBURTZ, et al. 2002. Effects of coenzyme Q_{10} in early Parkinson disease. Evidence of slowing of the functional decline. Arch. Neurol. **59:** 1541–1550.
39. RASCOL, O., D.J. BROOKS, A.D. KORCZYN, et al. 2000. A five-year study of the incidence of dyskinesia in patients with early Parkinson's disease who were treated with ropinirole or levodopa. N. Engl. J. Med. **342:** 1484–1491.
40. PARKINSON STUDY GROUP. 2000. Pramipexole versus levodopa as the initial treatment for Parkinson's disease: a randomized controlled trial. JAMA **284:** 1931–1938.

Physiology and Pathophysiology of Parkinson's Disease

CLEMENT HAMANI AND ANDRES M. LOZANO

Division of Neurosurgery, Toronto Western Hospital, University of Toronto, Toronto, Ontario, Canada

ABSTRACT: The behavior of neurons in the basal ganglia is severely disrupted in Parkinson's disease (PD). In nonhuman parkinsonian primate models, the disturbance in neurons in basal ganglia output structures include increased firing, bursting, an augmented synchrony, correlated activity, and a tendency towards loss of specificity in their receptive fields. This abnormal neuronal behavior, transmitted to the thalamus, cortex and brainstem, is thought to disrupt the functioning of the motor system and underlie the major motor manifestations of PD—tremor, rigidity, akinesia, gait, and postural disturbances. The mainstay of treatment has been to replace the missing dopamine with medication. With time and disease progression, however, dopamine replacement becomes less efficacious and new adverse effects, including the development of motor fluctuations and drug-induced involuntary movements or dyskinesias, emerge. When the patients reach this stage, surgical therapy becomes an option. Most surgical interventions are performed at the level of the thalamus, globus pallidus, and subthalamic nucleus, aiming at the disruption of the pathological activity that accompanies the Parkinson's deficiency state. With this abnormal neuronal activity neutralized, normal movements can in many cases be restored.

KEYWORDS: Parkinson's disease; surgery; subthalamic nucleus; globus pallidus; physiopathology; movement disorders

INTRODUCTION

It is estimated that approximately one million North Americans suffer from Parkinson's disease. To date, little is known about the etiology of this disorder; but some important clues are coming from a variety of sources, including genetic studies and studies of environmental toxins.[1,2] Despite these advances, the etiology of Parkinson's disease for most patients remains enigmatic.

The number of dopaminergic neurons in the substantia nigra varies from species to species[3–9] (TABLE 1). Humans have approximately 220,000 dopaminergic neurons in the substantia nigra of each hemisphere.[6] When more than 50% of these cells are lost, patients start to develop the signs and symptoms of the disease—tremor, rigidity, akinesia and bradykinesia (poverty and slowness of movement), as well as pos-

Address for correspondence: Andres Lozano, Toronto Western Hospital, West Wing 4-447, 399 Bathurst Street, Toronto, ON M5T 2S8, Canada. Voice: 416-603-6200; fax: 416-603-5298.
lozano@uhnres.utoronto.ca

Ann. N.Y. Acad. Sci. 991: 15–21 (2003). © 2003 New York Academy of Sciences.

TABLE 1. Number of nigral dopaminergic neurons in each hemisphere in various species

Species	Number of dopaminergic nigral neurons in each hemisphere	Reference
Mouse	10,000–15,000	3, 8
Rat	15,000–22,000	3, 5, 9
Primate	55,000–110,000	7
Human	120,000–290,000	3, 4, 6

tural and gait abnormalities. Treatment is directed mainly at replacing the dopamine deficiency in the form of dopamine agonists and levodopa therapy, which is the most effective medical therapy to date.[10,11] With disease progression and prolonged use of these drugs however, patients become less responsive to medications and start developing fluctuations in their response, oscillating between the "on" state, in which they display relatively good motor function, and the "off" state, in which they are mostly in an akinetic rigid condition. These fluctuations can occur in an unpredictable fashion, several times a day, and are not always time locked to medications. Moreover, with chronic drug usage a number of drug-related adverse effects emerge, at a rate of approximately 10% per year. Among these, drug-induced involuntary movements or dyskinesias are some of the most disabling. These side effects, combined with cognitive, psychiatric, gastrointestinal, and other disturbances, are the current important limits to our therapeutic armamentarium for symptomatic treatment for Parkinson's disease.

The first and most prominent manifestations of Parkinson's disease are the impairments in motor function (TABLE 2). With disease progression, however, a new set of problems emerge, including speech difficulties, cognitive dysfunction, depres-

TABLE 2. Major primary (motor) and secondary (nonmotor) manifestations of Parkinson's disease

Primary manifestations	Secondary manifestations
tremor	dementia
bradykinesia	depression
akinesia	sleep disturbances
rigidity	sensory complaints
postural instability	dysarthria
	dysphagia
	constipation and urinary dysfunction
	masked facies
	olfactory dysfunction
	sialorrhea
	seborrhea
	orthostatic hypotension

sion, sleep disturbances, constipation, bladder and sexual dysfunctions, and a series of autonomic problems that are outlined in TABLE 2.[2,12–14] Most of these problems are poorly or not responsive to dopaminergic replacement, suggesting that other neurotransmitter systems might be involved in their pathogenesis. In fact, there is increasing evidence for abnormalities in other neurotransmitter systems as well as for cell loss and degeneration that extends beyond the dopaminergic pathways. Indeed, the locus ceroeuleus catecholaminergic system, the raphe nuclei serotonergic system, and the cholinergic neurons from the nucleus basalis and a number of other areas, including the cortex, olfactory bulb, sympathetic ganglia, and the central sympathetic nervous system, are compromised in Parkinson's disease as well.[1,12,13,15] Degeneration in these diverse systems indicates that we are dealing with a disorder that extends beyond dopaminergic neurons, and both therapeutic maneuvers and pathogenic mechanisms have to take these associated conditions into account.

PATHOPHYSIOLOGY OF THE MAJOR PARKINSON'S DISEASE SYMPTOMS

How Does the Dopamine Deficiency State Lead to the Signs and Symptoms of PD?

In animal models and in humans with Parkinson's disease, the neurophysiologic consequences of dopamine deficiency are striking. A model of basal ganglia function in normal and dopamine deficiency states has been proposed (FIG. 1).[16,17] This model proposes that dopamine deficiency produces dysfunction in the striatum, leading to: (1) decreased activity in the direct pathway, from GABAergic striatal neurons to the internal segment of the globus pallidus (GPi) and substantia nigra pars reticulata (SNpr) and (2) increased drive through the indirect pathway, involving particularly the external segment of the globus pallidus (GPe) and subthalamic nucleus (STN). As a consequence, there is disruption of the activity in basal ganglia output structures (GPi and SNpr), which in turn disrupts the activity in brain stem motor areas, including the pedunculopontine nucleus and the thalamocortical motor system.[18] This disruption is thought to be responsible for the difficulty in initiation of movements and the poverty of motion that are characteristic of Parkinson's disease.[19–23] Although the model does reasonably well at explaining akinesia, it is does not adequately explain some of the other cardinal features of Parkinson's disease, such as tremor or rigidity.[24] Further, the model does not take into account that dopamine exerts its effects not only in the striatum but also throughout basal ganglia nuclei and at cortical levels.

The development of the nonhuman primate MPTP model of Parkinson's disease has made possible an examination of the behavior of neurons in normal and parkinsonian states, leading to significant insights into the disrupted activity that accompanies this condition.[25–27] Moreover, these new concepts have led to the reemergence of neurosurgery to treat medically refractory Parkinson's disease. The surgical approaches are producing striking symptomatic benefits in parkinsonian patients[28,29] and are providing a unique opportunity to examine cellular activity in the thalamus, globus pallidus, and subthalamic nucleus in Parkinson's disease.

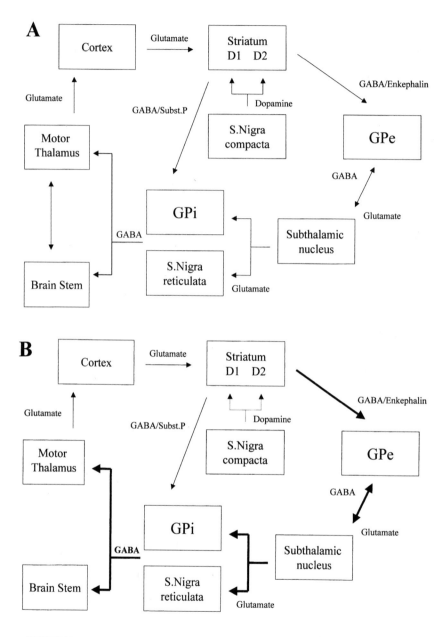

FIGURE 1. Proposed functional model of the basal ganglia in normal subjects **(A)** and patients with Parkinson's disease **(B)**. In **B**, the *width of the arrows* indicates the degree of overall functional change in activity as compared with the normal state. *Dotted lines* indicate the dysfunctional nigrostriatal dopamine system in Parkinson's disease. GPe, external segment of the globus pallidus; GPi, internal segment of the globus pallidus; S. Nigra, substantia nigra; Subst.P, substantia P.

NEUROSURGICAL PROCEDURES FOR PARKINSON'S DISEASE

The renaissance of surgery for movement disorders has come as a consequence of the unmet needs of a large number of patients who continue to be disabled despite the best available medical therapy, coupled with important technological advances in brain imaging and physiological recordings that have increased the accuracy and safety of surgery. By using these techniques, particularly microelectrode recordings, it has become possible to obtain direct measures of cellular activity of the basal ganglia in humans with Parkinson's disease and other movement disorders and to examine whether the pathological alterations seen in parkinsonian MPTP nonhuman primate models are also present in humans with Parkinson's disease.[30–37]

There is one main surgical strategy in current clinical use for the treatment of Parkinson's disease. It is the suppression of abnormal neural activity in basal ganglia circuits. This is achieved by either lesioning the involved structure or by the application of constant electrical stimulation, termed *deep-brain stimulation* or DBS, to block the pathological activity. These interventions occur at the level of the thalamus, globus pallidus, and subthalamic nucleus.

The overall surgical experience has made it clear that there are certain symptoms, including tremor, rigidity, and akinesia, that respond dramatically to surgery; while others respond less so, and yet an additional group is unresponsive. Levodopa-induced involuntary movements or dyskinesias are among the most effectively treated conditions. With surgical treatment one can anticipate reductions of up to 80–90% in these symptoms. Tremor improvement reaches 80% with any of the three targets previously described. Rigidity and akinesia scores improve by approximately 60%, as assessed with the Unified Parkinson's Disease Rating Scale, after bilateral deep-brain stimulation procedures. Gait and postural abnormalities are less responsive, although significant benefits can be observed. The effectiveness of surgical procedures seems to be equivalent whether lesions are performed or chronic deep-brain stimulation electrodes are implanted in the basal ganglia. Nevertheless, bilateral lesions lead to an unexpectedly high incidence of side effects, mostly deterioration in speech and cognitive effects. Because patients with Parkinson's disease are disabled by bilateral symptoms, deep-brain stimulation is becoming the procedure of choice as, in contrast to lesions, DBS is adjustable and reversible.[28,38,39]

An alternative surgical therapy, aiming at replacement of the missing neurotransmitter by transplantation of dopaminergic neurons, is under investigation.[40,41] To date however, these procedures provide only modest benefits and are associated with significant adverse effects, particularly due to the fact that dopamine release cannot be controlled. Therefore, transplants are not being used in clinical practice but are being studied in research protocols.

Shortcomings of Surgery

Despite these advances in therapy, there continues to be a number of signs and symptoms of Parkinson's disease that fail to respond to dopamine or surgery. The reason for this is likely related to coexisting pathological changes in other circuits and neurotransmitters that are also involved in the pathogenesis of the disease.

In conclusion, modern neurosurgery has allowed an examination of the neuronal activity that occurs in the brain of patients with Parkinson's disease. These studies have revealed prominent disruption in the activity of basal ganglia neurons. Surgical approaches alter, block, or neutralize this abnormal activity. In this sense, it appears that in physiological terms it is better to receive no neural activity from the motor component of the basal ganglia than to receive a pathological one. In other words,"no news is better than bad news."

To date, all surgical treatments are symptomatic, which means that we are treating only the symptoms of the disease without influencing its natural history. What is now needed are treatments that change the natural course of the disease, that slow it down or stop it. Future aspects of surgical treatment, including advancements in deep-brain stimulation, local delivery of neural active substances, the application of neurotrophins and stem cells, gene therapy, and molecular neurosurgery, are all promising strategies and can be considered bright lights in the horizon.

ACKNOWLEDGMENTS

C.H. is currently receiving a CAPES postdoctoral fellowship.

REFERENCES

1. LANG, A.E. & A.M. LOZANO. 1998. Parkinson's disease. First of two parts. N. Engl. J. Med. **339:** 1044–1053.
2. JELLINGER, K.A. 2001. The pathology of Parkinson's disease. Adv. Neurol. **86:** 55–72.
3. GERMAN, D.C., D.S. SCHLUSSELBERG & D.J. WOODWARD. 1983. Three-dimensional computer reconstruction of midbrain dopaminergic neuronal populations: from mouse to man. J. Neural. Transm. **57:** 243–254.
4. GERMAN, D.C., *et al.* 1989. Midbrain dopaminergic cell loss in Parkinson's disease: computer visualization. Ann. Neurol. **26:** 507–514.
5. GERMAN, D.C. & K.F. MANAYE. 1993. Midbrain dopaminergic neurons (nuclei A8, A9, and A10): three-dimensional reconstruction in the rat. J. Comp. Neurol. **331:** 297–309.
6. GRAYBIEL, A.M., E.C. HIRSCH & Y. AGID. 1990. The nigrostriatal system in Parkinson's disease. Adv. Neurol. **53:** 17–29.
7. EMBORG, M.E., *et al.* 1998. Age-related declines in nigral neuronal function correlate with motor impairments in rhesus monkeys. J. Comp. Neurol. **401:** 253–265.
8. NELSON, E.L., *et al.* 1996. Midbrain dopaminergic neurons in the mouse: computer-assisted mapping. J. Comp. Neurol. **369:** 361–371.
9. SMITH, Y. & J.Z. KIEVAL. 2000. Anatomy of the dopamine system in the basal ganglia. Trends Neurosci. **23:** S28–33.
10. JANKOVIC, J. 2000. Complications and limitations of drug therapy for Parkinson' disease. Neurology **55:** S2–6.
11. RASCOL, O., *et al.* 2002. Treatment interventions for Parkinson's disease: an evidence based assessment. Lancet **359:** 1589–1598.
12. SINGER, C., W.J. WEINER & J.R. SANCHEZ-RAMOS. 1992. Autonomic dysfunction in men with Parkinson's disease. Eur. Neurol. **32:** 134–140.
13. WOLTERS, E.C. 2000. Psychiatric complications in Parkinson's disease. J. Neural Transm. Suppl. (60): 1291–302.
14. WOLTERS, E.C. 2001. Psychiatric complications in the treatment of Parkinson's disease. Adv. Neurol. **86:** 385–393.
15. CHURCHYARD, A. & A.J. LEES. 1997. The relationship between dementia and direct involvement of the hippocampus and amygdala in Parkinson's disease. Neurology **49:** 1570–1576.
16. MINK, J.W. 1996. The basal ganglia: focused selection and inhibition of competing motor programs. Prog. Neurobiol. **50:** 381–425.

17. ALBIN, R.L., A.B. YOUNG & J.B. PENNEY. 1989. The functional anatomy of basal ganglia disorders. Trends Neurosci. **12:** 366–375.
18. PAHAPILL, P.A. & A.M. LOZANO. 2000. The pedunculopontine nucleus and Parkinson's disease. Brain **123** (Pt. 9): 1767–1783.
19. BERARDELLI, A., et al. 2001. Pathophysiology of bradykinesia in Parkinson's disease. Brain **124:** 2131–2146.
20. BLOEM, B.R., J.P. VAN VUGT & D.J. BECKLEY. 2001. Postural instability and falls in Parkinson's disease. Adv. Neurol. **87:** 209–223.
21. CANTELLO, R., et al. 1996. Pathophysiology of Parkinson's disease rigidity. Role of corticospinal motor projections. Adv Neurol. **69:** 129–133.
22. DELWAIDE, P.J., J.L. PEPIN & A. MAERTENS DE NOORDHOUT. 1990. [Parkinsonian rigidity: clinical and physiopathologic aspects]. Rev. Neurol. (Paris) **146:** 548–554.
23. YANAGISAWA, N., R. HAYASHI & H. MITOMA. 2001. Pathophysiology of frozen gait in Parkinsonism. Adv. Neurol. **87:** 199–207.
24. CARR, J. 2002. Tremor in Parkinson's disease. Parkinsonism Relat. Disord. **8:** 223–234.
25. BERGMAN, H., et al. 1998. Physiological aspects of information processing in the basal ganglia of normal and parkinsonian primates. Trends Neurosco. **21:** 32–38.
26. BERGMAN, H. & G. DEUSCHL. 2002. Pathophysiology of Parkinson's disease: from clinical neurology to basic neuroscience and back. Mov. Disord. **17** (Suppl. 3): S28–40.
27. DELONG, M.R. 1990. Primate models of movement disorders of basal ganglia origin. Trends Neurosci. **13:** 281–285.
28. LANG, A.E. & A.M. LOZANO. 1998. Parkinson's disease. Second of two parts. N. Engl. J. Med. **339:** 1130–1143.
29. LANG, A.E., et al. 1997. Posteroventral medial pallidotomy in advanced Parkinson's disease. N. Engl. J. Med. **337:** 1036–1042.
30. GURIDI, J., et al. 2000. Targeting the basal ganglia for deep brain stimulation in Parkinson's disease. Neurology **55:** S21–28.
31. GARONZIK, I.M., et al. 2002. Intraoperative microelectrode and semi-microelectrode recording during the physiological localization of the thalamic nucleus ventral intermediate. Mov. Disord. **17** (Suppl. 3): S135–144.
32. HUTCHISON, W.D., et al. 1994. Differential neuronal activity in segments of globus pallidus in Parkinson's disease patients. Neuroreport **5:** 1533–1537.
33. HUTCHISON, W.D., et al. 1998. Neurophysiological identification of the subthalamic nucleus in surgery for Parkinson's disease. Ann. Neurol. **44:** 622–628.
34. LOZANO, A.M., et al. 1995. Effect of GPi pallidotomy on motor function in Parkinson's disease. Lancet **346:** 1383–1387.
35. MAGNIN, M., A. MOREL & D. JEANMONOD. 2000. Single-unit analysis of the pallidum, thalamus and subthalamic nucleus in parkinsonian patients. Neuroscience **96:** 549–564.
36. LENZ, F.A., et al. 1988. Single unit analysis of the human ventral thalamic nuclear group: correlation of thalamic "tremor cells" with the 3–6 Hz component of parkinsonian tremor. J. Neurosci. **8:** 754–764.
37. LENZ, F.A., et al. 1988. Single-unit analysis of the human ventral thalamic nuclear group: somatosensory responses. J. Neurophysiol. **59:** 299–316.
38. LANOTTE, M.M., et al. 2002. Deep brain stimulation of the subthalamic nucleus: anatomical, neurophysiological, and outcome correlations with the effects of stimulation. J. Neurol. Neurosurg. Psychaitry **72:** 53–58.
39. OBESO, J.A., et al. 2000. Pathophysiologic basis of surgery for Parkinson's disease. Neurology **55:** S7–12.
40. OLANOW, C.W., T. FREEMAN & J. KORDOWER. 2001. Transplantation of embryonic dopamine neurons for severe Parkinson's disease. N. Engl. J. Med. **345:** 146; discussion 147.
41. ISACSON, O., et al. 2001. Improved surgical cell therapy in Parkinson's disease. Physiological basis and new transplantation methodology. Adv. Neurol. **86:** 447–454.

PET Studies on the Function of Dopamine in Health and Parkinson's Disease

DAVID J. BROOKS

MRC Clinical Sciences Centre and Division of Neuroscience,
Faculty of Medicine, Imperial College, London, UK

ABSTRACT: Positron emission tomography (PET) can detect the presence of striatal, pallidal, midbrain, and cortical dopamine terminal dysfunction *in vivo* in Parkinson's disease (PD). In addition, dopamine release during motor tasks can be assessed as reflected by changes in receptor availability to PET ligands. Furthermore, the functional effects of focal dopamine replacement via implantation of fetal cells or glia-derived neurotrophic factor (GDNF) infusion into putamen can be monitored. In this review, the insight that PET has given us concerning the role of dopamine in motor control is presented, and the functional substrates underlying PD symptomatologies are discussed.

KEYWORDS: Parkinson; dopamine; serotonin; motor; PET; activation; GDNF

INTRODUCTION

Functional imaging allows four potential approaches to determining possible roles of dopamine in control of motor functions: First, loss of dopamine terminal function, as reflected by levels of striatal and extrastriatal ^{18}F-dopa uptake or dopamine transporter (DAT) ligand binding, can be correlated with disability and cognitive performance. Second, the locomotor and behavioral responses to focal striatal replacement of dopaminergic tone with implants of fetal mesencephalic cells or local neurotropic factor infusions can be correlated with dopaminergic function. Third, alterations in the patterns of resting and activated blood flow and metabolism in PD and their normalization following dopaminergic replacement can be monitored. Fourth, dopamine release in striatal and cortical areas during task performance or following pharmacological challenges can be measured indirectly *in vivo* as reflected by reductions in dopamine receptor availability to antagonists such as ^{11}C-raclopride. Based on microdialysis studies, it has been estimated that a 1% change in striatal ^{11}C-raclopride binding corresponds to at least an 8% change in synaptic dopamine levels.[1]

Dopamine fibers arise from the substantia nigra compacta and the ventral tegmentum (VTA) of the midbrain and project to dorsal (caudate, putamen) and ventral (caudate, putamen, nucleus accumbens, olfactory tubercle) striatum. There is a less-

Address for correspondence: David J. Brooks, M.D., D.Sc., F.R.C.P., F.Med.Sci., Hartnett Professor of Neurology, Cyclotron Building, Hammersmith Hospital, Du Cane Rd., London W12 0NN, UK.

david.brooks@csc.mrc.ac.uk

Ann. N.Y. Acad. Sci. 991: 22–35 (2003). © 2003 New York Academy of Sciences.

er output to frontal cortex, amygdala, and the anterior cingulate area. Our understanding about the precise role that dopamine plays in motor control and cognition is still limited. Awake animal studies have suggested that burst release of dopamine alerts animals to novel and rewarding stimuli, burst firing of dopamine neurons being correlated with the presence of an incentive rather than with movement per se.[2,3] Unexpected rewards are most effective in inducing phasic firing of dopamine neurons. As conditioning to a stimulus reliably predicts the presence of a reward, firing of dopamine neurons on reward presentation becomes attenuated, while firing on presentation of the conditioning stimulus increases.[4] Once conditioning is complete and timing of the reward on stimulus presentation becomes entirely predictable, dopamine neurons cease to fire on presentation of the conditioning stimulus. Phasic firing is then observed only if an unexpected reward occurs, and depression of activity is seen if a predicted reward fails to occur. These observations suggest that dopamine neurons are reacting to errors in reward prediction rather than presentation of the reward per se. This in turn suggests that they act to reinforce rewarding patterns of behavior and so play a primary role in conditional motor learning.

Dopamine, however, does not simply mediate rewarded behavior but almost certainly facilitates conditional learning in general.[5] When rats are aversively conditioned to auditory and visual stimuli with an electric foot shock, the first presentation of the foot shock with the conditioning stimulus results in an increase in frontal dopamine release, while ventral striatal dopamine levels remain unaltered.[6] Successful aversive conditioning, then, results in progressive increases in ventral striatal dopamine release, while frontal dopamine release diminishes. These findings support the concept that dopamine release in striatum reinforces learning but suggest the frontal dopamine release is concerned more with alerting animals to novel circumstances and mediating selective attention.[7]

Trying to dissociate the functional roles of basal ganglia and frontal dopamine release is probably inappropriate, as the basal ganglia and frontal areas are relays in a system of parallel distributed corticosubcortical loops. At least five separate loops link the basal ganglia via the ventral and dorsomedial thalamus to cortical premotor and prefrontal areas.[8] These include supplementary motor area (SMA)–putamen; dorsolateral prefrontal cortex (DLPFC)–dorsal caudate; orbitofrontal cortex (OFC) –ventral striatal; and anterior cingulate cortex (ACA)–ventral striatal loops. These loops appear to be spatially segregated based on the findings of anterograde and retrograde tracer experiments in nonhuman primates.[9] It has been proposed that tonic background dopamine release in the basal ganglia may act to "bind" or focus and filter the individual functions of these segregated loops.[7]

The pathology of Parkinson's disease (PD) targets the dopamine cells in the substantia nigra in association with the formation of neuronal Lewy inclusion bodies. Midbrain tegmental dopamine neurons projecting to anterior cingulate, orbitofrontal cortex, and amygdala are involved to a lesser extent. Serotonergic cells in the median raphe and noradrenergic cells in the locus ceruleus also degenerate, as do other pigmented and brain stem nuclei including the locus coeruleus and nucleus basalis.[10] Loss of cells from the substantia nigra in PD results in profound dopamine depletion in the striatum, lateral nigral projections to putamen being most affected.[11,12] While the pathology of PD targets subcortical nuclei, anterior cingulate and association neocortex can also show Lewy body degeneration; and currently it remains uncertain whether dementia of Lewy body type and PD represent ends of a spectrum.[13]

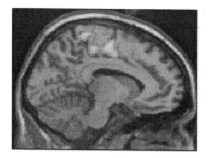 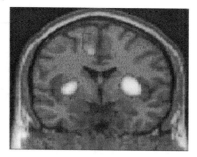

FIGURE 1. A statistical parametric map superimposed on an MRI template showing bilateral putamen, cingulate, and motor cortex loss of dopamine storage in early hemi-PD.

FOCAL STRIATAL REPLACEMENT OF DOPAMINE IN PD

Visual inspection of ^{18}F-dopa positron emission tomography (PET) images of patients with early Parkinson's disease gives the impression that loss of dopamine terminal function is confined to nigrostriatal projections. Using statistical parametric mapping (SPM) to compare mean dopamine storage capacity at a voxel level between early PD cases and age-matched normal subjects, however, reveals early motor cortex and anterior cingulate terminal dysfunction (see FIG. 1). This emphasises that PD does not simply provide a natural lesion model for basal ganglia dysfunction. As the disease advances, progressive loss of striatal, cingulate, and frontal dopamine storage is seen. Significant inverse correlations between disability scores rated with the Unified Parkinson's Disease Rating Scale (UPDRS) and putamen, midbrain, and anterior cingulate ^{18}F-dopa influx constants (Ki) are evident across the mild-to-advanced range of PD (FIG. 2. This raises the question, how great an influence does frontal loss of dopamine have in actuality on locomotor and behavioral function in PD?

One approach to answer this question is simply to correlate scores on behavioral tasks with regional levels of brain ^{18}F-dopa uptake in PD. When correct scores on the Tower of London task were compared with regional brain dopamine storage in PD, only individual right head of caudate nucleus Ki's showed a significant correlation with efficiency of spatial planning.[14] This finding implies that adequate levels of caudate dopamine are crucial for performance of spatial executive tasks. However, one cannot rule out a role of frontal dopamine even though no correlation was seen with either cingulate or prefrontal Ki levels, as these signals are relatively low (only 20% of caudate levels in normal subjects).

A more novel way of approaching the problem is to examine the behavioral effects of focal striatal replacement of dopamine using implants of human fetal mesencephalic cells or intraputamenal infusions of neurotropic factors such as glia-derived neurotrophic factor (GDNF). Several open series and a double-blind controlled trial of the efficacy of transplants in advanced PD have demonstrated significant increases in striatal ^{18}F-dopa storage after grafting in PD, which correlate with improved UPDRS scores.[15] It has also been shown that grafts survive in man for over 10 years and release normal levels of dopamine after an amphetamine challenge.[16]

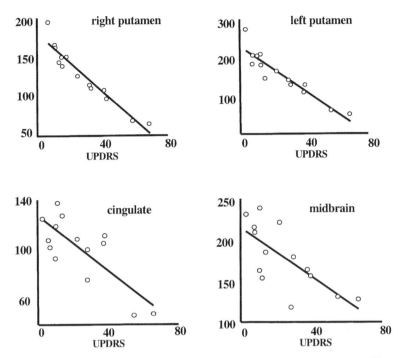

FIGURE 2. Inverse correlations between putamen, cingulate, and midbrain ^{18}F-dopa uptake and off UPDRS scores in PD.

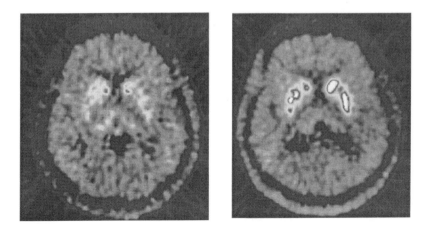

FIGURE 3. ^{18}F-dopa PET in PD before **(left)** and after **(right)** dopamine cell implantation.

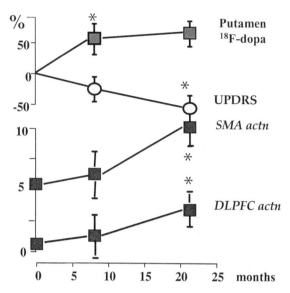

FIGURE 4. Recovery of PD cortical activation vs. dopamine function after grafting. Serial putamen ^{18}F-dopa Ki values, off UPDRS scores, and percentage increases in supplementary motor area and dorsolateral prefrontal activation measured with H_2[15]O PET in four transplanted PD patients. *$P < 0.05$.

Piccini and coworkers have studied the effects of implanting head of caudate and putamen bilaterally with human fetal mesencephalic cells[17] (see FIG. 3). At 6.5 months after transplantation mean striatal dopamine storage capacity, as measured by ^{18}F-dopa PET, was significantly elevated in these patients (putamen 78%, caudate 27%). This was associated with a nonsignificant mean 12-point clinical improvement on the UPDRS (see FIG. 4). At 18 months postsurgery there was further significant clinical improvement (24 points compared with baseline) in the absence of further increases in striatal ^{18}F-dopa uptake, suggesting that the graft had developed more effective connections.

PD patients, when withdrawn from medication, show a characteristic impairment of activation of striatomesial premotor-prefrontal projections during performance of motor tasks.[18] It has been demonstrated that replacement of dopaminergic tone by giving oral levodopa or subcutaneous apomorphine, a D1/D2 agonist, functionally restores cortical activation in PD[19–22] along with reduction of akinesia. More recently, the effects of focally implanting the striatum with fetal dopaminergic cells on movement-related premotor and prefrontal activation in PD have been studied.[17] Four PD patients who received bilateral human fetal mesencephalic transplants into caudate and putamen were studied with H_2[15]O PET at baseline and over two years following surgery. At baseline, H_2[15]O PET studies showed reduced premotor and absent prefrontal activation during performance of a paced motor task where the patient moved a joystick in freely chosen directions. At six months there was no significant change in cortical activation, but by 18 months mesial premotor and dorsal prefrontal activation had significantly improved (FIG. 4). These observations suggest that dorsal striatal grafts of dopamine cells in PD are effective in restoring levels of dorsal premotor and prefrontal activation and improving executive behavior. Additionally, graft function goes beyond that of a simple dopamine delivery system, and integration of the grafted neurons into the host brain is necessary in order to produce substantial clinical recovery in PD. This strengthens the argument that frontal dopamine loss, though present in PD, may be less critical than striatal loss for mediating dorsal prefrontal executive behaviors.

GDNF is a potent neurotrophic factor known to prevent the degeneration of dopamine neurons in rodent and primate models of PD where nigral degeneration is toxically induced. Gill and colleagues have recently examined the safety and efficacy of infusing GDNF directly into the posterior putamen of five patients with PD via in-dwelling catheters.[23] All patients tolerated constant GDNF delivery at a final level of 14 μg/day (6 mL/hour) into the posterior dorsal putamen via mechanical pumps for over one year, unilaterally in one and bilaterally in four patients, without serious side effects. Significant improvements were found in UPDRS subscores: 39% and 61% improvements in the off-medication motor III and activities of daily living II subscales, respectively, at 12 months. No change in cognitive status was detected on a battery of behavioral tests. Regions of interest placed in the immediate vicinity of the catheter tip showed 18–24% increases in putaminal ^{18}F-dopa Ki, which were confirmed with statistical parametric mapping. Additionally, SPM detected 16–26% increases in nigral dopamine storage, suggesting that retrograde transport of GDNF had occurred. These findings imply that local GDNF infusion appears to be safe and represents a potential restorative therapy for PD when applied directly to striatum.

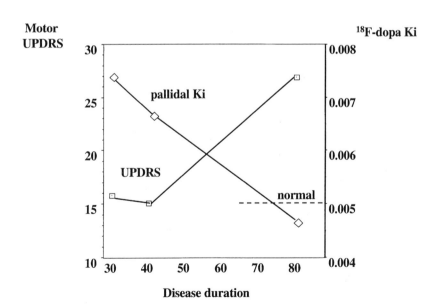

FIGURE 5. Levels of internal pallidal ^{18}F-dopa Ki versus off motor UPDRS scores in PD. While pallidal ^{18}F-dopa uptake is raised, the UPDRS score is maintained low but rapidly rises with fluctuations when pallidal ^{18}F-dopa uptake falls below normal.

Interestingly, dramatic improvements in basic locomotor functions were achieved with a neurotropic effect targeting primarily posterior dorsal putamen. Similar observations have been reported when implants of fetal mesenecephalic tissue are limited to posterior putamen alone.[24]

THE ROLE OF PALLIDAL DOPAMINE

While striatal and frontal brain regions show loss of ^{18}F-dopa uptake in early PD, this is by no means true of all areas. Recently, the internal pallidum, which receives dopamine projections from medial nigral cells at around 20% the level of the striatum, has been shown to increase its ^{18}F-dopa uptake by 25% in early PD[25] (FIG. 5). In contrast, PD patients with fluctuating responses to levodopa show reduced pallidal ^{18}F-dopa uptake. These findings suggest that increased internal pallidal dopamine storage may be a compensatory mechanism to loss of striatal dopamine tone, helping to maintain a fluent output from the basal ganglia and keep UPDRS disability scores at a low level. When both putamen and pallidal dopamine levels fall below normal, then basal ganglia output becomes unpredictable due to the double hit, leading to a rapid rise in UPDRS ratings and fluctuating treatment responses.

DOPAMINE AND THE CARDINAL SYMPTOMS OF PD

Several series have shown a correlation between putamen ^{18}F-dopa uptake in PD and ratings of both bradykinesia and rigidity. Similar results have been obtained with PET and single-photon computed tomography (SPECT) markers of terminal dopamine transporter binding. A consistent finding of these studies has been the lack of a correlation between severity of rest tremor and levels of striatal dopaminergic integrity. In animal models, a pure lesion of nigrostriatal dopaminergic projections is associated with rigidity and bradykinesia but not tremor. Lesions of cerebellar connections in the presence of harmaline lead to a postural 4–8-Hz tremor with essential characteristics; but in order to produce a 3–5-Hz tremor it is necessary to lesion the midbrain, interrupting cerebellar-thalamic, rubrospinal, and nigrostriatal connections along with serotonergic projections from the median raphe.

Midbrain 5-HT$_{1A}$ binding can be measured *in vivo* with ^{11}C-WAY 100635 PET and provides a functional measure of the integrity of both the serotonergic system and the tegmentum (FIG. 6a). Doder and coworkers[26] have studied 23 PD patients and 8 age-matched healthy volunteers with ^{11}C-WAY 100635 PET and found a mean 25% reduction in the midbrain raphe 5-HT$_{1A}$ binding potential in patients with PD compared to healthy volunteers ($P < 0.01$) (FIG. 6b). UPDRS composite ($P < 0.01$) and rest ($P < 0.001$) tremor scores both correlated significantly with 5-HT$_{1A}$ binding in the raphe, but not rigidity or bradykinesia. These findings confirm that serotonergic neurotransmission is decreased in PD and also show an association between 5-HT$_{1A}$ receptor availability in the raphe and severity of tremor in PD. This may indicate a role of the serotonergic system in the generation of rest tremor; it is known, for instance, that HT$_{1A}$ blockers such as propranolol can relieve tremor. However, it is equally possible that these findings simply reflect the presence of additional tegmental pathology required on top of nigrostriatal disruption to cause rest tremor in PD patients.

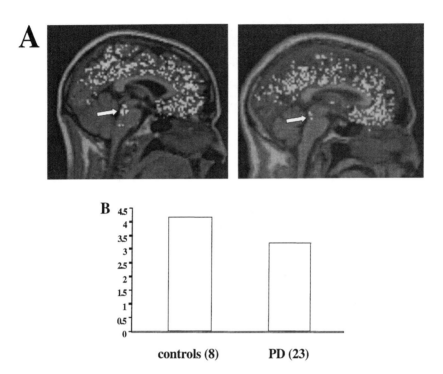

FIGURE 6. (A) ^{11}C-WAY100635 PET showing a 25% reduction in median raphe sero-tonin HT_{1A} binding in PD. Scan on **left** shows healthy volunteer; scan on **right** shows PD patient. **(B)** Bar graph showing the reduction in in midbrain raphe 5-HT_{1A} binding potential in PD patients as compared to age-matched healthy volunteers. $P < 0.01$.

DOPAMINE ACTIVATION STUDIES

Imaging changes in neuroceptor availability to PET ligands can be used to indi-rectly detect synaptic neurotransmitter fluxes in the living human brain.[1] When en-dogenous dopamine (DA) binds to D2 receptors, it competes with the reversible antagonist ^{11}C-raclopride (FIG. 7). This phenomenon allows synaptic DA levels to be estimated indirectly from changes in tracer D2 receptor binding potentials. It has been estimated that a 10% reduction in availability of D2 receptors for ^{11}C-raclo-pride binding reflects a fivefold increase in synaptic DA levels.[1] In reality the situa-tion is probably more complex than this, as binding of DA may lead to temporary internalization of D2 receptors.[27,28] However, internalization of D2 receptors fol-lowing DA release does not invalidate the ^{11}C-raclopride PET approach, as the ligand can bind only to D2 receptors on the cell surface, its low lipophilicity prevent-ing diffusion through plasma membranes into the cell cytoplasm.[29]

Elevation of DA synaptic concentrations can be achieved *in vivo* by administering inhibitors of the DA transporter such as methylphenidate,[30] or DA releasers such as

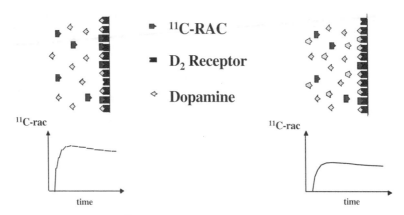

FIGURE 7. Two-scan ^{11}C-raclopride study showing competition between dopamine and ^{11}C-raclopride for D2 sites. (**Left**) scan 1: baseline; (**right**) scan 2: activation.

amphetamine.[1,31,32] Consequent falls in striatal ^{11}C-raclopride and ^{123}I-IBZM binding have been demonstrated in PET and SPECT studies (FIG. 8a). Piccini and colleagues have compared, using methamphetamine (MA) challenges and ^{11}C-raclopride PET, the levels of induced increases in synaptic DA in striatal and cortical structures in six normal subjects and six advanced PD patients.[33] A 0.3-mg/kg MA challenge induced significant 17% and 25% reductions in caudate and putamen ^{11}C-raclopride binding potentials (BP) in the normal subjects. Significant lesser reductions in ^{11}C-raclopride caudate and putamen BP following MA were observed in the PD patients (8% in caudate and 7% in putamen) (FIG. 8b). In individual PD patients there was a correlation between the percentage decrease in putamen ^{11}C-raclopride BP induced by MA and both putamen ^{18}F-dopa Ki values ($P = 0.005$) and motor disability rated with the UPDRS when withdrawn from medication ($P = 0.03$). Localization of significant changes in ^{11}C-raclopride binding after MA at a voxel level with statistical parametric mapping (SPM) identified striatal, dorsal, and ventrolateral prefrontal and orbitofrontal DA release in both normal subjects and PD patients. While amphetamine-induced striatal DA release was 60% reduced in PD, frontal DA release remained at a normal level. These findings provide further *in vivo* evidence that reduced striatal rather than frontal DA release is likely to be most relevant to the locomotor and cognitive disabilities associated with Parkinson's disease.

Methamphetamine and related psychostimulant drugs induce in humans heightened energy and a euphoric sense of well being through a mechanism thought to involve release of presynaptic DA. The concept that the behavioral effects of MA and similar drugs is due to their ability to increase extracellular DA in the dopaminergic mesocorticolimbic system, particularly in the nucleus accumbens, has been postulated since the 1980s.[34] While Laruelle *et al.*[31] and Volkow *et al.*[30] explored the effects of D-amphetamine and methylphenidate on brain DA release in humans in pioneering studies, a limitation was that measurements were made only in striatum. Consequently, this was the only region in which a correlation between behavioral effects of the drugs and release of DA could be reported.

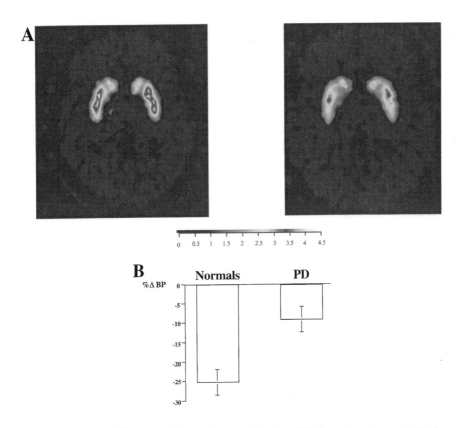

FIGURE 8. (A) ^{11}C-raclopride uptake: normal subject (D2 dopamine site availability). PET scans showing a 25% fall in striatal ^{11}C-raclopride binding after metamphetamine in a normal subject (**right** scan); placebo shown in **left** scan. (B) Percent decrease in ^{11}C-raclopride binding potentials after metamphetamine in normals and PD. In PD metamphetamine-induced decreases in striatal ^{11}C-raclopride binding are 40% of normal.

Piccini and colleagues have subsequently studied the relationship between subjective emotional experience induced in humans by methamphetamine and DA release in different components of the mesolimbic system.[35] No significant differences were found in the magnitude of self-reported euphoria and behavioral changes after methamphetamine in normal volunteers and PD patients. However, while in the normal subjects the magnitude of behavioral changes correlated with degrees of DA release in ventral striatum, a region containing the nucleus accumbens, and in prefrontal cortex, in the patient group behavioral changes correlated with the release of DA in prefrontal cortex only. These findings represent the first demonstration that methamphetamine induces endogenous DA release in frontal areas and that this release is associated with the stimulant effects of the drug. The similar effects observed in normals and in PD patients despite their severe reduction of striatal DA point to a direct role of prefrontal cortex and of prefrontal cortical DA in the reinforcing effects of psychostimulant drugs in humans.

DOPAMINE RELEASE DURING MOTOR TASKS

Koepp and colleagues[36] were the first to report a reduction of striatal ^{11}C-raclopride binding during performance of behavioral task. These workers asked subjects to play a video game, and they were financially rewarded according to their level of success. Subjects had to navigate a tank through a battlefield with a computer mouse, shoot at and avoid the shells of enemy tanks, and collect flags. If all flags were collected, they progressed to a higher level. The control task was watching a blank computer display. There were mean 7.5% and 12.8% reductions in dorsal and ventral striatal ^{11}C-raclopride binding during task performance, and individual reductions correlated significantly with the level of financial reward. These findings suggest that ventral striatal levels of dopamine at least doubled during participation in the video game and were increased to a greater extent than dorsal levels in this rewarded paradigm. However, the presence of dorsal striatal ^{11}C-raclopride binding reductions suggested that nonmotivational learning per se may also require dopamine release.

A difficulty with interpreting the findings of the above study is that appetitive stimuli, reinforcement of learning, motor coordination, and response selection were all features. Graybiel and colleagues[37] have shown that learning is impaired in monkeys after adminstration of the nigral toxin MPTP. Lawrence and Brooks,[38] therefore, investigated whether increased dopamine release could be detected during acquisition of a novel sequence of finger movements by trial and error, as previously decribed, compared with performance of prelearned sequential finger movements. Finger movements were paced by a tone at the same frequency in both tasks. The average number of novel eight-move sequences learned by each subject during the 50-minute ^{11}C-raclopride PET study was 14, and during task performance there was a significant additional 5% fall in dorsal putamen and 4% fall in caudate ^{11}C-raclopride binding relative to performance of prelearned sequential finger movements. This finding demonstrates that dopamine release does occur in dorsal putamen during unrewarded motor tasks such as sequence learning and is line with the view that dopamine acts to reinforce motor learning as well as to alert to the presence of rewarding stimuli.

This raises the question as to whether simple finger movements induce release of dopamine. Goerendt and coworkers[39] used ^{11}C-raclopride PET to investigate levels of striatal dopamine release by healthy volunteers and PD patients during performance of a prelearned sequence of finger movements. Five healthy volunteers and six patients with early unilateral PD were studied. Prelearned sequential finger movements in healthy volunteers significantly decreased ^{11}C-raclopride binding bilaterally in the dorsal putamen by 8–11% and ipsilaterally by 12% in the caudate. PD patients showed no significant reduction of putamen ^{11}C-raclopride binding during successful performance of this task, but a 5% reduction was detected in the caudate contralateral to the affected limbs. These findings, therefore, suggest that even unrewarded prelearned sequential finger movements are associated with significant putamen and caudate dopamine release in normal volunteers. Endogenous striatal dopamine release can also be detected during this task in Parkinson's disease, but only at a low level and in the caudate, where dopamine levels are most preserved.

CONCLUSIONS

- Striatal dopamine release can be detected with PET during unrewarded actions such as performance of learned sequential finger movements. Active motor learning and the presence of an incentiuve lead to further increases.
- Loss of putamen dopamine in PD correlates with severity of akinesia and rigidity but not rest tremor, which correlates with loss of midbrain raphe serotonin HT_{1A} binding.
- Reduced pallidal dopamine in PD is associated with loss of the honeymoon phase to levodopa medication and onset of motor fluctuations.
- In PD frontal dopamine release following an amphetamine challenge appears to be preserved, and levels correlate well with induced euphoria.
- Striatal implants of fetal mesencephalic tissue restore cortical activation, while direct GDNF infusion into posterior putamen increases dopamine storage and improves locomotor function.

REFERENCES

1. BREIER, A., T.P. SU, R. SAUNDERS, et al. 1997. Schizophrenia is associated with elevated amphetamine-induced synaptic dopamine concentrations: evidence from novel positron emission tomography method. Proc. Natl. Acad. Sci. USA **94:** 2569–2574.
2. SCHULTZ, W. 1998. Predictive reward signal of dopamine neurons. J. Neurophysiol. **80:** 1–27.
3. SCHULTZ, W. 2000. Multiple reward signals in the brain. Nat. Rev. Neurosci. **1:** 199–207.
4. MIRENOWICZ, J. & W. SCHULTZ. 1996. Preferential activation of midbrain dopamine neurons by appetitive rather than aversive stimuli. Nature **379:** 449–451.
5. TAYLOR, A.E., J.A. SAINT-CYR & A.E. LANG. 1986. Frontal lobe dysfunction in Parkinson's disease. Brain **109:** 845–883.
6. WILKINSON, L.S., T. HUMBY, A.S. KILLCROSS, et al. 1998. Dissociations in dopamine release in medial prefrontal cortex and ventral striatum during the acquisition and extinction of classical aversive conditioning in the rat. Eur. J. Neurosci. **10:** 1019–1026.
7. WICHMAN, T. & M.R. DELONG. 1999. Oscillations in the basal ganglia. Nature **400:** 621–622.
8. ALEXANDER, G.E. & D. CRUTCHER. 1990. Functional architecture of basal ganglia circuits: neural substrates of parallel processing. TINS **13:** 266–271.
9. MIDDLETON, F.A.S.P.L. 1997. New concepts about the organization of basal ganglia output. Adv. Neurol. **74:** 57–68.
10. JELLINGER, K. 1987. The pathology of parkinsonism. In Movement Disorders 2. C.D. Marsden & S. Fahn, Eds.: 124–165. Butterworth. London.
11. FEARNLEY, J.M. & A.J. LEES. 1991. Aging and Parkinson's disease: substantia nigra regional selectivity. Brain **114:** 2283–2301.
12. KISH, S.J., K. SHANNAK & O. HORNYKIEWICZ. 1988. Uneven pattern of dopamine loss in the striatum of patients with idiopathic Parkinson's disease. N. Engl. J. Med. **318:** 876–880.
13. BYRNE, E.J., J. LOWE, R.B. GODWIN-AUSTEN, et al. 1987. Dementia of Parkinson's disease associated with diffuse cortical Lewy bodies. Lancet. **i:** 501.

14. CHEESMAN, A.L., S.J.G. LEWIS, R. BARKER, et al. 2002. Right caudate dopamine storage correlates with spatial planning in Parkinson's disease. Neurology **58** (Suppl. 3): A487.
15. LINDVALL, O. 1999. Cerebral implantation in movement disorders: state of the art. Mov. Disord. **14:** 201–205.
16. PICCINI, P., D.J. BROOKS, A. BJORKLUND, et al. 1999. Dopamine release from nigral transplants visualised in vivo in a Parkinson's patient. Nat. Neurosci. **2:** 1137–1140.
17. PICCINI, P., O. LINDVALL, A. BJORKLUND, et al. 2000. Delayed recovery of movement-related cortical function in Parkinson's disease after striatal dopaminergic grafts. Ann. Neurol. **48:** 689–695.
18. BROOKS, D.J. 2001. Functional imaging studies on dopamine and motor control J. Neural Transm. **108:** 1283–1298.
19. RASCOL, O., U. SABATINI, F. CHOLLET, et al. 1992. Supplementary and primary sensory motor area activity in Parkinson's disease. Regional cerebral blood flow changes during finger movements and effects of apomorphine. Arch. Neurol. **49:** 144–148.
20. RASCOL, O., U. SABATINI, F. CHOLLET, et al. 1994. Normal activation of the supplementary motor area in patients with Parkinson's disease undergoing long-term treatment with levodopa. J. Neurol. Neurosurg. Psychiat. **57:** 567–571.
21. BROOKS, D.J., I.H. JENKINS & R.E. PASSINGHAM. 1993. Positron emission tomography studies on regional cerebral control of voluntary movement. In Role of the Cerebellum and Basal Ganglia in Voluntary Movement. N. Mano, I. Hamada & M.R. DeLong, Eds.: 267–274. Excerpta Medica. Amsterdam.
22. JENKINS, I.H., W. FERNANDEZ, E.D. PLAYFORD, et al. 1992. Impaired activation of the supplementary motor area in Parkinson's disease is reversed when akinesia is treated with apomorphine. Ann. Neurol. **32:** 749–757.
23. GILL, S.S., N.K. PATEL, K. O'SULLIVAN, et al. 2002. Intraparenchymal putaminal administration of glial-derived neurotrophic factor in the treatment of advanced Parkinson's disease. Neurology **58** (Suppl. 3): A241.
24. HAUSER, R.A., T.B. FREEMAN, B.J. SNOW, et al. 1999. Long-term evaluation of bilateral fetal nigral transplantation in Parkinson disease. Arch. Neurol. **56:** 179–187.
25. WHONE, A.L., R.Y. MOORE, P. PICCINI & D.J. BROOKS. 2001. Compensatory changes in the globus pallidus in early Parkinson's disease: an F-18-dopa PET study. Neurology **56** (Suppl. 3): A72–A73.
26. DODER, M., E.I. RABINER, N. TURJANSKI, et al. 2001. Functional imaging of tremor in Parkinson's disease with [C- 11]-WAY 100635 PET. Neurology **56** (Suppl. 3): A271–A272.
27. CHUGANI, D.C., R.F. ACKERMANN & M.E. PHELPS. 1988. In vivo 3H-spiperone binding: evidence for accumulation in corpus striatum by agonist mediated receptor internalisation J. Cereb. Blood Flow Metabol. **8:** 291–303.
28. MURIEL, M.P., V. BERNARD, A.I. LEVEY, et al. 1999. Levodopa induces a cytoplasmic localisation of D1 dopamine receptors in striatal neurons in Parkinson's disease. Ann. Neurol. **46:** 103–111.
29. LARUELLE, M. 2000. Imaging synaptic neurotransmission with in vivo binding competition techniques: a critical review. J. Cereb. Blood Flow Metab. **20:** 423–451.
30. VOLKOW, N.D., G.-J. WANG, J.S. FOWLER, et al. 1994. Imaging endogenous dopamine competition with [^{11}C]raclopride in the human brain. Synapse **16:** 255–262.
31. LARUELLE, M., C.D. D'SOUZA, R.M. BALDWIN, et al. 1997. Imaging D2 receptor occupancy by endogenous dopamine in humans. Neuropsychopharmacology **17:** 162–174.
32. GINOVART, N., L. FARDE, C. HALLDIN & C.G. SWAHN. 1999. Changes in striatal D2-receptor density following chronic treatment with amphetamine as assessed with PET in nonhuman primates. Synapse **31:** 154–162.
33. PICCINI, P., N. PAVESE, O. LINDVALL, et al. 2000. Endogenous dopamine release correlates with dopamine storage in patients with Parkinson's disease: an ^{11}C-raclopride and ^{18}F-dopa PET study. (Abstr.) Neurology **54** (Suppl. 3): A329.
34. IVERSEN, L.L. 1996. Smoking...harmful to the brain. Nature **382:** 206–207.
35. PICCINI, P., N. PAVESE & D.J. BROOKS. 2002. Effects of methamphetamine on mood correlate with endogenous dopamine release in frontal areas. Neurology **58** (Suppl. 3): A357.

36. KOEPP, M.J., R.N. GUNN, A.D. LAWRENCE, *et al.* 1998. Evidence for striatal dopamine release during a video game. Nature **393:** 266–268.
37. GRAYBIEL, A.M., T. AOSAKI, A.W. FLAHERTY, *et al.* 1994. The basal ganglia and adaptive motor control. Science **265:** 1826–1831.
38. LAWRENCE, A.D. & D.J. BROOKS. 1999. Neural correlates of reward processing in the human brain: a PET study. (Abstr.) Neurology **52** (Suppl. 2): A307.
39. GOERENDT, I.K., C. MESSA, A.D. LAWRENCE, *et al.* Dopamine release during sequential finger movements in health and Parkinson's disease: a PET study. Brain. In press.

Midbrain Dopaminergic Neurons

Determination of Their Developmental Fate by Transcription Factors

HORST H. SIMON, LAVINIA BHATT, DANIEL GHERBASSI, PAOLA SGADÓ, AND LAVINIA ALBERÍ

Center for Neuroscience, Department of Neuroanatomy, University of Heidelberg, 69120 Heidelberg, Germany

ABSTRACT: Midbrain dopaminergic neurons are the main source of dopamine in the mammalian central nervous system and are associated with one of the most prominent human neurological disorders, Parkinson's disease. During development, they are induced in the ventral midbrain by an interaction between two diffusible factors, SHH and FGF8. The local identity of this part of the midbrain is probably determined by the combinatorial expression of three transcription factors, *Otx2*, *Pax2*, and *Pax5*. After the last cell division, the neurons start to express transcription factors that control further differentiation and the manifestation of cellular properties characteristic for adult dopaminergic neurons of the substantia nigra compacta and the ventral tegmentum. The first to appear is the LIM-homeodomain transcription factor, *Lmx1b*. It is essential for the survival of these neurons, and it regulates the expression of another transcription factor, *Pitx3*, an activator of tyrosine hydroxylase. *Lmx1b* is followed by the orphan steroid receptor *Nurr1*. It is essential for the expression of the dopaminergic phenotype. Several genes involved in dopamine synthesis, transport, release, and reuptake are regulated by *Nurr1*. This requirement is specific to the midbrain dopaminergic neurons, since other populations of the same neurotransmitter phenotype develop normally in absence of the gene. A day after *Nurr1*, two homeodomain transcription factors, *engrailed-1* and *-2*, are expressed. In animals deficient in the two genes, the midbrain dopaminergic neurons are generated, but then fail to differentiate and disappear very rapidly. Interestingly, *α-synuclein*, a gene recently linked to familial forms of Parkinson's disease, is regulated by *engrailed-1* and *-2*.

KEYWORDS: substantia nigra; ventral tegmentum; Parkinson's disease; dopaminergic neurons; *Nurr1*; *engrailed*; *Lmx1b*; neuronal specification

Neurogenesis is a gradual process that transforms undefined neuroepithelial cells into fully differentiated neurons. It can be roughly divided into two phases: an early phase, when the precursor cells are proliferating and slowly adopt a successively more restricted cell fate; and a later phase, when the neurons are postmitotic and ful-

Address for correspondence: Horst H. Simon, Center for Neuroscience, Department of Neuroanatomy, University of Heidelberg, Im Neuenheimer Feld 307, 69120 Heidelberg, Germany. Voice: +49 6221 548342; fax: +49 6221 545605.

horst.simon@urz.uni-heidelberg.de

Ann. N.Y. Acad. Sci. 991: 36–47 (2003). © 2003 New York Academy of Sciences.

ly committed to a specific cell type, but not all adult properties are yet established. The most visible sign of the first phase is the appearance of regional subdivisions, like the fore-, mid- and hindbrain,[1] in the expanding neuroepithelium. During the second phase, examples of continuous differentiation are the outgrowth of axons and dendrites, the initiation of neurotransmitter synthesis, and the establishment of synaptic connections. The individual differentiation steps are often controlled by diffusible inductive and instructive signals,[2-4] to which the proliferating neuroepithelial cells and the postmitotic neurons respond in a concentration-dependent manner. Frequently, the first sign that a given cell has been further committed to the next step of differentiation is the up- or downregulation of transcription factors.[5]

Midbrain dopaminergic (mDA) neurons develop in this way. They are the largest source of dopamine in the mammalian central nervous system, located in three distinct nuclei, the ventral tegmental area (VTA), the substantia nigra compacta (SNC), and the retrorubral field.[6] Axons arising from DA neurons of the VTA form the mesolimbic pathway, innervating the nucleus accumbens and the olfactory tubercle. It has been speculated that changes in the limbic system are related to schizophrenia and other behavioral disorders.[7] Neurons of the SNC almost exclusively innervate the dorsal striatum forming the nigrostriatal pathway. They have been implicated in one of the most prominent human neurodegenerative disorders, Parkinson's disease (PD). A slow, progressive degeneration of DA neurons in the SNC leads to a diminished release of dopamine in the striatum. When a minimal threshold of dopamine is attained, the clinical symptoms of PD appear. They are caused by an excessive inhibition of brain stem and thalamocortical neurons involved in motor behavior.[8] The best known symptoms are resting tremor, muscular rigidity, difficulties in initiating movement, and loss of postural reflex.[9] Neuronal loss during PD is most prominent in nigral mDA neurons,[10] suggesting a specific vulnerability of this population. This idea is further supported by the unique toxicity of molecules like 6-hydroxydopamine, MPTP, and rotenone.[11] In recent years, a significant amount of scientific resources have been dedicated to identifying the molecules that cause this vulnerability. This ongoing work has led among other results to the identification of several independent developmental cascades that are essential for the generation of fully differentiated adult mDA neurons. These results are particularly important in the light of current research with the objective of generating these cells from embryonic[12-14] or adult[15,16] stem cells for new therapeutical approaches to PD.

EARLY EMBRYOGENESIS

The central nervous system arises from the neuroectoderm, which is generated briefly after gastrulation due to a series of inductive events. The neuroectoderm soon begins to thicken and subsequently rolls up along its rostrocaudal axis to form the neural tube that partitions at its rostral end into the basic subdivisions of the vertebrate brain, the fore-, mid- and hindbrain.[1,17] This rostrocaudal patterning is followed by the dorsoventral polarization of the neural tube,[18,19] which is induced by two antipodal diffusible signals. These are the ventralizing sonic hedgehog (SHH), which emanates from the notochord and floor plate, and the dorsalizing bone morphogenetic proteins (BMPs), which are first released by nonepidermal ectoderm and later by roof plate cells.[18] During this period of development, the expression do-

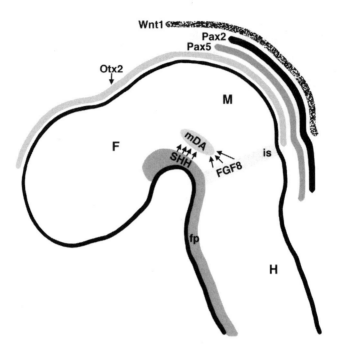

FIGURE 1. Expression pattern of *Otx2*, *Pax2*, *Pax5*, and *Wnt-1* at E8 and E9 of mouse development. The simplified scheme of the expression domains of *Otx2*, *Pax2*, *Pax5*, and *Wnt-1*, which are represented by *bars* above the embryo, shows an overlap of all four genes in the midbrain rostral to the isthmus. This is the region where the mDA neurons are induced by an interaction between SHH and FGF8. The scheme does not reflect the dynamic nature of the expression pattern at these ages. SHH = sonic hedgehog, FGF8 = fibroblast growth factor 8, fp = floor plate, is = isthmus, F = forebrain, M = midbrain, H = hindbrain.

mains of transcription factors begin to delineate the region that will give rise to mDA neurons. Probably the first to do so is the homeobox transcription factor *Otx2*, which initially appears in all three germ layers, regresses during further development, and from E7 onwards (mouse) defines the anterior neuroectoderm that will give rise to the fore- and midbrain. Shortly thereafter, *Pax2* appears in the developing midbrain, followed by *Pax5* at the same location. In parallel to *Pax2*, the secreted molecule *Wnt1* is expressed (FIG.1). Homozygous mutant mice null for *Otx2*, *Wnt1*, and the double mutants for *Pax2/5* all show the same phenotype with respect to the midbrain—a complete deletion of it.[20–23] A consequence of midbrain deletion in *Wnt1*–/– mutants is the lack of all mDA neurons (FIG. 2). This is very likely also the case in *Otx2*-null mutants since the fore-, mid-, and anterior hindbrain are deleted. A dependence of *Pax2*, *Pax5*, and *Wnt1* on each other after the initial onset of their expression suggests the same for the *Pax2/5* double mutants.[24] Further evidence that the *Otx2*, *Pax2*, and *Pax5* expression domain is the source for mDA neurons is provided by explant culture experiments and the analysis of transgenic mice.[25–27] The mDA neurons are induced at E9 (rat) by the combinatorial action of SHH and the fibroblast growth factor 8 (FGF8), released by the floor plate and isthmus, respec-

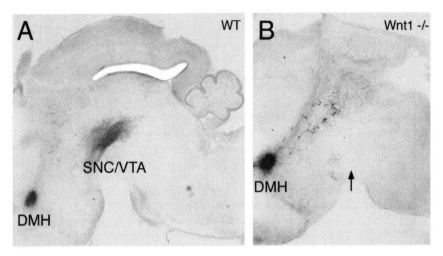

FIGURE 2. Total loss of mDA neurons in *Wnt1*-null mutant. Midsagittal brain sections of P0 wild-type and *Wnt1−/−* mutant mouse stained against TH. (**A**) TH-positive cell bodies of SNC and VTA are detectable in the ventral midbrain of the wild type, whereas (**B**) the mutant mice have lost all mDA neurons (*arrow*). Staining in the dorsomedial hypothalamic nucleus (DMH) demonstrates that other dopaminergic populations are not affected.

tively. The floor plate spans almost the entire rostral-to-caudal neuroaxis, and the isthmus releases FGF8 into the midbrain and into the hindbrain. However, only a very restricted area of the developing neural tube, the midbrain directly anterior to the isthmus, is capable of generating DA neurons characteristic for the SNC and VTA. Further evidence was provided by the analysis of transgenic mice that express *HNF3β* under the *En2* promoter enhancer. These mice form an ectopic dorsal *SHH*-expressing floor plate in the midbrain and the anterior hindbrain, leading to an ectopic induction of mDA neurons in the midbrain tissue, but not in the hindbrain. These findings demonstrated that only the tissue rostral to the isthmus is competent to form mDA neurons. The developmental stage when the mDA neurons are generated corresponds to the timing of the *Otx2*, *Pax2*, and *Pax5* expression; and the region of the neural tube where the induction takes place is the area where these three transcription factors overlap. All this strongly suggests that the combination of the three specifies the region along the rostrocaudal axis of the neural tube where mDA can be generated, but the final conclusive experiments are still missing. If this hypothesis is true, a caudal shift of the *Otx2* domain should increase the amount of mDA neurons or at least reallocate them in the posterior direction.[28]

POSTMITOTIC DIFFERENTIATION OF MIDBRAIN DOPAMINERGIC NEURONS

Studies using tritiated thymidine on rat fetuses showed that the majority of mDA neurons become postmitotic at around E13 to E15.[29] This corresponds to approximately E11 to E13 in mouse (from here on we will use mouse embryonic ages even if rat studies are mentioned, setting mouse age at rat − 2 days). Twelve to 24 hours later tyrosine hydroxylase (TH), the rate-limiting enzyme of dopamine synthesis, is detectable by conventional immunohistochemistry.[30] The exact start point of the *TH* expression is, however, controversial. Studies using an acrolein-based fixative were able to identify TH-positive cells on the ventricular side of the ventral midbrain as early as E8.5 to E9, suggesting that mDA neurons express *TH* before or shortly after they become postmotic.[31] All in all, the mDA neurons belong to one of the first neuronal populations generated in the developing CNS.[32] After becoming postmitotic, the next major developmental step is the formation of axonal connections to the basal ganglia and the frontal cortex. The first thin processes resembling axons are detectable with an antibody against dopamine at E11.[33] A day later, thick axonal bundles that have passed the diencephalons begin to enter the ventral telencephalon, where the forefront of the bundle reaches the ganglionic eminence and bends towards the cortical anlage. The formation of axonal terminals and the transient striosomal patterning begin at E18. Some of these differentiation steps are associated with the appearance of transcription factors, which probably regulate the individual events. Three independent regulatory pathways involved in the differentiation of the mDA neurons have been identified to date. The key transcription factors for these regulatory pathways are *Nurr1*, the *engrailed* genes, and *Lmx1b*.

THE ORPHAN STEROID RECEPTOR *Nurr1*

Nurr1 (also known as RNR1, Not, or HZF-1) was first recognized by its expression in the brain[34] and regenerating liver.[35] Its sequence suggests that it is an orphan nuclear receptor with a yet-unidentified ligand and acts as a ligand-activated transcription factor. It appears in the marginal and mantle zone of the ventral midbrain at E10.5, at the location where mDA neurons are generated, but 24 hours before they express any phenotypic markers such as *TH*.[36] From this age continuing into adulthood, *Nurr1* is expressed in at least 95% of all *TH*-positive midbrain neurons.[37] The targeted deletion of *Nurr1* by homologous recombination leads to mutant mice that seem to develop normally during embryogenesis but are unable to feed and die shortly after birth.[15,36,38] Detailed analysis of these mutant mice demonstrated that *Nurr1* controls the most prominent feature of mDA neurons, the use of dopamine as their neurotransmitter. Several genes that are involved in synthesis, axonal transport, storage, release, or reuptake of dopamine are not expressed in the mutant neurons. These genes are *TH*, *AADC* (aromatic aminoacid decarboxylase), *VMAT* (vesicle membrane–associated transporter), and *DAT* (dopamine transporter).[36,38,39] Surprisingly, this requirement of *Nurr1* for the expression of the dopaminergic phenotype is restricted to mDA neurons alone. Furthermore, the use of *Nurr1*-independent markers for mDA neurons, such as *AHD2*, *En1*, and a *Nurr1* riboprobe 5′ to the deletion, revealed that the cells otherwise develop normally in the mutant embryos until E15.5. From this point of embryogenesis, the reports of two groups who analyzed the mutant phenotype contradict each other. One group claims a role of *Nurr1* in the migration, striatal target innervation, and survival of these cells.[40] The DA neurons in the *Nurr1* mutants were abnormally distributed, no axons were traceable from the striatum, and a high amount of apoptotic nuclei were present in the ventral midbrain. The other group, doing essentially the same experiments, was unable to observe any of these alterations.[41] However, the two groups agreed in one respect, that there are still some mDA neurons left in the *Nurr1* mutant mice at birth. An explanation for these different observations could be that the investigated mutant mice are the results of two separate experiments using different constructs. The first group removed exons 2, 3, and part of 4, whereas the second group removed only exon 3. It is therefore plausible that a partial Nurr1 protein is still translated in the latter case, resulting in a weaker phenotype.

THE HOMEODOMAIN TRANSCRIPTION FACTORS
Engrailed-1 AND *Engrailed–2*

The mammalian *engrailed* genes, *En1* and En2, are homeodomain transcription factors that were originally cloned on the basis of their sequence similarity to *Drosophila engrailed*.[42,43] As in insects, they have two distinct ontogenetic roles: during early embryogenesis they take part in the regionalization of the embryo,[44–47] whereas during later embryogenesis they are involved in the specification of neuronal phenotypes.[48–51] Both *engrailed* genes appear at E8 in the anterior mouse neuroectoderm as patches, which subsequently fuse to mark a band of cells that will later give rise to the border region between midbrain and hindbrain. Between E11 and E12, the two genes emerge in postmitotic mDA neurons and are then continuously expressed throughout the entire life of these cells (FIG. 3).[51–53] Mice homozygous for an *En1*-null mutation die at birth and show a deletion of the inferior colliculus and parts of the cerebellum; both these brain areas arise from the midbrain neuroepithelium, which expresses *En1* during early embryogenesis.[47] The *En2* mutant phenotype is comparatively subtle despite the overlapping expression with *En1* in the midbrain. These mice are viable and fertile, and show only a minor defect in cerebellar foliation.[54,55] Neither of the two *engrailed* mutant strains, however, show a significant phenotype with respect to mDA neurons. The requirement for the *engrailed* genes is apparent only in mutant mice deficient for both *En1* and *En2*. Like the *En1*-null mutants, the *engrailed* double mutants die at birth and exhibit a deletion of the midbrain and anterior hindbrain. The phenotype with respect to mDA neurons is, however, significantly different. The neurons are generated in the ventral midbrain and start to express *TH*, but then fail to further differentiate and disappear. By E14, they are no longer detectable (FIG. 4D). Use of an *En-1/tau-LacZ* knock-in mouse as an autonomous marker demonstrated that the cells are lost in the double-mutant animals, unlike the *Nurr1* mutant mice, where only the neurotransmitter phenotype is changed. Since the *engrailed* double-mutant mice show a deletion of the midbrain and anterior hindbrain,[51,56] two scenarios are possible. Either the genes are cell-autonomously required for the survival or, due to the missing midbrain tissue, an essential external support is absent in the mutant mice (non-cell-autonomous). Such questions are best addressed by experiments that mix wild-type and mutant cells. *Engrailed* double-mutant ES cells were injected into wild-type blastula and the chimeras raised to adulthood. These animals showed a normal brain morphology but a significant loss of DA neurons in the SNC and VTA, clearly demonstrating that the *engrailed* genes are cell autonomously required for the survival of these cells (unpublished data). Furthermore, the mutant analysis also provided evidence that the expression of α-*synuclein* may be regulated by the two *engrailed* genes. α-*Synuclein*

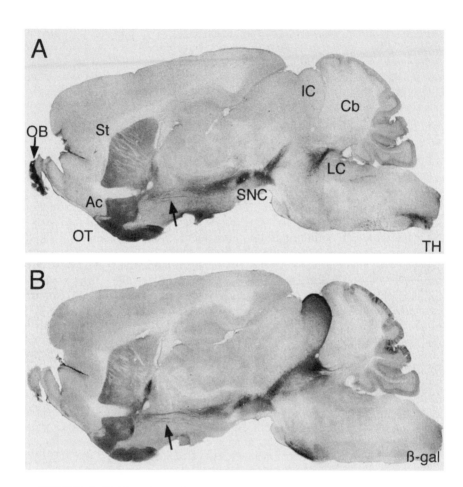

FIGURE 3. *En1* is expressed by mDA neurons. Sagittal brain section immunostained against TH (**A**) and β-gal (**B**) of adult mouse, where En1 was replaced by tau-lacZ in one allele. (**A,B**) Cell bodies in the VTA and the SNC, their axons (*arrow*), and their axonal terminals in the dorsal striatum (St), the nucleus accumbens (Ac), and the olfactory tubercle (OT) are stained by the antibodies against TH and β-gal. (**A**) TH expression is also observed in the locus coeruleus (LC) and the olfactory bulb (OB) and (**B**) β-gal expression in the inferior colliculus (IC) and the superior olive, which corresponds to the normal En1 expression pattern. NOTE: the normal nuclear distribution of the transcription factor En1 is represented in the tau-LacZ mouse by the cytoplasmic β-gal that is found in the cell bodies and the axons. Cb = cerebellum.

appears at around E12, an age when the cells are still present in the *engrailed* double-mutant embryos. The *En1* single mutant exhibits a significant reduction of the α-*synuclein* expression, and it is totally absent in the remaining mDA neurons of the double mutant.[51] Interestingly, two human point mutations in the α-*synuclein* gene have been recently linked to a familial form of PD.[57,58]

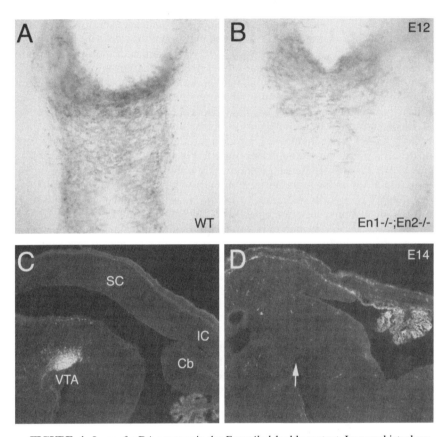

FIGURE 4. Loss of mDA neurons in the *Engrailed* double mutant. Immunohistochemistry against TH on whole mounts of E12 embryo brains **(A,B)** and midsagittal sections of E14 embryo head **(C,D)** of wild type **(A,C)** and En1–/–; En2–/– mutant **(B,D)**. **(A)** Wholemount staining of wild type reveals TH-positive cells in the ventral midbrain that will give rise to the dopaminergic neurons of the SNC and VTA. **(B)** TH-positive cells are also present in the ventral midbrain of engrailed double mutants; however, the amount of cells is significantly smaller than in the wild type. **(C)** Two days later at E14, the dopaminergic neurons, which begin to adopt an adult distribution, are detectable in the wild-type ventral midbrain. Cb = cerebellum; IC = inferior colliculus; SC = superior colliculus; VTA = ventral tegmental area. **(D)** The E14 mutant brain at the same plane of section shows no dopaminergic neurons at this position (*arrow*).

THE LIM-HOMEODOMAIN TRANSCRIPTION FACTOR 1B (*Lmx1b*) AND THE PITUITARY HOMEOBOX 3 (*Pitx3*)

Lmx1b is a member of the LIM-homeodomain family of proteins. It is expressed in a wide range of different tissues and has been implicated in the development of diverse structures such as skeleton, eye, kidney, and limb.[59] In humans, loss-of-function mutations lead to nail patella syndrome,[60] defects that are very similar to those seen in mice homozygous for the *Lmx1b* null mutation.[59] Its role in the development of mDA neurons has recently come to light. It is expressed in the neural tube as early as E7.5, including the region of the ventral midbrain that gives rise to dopamine cells.[61] At least from E16 continuing into adulthood, it is colocalized with *TH* and *Pitx3* (see below) in the ventral midbrain. The specificity of this expression was confirmed by unilateral injection of 6-hydroxydopamine into the striatum. The functional deletion of *Lmx1b* by homologous recombination has a profound effect on mDA neurons. Only a small amount of TH-positive cells are detectable in the ventral midbrain at E12.5, and they entirely disappear a few days later. Additionally, the expression of *Pitx3* is affected in these embryos. The wild-type expression of *Pitx3* in the ventral midbrain always matches the distribution of *TH*; however, in the *Lmx1b* mutant embryos fewer cells were positive for *Pitx3* than for *TH*, suggesting a regulatory role of *Lmx1b*. Unfortunately, the published data are rather limited, and it is an open question whether the ablation of mDA neurons in the mutant is due to a cell-autonomous requirement of *Lmx1b* in the neurons or is an effect of the large midbrain deficit also observed in the mutant animals. In the chicken, the expression of *Lmx1b* is followed by the expression of *Wnt1*; and gain-of-function experiments using a replication-competent retroviral vector (Lmx1b/RCAS) suggest that *Lmx1b* is required for the onset and maintenance of the *Wnt1* expression.[62] If this interaction also exists in mouse, then the *Lmx1b* mutant phenotype with respect to the mDA neurons is likely to be a consequence of the lack of *Wnt1* expression in the midbrain (FIG. 2); this argues against the notion of a cell-autonomous requirement of *Lmx1b*. Furthermore, it is still unresolved whether the cells that express *Lmx1b* in the ventral midbrain during early embryogenesis are the precursor cells of adult mDA neurons or this expression is purely coincidental.

   Pitx3, also sometimes called *Ptx3*, (paired-like homeodomain transcription factor 3 or pituitary homeobox 3) is a homeodomain containing transcription factor with binding activity to DNA similar to the *Drosophila bicoid*. It is uniquely expressed in the brain by mDA neurons from E11.5 onwards and is maintained throughout the entire life of the animal.[63] Its relevance is connected to the appearance of *TH* just briefly after *Pitx3* is detected and the presence of a conserved *bicoid* response element (GGCTTT) just a few bases upstream of the TATA box of the TH gene in the rat, mouse, and human.[64] Gel shift experiments demonstrated an affinity of *Pitx3* to this response element. Moreover, transient transfection experiments showed a cell type–dependent 8- to 12-fold increase of *TH* promoter activity when the Pitx3 protein was present. However, such *in situ* studies are only suggestive, and the precise role of *Pitx3* in the development of the mDA neurons still needs to be determined. It is likely that the analysis of the Aphakia mutant mice, which has been recently linked to a deletion in the *Pitx3* gene,[65,66] may provide evidence pointing to its biological function.

REFERENCES

1. LUMSDEN, A. & R. KRUMLAUF. 1996. Patterning the vertebrate neuraxis. Science **274:** 1109–1115.
2. MCALLISTER, A.K., L.C. KATZ & D.C. LO. 1999. Neurotrophins and synaptic plasticity. Annu. Rev. Neurosci. **22:** 295–318.

3. MARTI, E. & P. BOVOLENTA. 2002. Sonic hedgehog in CNS development: one signal, multiple outputs. Trends Neurosci. **25:** 89–96.
4. KENNEDY, T.E. 2000. Cellular mechanisms of netrin function: long-range and short-range actions. Biochem. Cell Biol. **78:** 569–575.
5. EDLUND, T. & T.M. JESSELL. 1999. Progression from extrinsic to intrinsic signaling in cell fate specification: a view from the nervous system. Cell **96:** 211–224.
6. NELSON, E.L., *et al.* 1996. Midbrain dopaminergic neurons in the mouse: computer-assisted mapping. J. Comp. Neurol. **369:** 361–371.
7. MEYER-LINDENBERG, A., *et al.* 2002. Reduced prefrontal activity predicts exaggerated striatal dopaminergic function in schizophrenia. Nat. Neurosci. **5:** 267–271.
8. OBESO, J.A., *et al.* 2000. Pathophysiology of the basal ganglia in Parkinson's disease. Trends Neurosci. **23:** S8–19.
9. JENNER, P., A.H. SCHAPIRA & C.D. MARSDEN. 1992. New insights into the cause of Parkinson's disease. Neurology **42:** 2241–2250.
10. HIRSCH, E.C., *et al.* 1997. Neuronal vulnerability in Parkinson's disease. J. Neural Transm. Suppl. **50:** 79–88.
11. BEAL, M.F. 2001. Experimental models of Parkinson's disease. Nat. Rev. Neurosci. **2:** 325–334.
12. LEE, S.H., *et al.* 2000. Efficient generation of midbrain and hindbrain neurons from mouse embryonic stem cells. Nat. Biotechnol. **18:** 675–679.
13. KAWASAKI, H., *et al.* 2000. Induction of midbrain dopaminergic neurons from ES cells by stromal cell-derived inducing activity. Neuron **28:** 31–40.
14. ROLLETSCHEK, A., *et al.* 2001. Differentiation of embryonic stem cell-derived dopaminergic neurons is enhanced by survival-promoting factors. Mech. Dev. **105:** 93–104.
15. SAKURADA, K., *et al.* 1999. Nurr1, an orphan nuclear receptor, is a transcriptional activator of endogenous tyrosine hydroxylase in neural progenitor cells derived from the adult brain. Development **126:** 4017–4026.
16. LIE, D.C., *et al.* 2002. The adult substantia nigra contains progenitor cells with neurogenic potential. J. Neurosci. **22:** 6639–6649.
17. RUBENSTEIN, J.L. & P.A. BEACHY. 1998. Patterning of the embryonic forebrain. Curr. Opin. Neurobiol. **8:** 18–26.
18. LEE, K.J. & T.M. JESSELL. 1999. The specification of dorsal cell fates in the vertebrate central nervous system. Annu. Rev. Neurosci. **22:** 261–294.
19. SIMON, H., A. HORNBRUCH & A. LUMSDEN. 1995. Independent assignment of antero-posterior and dorso-ventral positional values in the developing chick hindbrain. Curr. Biol. **5:** 205–214.
20. ACAMPORA, D., *et al.* 1995. Forebrain and midbrain regions are deleted in Otx2-/- mutants due to a defective anterior neuroectoderm specification during gastrulation. Development **121:** 3279–3290.
21. ANG, S.L., *et al.* 1996. A targeted mouse Otx2 mutation leads to severe defects in gastrulation and formation of axial mesoderm and to deletion of rostral brain. Development **122:** 243–252.
22. SCHWARZ, M., *et al.* 1997. Conserved biological function between Pax-2 and Pax-5 in midbrain and cerebellum development: evidence from targeted mutations. Proc. Natl. Acad. Sci. USA **94:** 14518–14523.
23. MCMAHON, A.P. & A. BRADLEY. 1990. The Wnt-1 (int-1) proto-oncogene is required for development of a large region of the mouse brain. Cell **62:** 1073–1085.
24. RHINN, M. & M. BRAND. 2001. The midbrain-hindbrain boundary organizer. Curr. Opin. Neurobiol. **11:** 34–42.
25. HYNES, M., *et al.* 1995. Control of neuronal diversity by the floor plate: contact-mediated induction of midbrain dopaminergic neurons. Cell **80:** 95–101.
26. HYNES, M., *et al.* 1995. Induction of midbrain dopaminergic neurons by Sonic hedgehog. Neuron **15:** 35–44.
27. YE, W., *et al.* 1998. FGF and Shh signals control dopaminergic and serotonergic cell fate in the anterior neural plate. Cell **93:** 755–766.
28. BROCCOLI, V., E. BONCINELLI & W. WURST. 1999. The caudal limit of Otx2 expression positions the isthmic organizer. Nature **401:** 164–168.

29. ALTMAN, J. & S.A. BAYER. 1981. Development of the brain stem in the rat. V. Thymidine-radiographic study of the time of origin of neurons in the midbrain tegmentum. J. Comp. Neurol. **198:** 677–716.
30. FOSTER, G.A., *et al.* 1988. Ontogeny of the dopamine and cyclic adenosine-3':5'-monophosphate-regulated phosphoprotein (DARPP-32) in the pre- and postnatal mouse central nervous system. Int. J. Dev. Neurosci. **6:** 367–386.
31. DI PORZIO, U., *et al.* 1990. Early appearance of tyrosine hydroxylase immunoreactive cells in the mesencephalon of mouse embryos. Int. J. Dev. Neurosci. **8:** 523–532.
32. SECHRIST, J. & M. BRONNER-FRASER. 1991. Birth and differentiation of reticular neurons in the chick hindbrain: ontogeny of the first neuronal population. Neuron **7:** 947–963.
33. VOORN, P., *et al.* 1988. The pre- and postnatal development of the dopaminergic cell groups in the ventral mesencephalon and the dopaminergic innervation of the striatum of the rat. Neuroscience **25:** 857–887.
34. LAW, S.W., *et al.* 1992. Identification of a new brain-specific transcription factor, NURR1. Mol. Endocrinol. **6:** 2129–2135.
35. SCEARCE, L.M., *et al.* 1993. RNR-1, a nuclear receptor in the NGFI-B/Nur77 family that is rapidly induced in regenerating liver. J. Biol. Chem. **268:** 8855–8861.
36. ZETTERSTRÖM, R.H., *et al.* 1997. Dopamine neuron agenesis in Nurr1-deficient mice. Science **276:** 248–250.
37. BACKMAN, C., *et al.* 1999. A selective group of dopaminergic neurons express Nurr1 in the adult mouse brain. Brain Res. **851:** 125–132.
38. CASTILLO, S.O., *et al.* 1998. Dopamine biosynthesis is selectively abolished in substantia nigra/ventral tegmental area but not in hypothalamic neurons in mice with targeted disruption of the Nurr1 gene. Mol. Cell. Neurosci. **11:** 36–46.
39. SAUCEDO-CARDENAS, O., *et al.* 1998. Nurr1 is essential for the induction of the dopaminergic phenotype and the survival of ventral mesencephalic late dopaminergic precursor neurons. Proc. Natl. Acad. Sci. USA **95:** 4013–4018.
40. WALLEN, A., *et al.* 1999. Fate of mesencephalic AHD2-expressing dopamine progenitor cells in NURR1 mutant mice. Exp. Cell Res. **253:** 737–746.
41. WITTA, J., *et al.* 2000. Nigrostriatal innervation is preserved in Nurr1-null mice, although dopaminergic neuron precursors are arrested from terminal differentiation. Mol. Brain Res. **84:** 67–78.
42. JOYNER, A.L., *et al.* 1985. Expression during embryogenesis of a mouse gene with sequence homology to the Drosophila engrailed gene. Cell **43:** 29–37.
43. JOYNER, A.L. & G.R. MARTIN. 1987. En-1 and En-2, two mouse genes with sequence homology to the Drosophila engrailed gene: expression during embryogenesis [published erratum appears in 1987. Genes Dev. **1**(5): 521]. Genes Dev. **1:** 29–38.
44. KORNBERG, T., *et al.* 1985. The engrailed locus of Drosophila: in situ localization of transcripts reveals compartment-specific expression. Cell **40:** 45–53.
45. KORNBERG, T. 1981. Engrailed: a gene controlling compartment and segment formation in Drosophila. Proc. Natl. Acad. Sci. USA **78:** 1095–1099.
46. TABATA, T., *et al.* 1995. Creating a Drosophila wing de novo, the role of engrailed, and the compartment border hypothesis. Development **121:** 3359–3369.
47. WURST, W., A.B. AUERBACH & A.L. JOYNER. 1994. Multiple developmental defects in Engrailed-1 mutant mice: an early mid-hindbrain deletion and patterning defects in forelimbs and sternum. Development **120:** 2065–2075.
48. LUNDELL, M.J., *et al.* 1996. The engrailed and huckebein genes are essential for development of serotonin neurons in the Drosophila CNS. Mol. Cell. Neurosci. **7:** 46–61.
49. CONDRON, B.G., N.H. PATEL & K. ZINN. 1994. Engrailed controls glial/neuronal cell fate decisions at the midline of the central nervous system. Neuron **13:** 541–554.
50. SAUERESSIG, H., J. BURRILL & M. GOULDING. 1999. Engrailed-1 and netrin-1 regulate axon pathfinding by association interneurons that project to motor neurons. Development **126:** 4201–4212.
51. SIMON, H.H., *et al.* 2001. Fate of midbrain dopaminergic neurons controlled by the engrailed genes. J. Neurosci. **21:** 3126–3134.

52. DAVIS, C.A. & A.L. JOYNER. 1988. Expression patterns of the homeo box-containing genes En-1 and En-2 and the proto-oncogene int-1 diverge during mouse development. Genes Dev. **2:** 1736–1744.
53. GARDNER, C.A. & K.F. BARALD. 1992. Expression patterns of engrailed-like proteins in the chick embryo. Dev. Dyn. **193:** 370–388.
54. MILLEN, K.J., *et al.* 1994. Abnormal embryonic cerebellar development and patterning of postnatal foliation in two mouse Engrailed-2 mutants. Development **120:** 695–706.
55. JOYNER, A.L., *et al.* 1991. Subtle cerebellar phenotype in mice homozygous for a targeted deletion of the En-2 homeobox. Science **251:** 1239–1243.
56. LIU, A. & A.L. JOYNER. 2001. EN and GBX2 play essential roles downstream of FGF8 in patterning the mouse mid/hindbrain region. Development **128:** 181–191.
57. KRUGER, R., *et al.* 1998. Ala30Pro mutation in the gene encoding alpha-synuclein in Parkinson's disease. Nat. Genet. **18:** 106–108.
58. POLYMEROPOULOS, M.H., *et al.* 1997. Mutation in the alpha-synuclein gene identified in families with Parkinson's disease. Science **276:** 2045–2047.
59. CHEN, H., *et al.* 1998. Limb and kidney defects in Lmx1b mutant mice suggest an involvement of LMX1B in human nail patella syndrome. Nat. Genet. **19:** 51–55.
60. KNOERS, N.V., *et al.* 2000. Nail-patella syndrome: identification of mutations in the LMX1B gene in Dutch families. J. Am. Soc. Nephrol. **11:** 1762–1766.
61. MIDT, M.P., *et al.* 2000. A second independent pathway for development of mesencephalic dopaminergic neurons requires Lmx1b. Nat. Neurosci. **3:** 337–341.
62. ADAMS, K.A., *et al.* 2000. The transcription factor Lmx1b maintains Wnt1 expression within the isthmic organizer. Development **127:** 1857–1867.
63. SMIDT, M.P., *et al.* 1997. A homeodomain gene Ptx3 has highly restricted brain expression in mesencephalic dopaminergic neurons. Proc. Natl. Acad. Sci. USA **94:** 13305–13310.
64. CAZORLA, P., *et al.* 2000. A response element for the homeodomain transcription factor Ptx3 in the tyrosine hydroxylase gene promoter. J. Neurochem. **74:** 1829–1837.
65. RIEGER, D.K., *et al.* 2001. A double-deletion mutation in the Pitx3 gene causes arrested lens development in aphakia mice. Genomics **72:** 61–72.
66. SEMINA, E.V., *et al.* 2000. Deletion in the promoter region and altered expression of Pitx3 homeobox gene in aphakia mice. Hum. Mol. Genet. **9:** 1575–1585.

Transcriptional Control of Dopamine Neuron Development

ÅSA WALLÉN AND THOMAS PERLMANN

The Ludwig Institute for Cancer Research and Department of Cell and Molecular Biology, Karolinska Institutet, SE-171 77 Stockholm, Sweden

ABSTRACT: Recent studies have identified several factors that influence the development of midbrain dopamine (DA) neurons. The identity of early proliferating DA progenitor cells are specified by the secreted factors sonic hedgehog and fibroblast growth factor 8, derived from the floor plate of the ventral midline and the mid/hindbrain border, respectively. While transcription factors specifically expressed in the proliferating DA progenitor cells remain to be identified, several transcription factors important for postmitotic DA cell development have been characterized. These include Nurr1, Lmx1b, Pitx3, and En1/En2. The studies of these transcription factors have not only increased the understanding of how DA neurons are generated *in vivo*, but also allowed the development of new strategies using stem cells for engineering DA neurons *in vitro*, results that may have significance in future therapies of patients with Parkinson's disease.

KEYWORDS: dopamine neuron; development; progenitor cell; stem cell; Parkinson's disease; transcription factor; nuclear receptor; Nurr1; Pitx3; Lmx1b; engrailed

ORGANIZATION OF DOPAMINE NEURONS

The original identification and localization of the brain dopamine (DA) cell groups was done by the Falck-Hillarp histofluorescence method,[1] which is based on the visualization of fluorescent monoamines upon formaldehyde treatment. It was shown that DA cells are localized in the diencephalon (part of the forebrain), in the mesencephalon (midbrain), and in the olfactory bulb and retina.[2,3] The most prominent DA cell group resides in the ventral part of the mesencephalon, which contains approximately 75% of the total number of brain DA cells. Within the ventral midbrain, the DA neurons are located in the lateral groups of the retrorubral field (RRF) and the substantia nigra pars compacta (SNc) as well as the medially located ventral tegmental area (VTA). Based on the initial mapping studies, these cell groups are also commonly referred to as A8, A9, and A10, respectively.[2] The DA neurons

Address for correspondence: Thomas Perlmann, The Ludwig Institute, Box 240, Karolinska Institutet, SE-17177 Stockholm, Sweden. Voice: +46-8-728-7106; fax: +46-8-332-812; or Åsa Wallén, AstraZeneca R&D, Transgenics and Comparative Genomics, SE-42183 Mölndal, Sweden. Voice: +46-31-7065532; fax: +46-31-7763705.
thomas.perlmann@licr.ki.se
asa.wallen@astrazeneca.com

Ann. N.Y. Acad. Sci. 991: 48–60 (2003). © 2003 New York Academy of Sciences.

project to different forebrain areas, forming the mesotelenecephalic system, where the target neurons are localized in the striatal, limbic, and cortical areas. The SNc neurons project to the dorsolateral striatum, the caudate putamen, forming the nigrostriatal pathway involved in the control of voluntary movement. The neurons of the VTA project via the median forebrain bundle to the ventromedial striatum and the subcortical and cortical areas, forming the mesolimbocortical system, which is involved in emotional behavior and mechanisms of natural motivation and reward. Finally, RRF neurons project to the SNc and VTA and seem to be involved in interconnecting these two areas. They also project to the dorsal striatum via the nigrostriatal pathway.[4,5]

SPECIFICATION OF A PROLIFERATING DOPAMINE PROGENITOR CELL

The mesencephalic DA neurons are generated in the immediate vicinity of two organizing centers, the mid/hindbrain boundary (MHB; also called the isthmus organizer) and the floor plate, a specialized cell type that lies along the CNS ventral midline. Expression of tyrosine hydroxylase (TH), the rate-limiting enzyme of DA synthesis and a frequently used marker for DA neurons, can be detected from approximately embryonic day (E) 11 in the mouse midbrain. TH initially appears rostrally of the MHB and close to the ventral midline.[6] Several studies show that proliferating DA progenitor cells are specified well before E11 by the combined actions of two secreted signaling proteins, sonic hedgehog (Shh) and fibroblast growth factor 8 (Fgf8).[7,8] Shh is secreted from the floor plate and is instructive in positional information along the dorsoventral axis at many levels of the developing CNS.[9–14] Fgf8 is locally produced in the narrow domain corresponding to the MHB.[15–17] *Shh* and *Fgf8* expression domains intersect in the ventral MHB, and the combined signaling by these two proteins leads to the induction of DA progenitor cells rostrally of the MHB. Interestingly, Shh and Fgf8, together with Fgf4, are also required for specification of serotonergic neurons located caudally of the MHB.[17] A schematic illustration of the location of Shh, Fgf4, Fgf8, DA, and serotonergic neurons in the early mouse brain is shown in FIGURE 1.

Remarkably, only one marker specific for the proliferating DA progenitor cells has been reported. Aldh1 (previously named AHD2), an aldehyde dehydrogenase capable of metabolizing retinaldehyde into retinoic acid,[18] is expressed in the ventral midbrain already at E9.5.[19] Its expression is confined to proliferating cells of the ventral midbrain neuroepithelium, but it continues to be expressed after cells have stopped proliferating and is later colocalized with postmitotic markers including TH.[20] These findings raise the possibility that retinoic acid is an additional early signal involved in DA cell differentiation. However, although retinoids have been shown to promote maturation of a dopaminergic cell line,[21] any clear data supporting a role in DA cell development *in vivo* remains to be presented.

Several transcription factors are expressed in the early midbrain neuroepithelium, but their expression patterns are not confined to the domain of DA progenitor cells. These factors include engrailed (En1 and En2), Lmx1b, Otx2, and Gbx2.[6] This early expression is a reflection of their roles in the establishment and patterning of the mid/hindbrain region rather than of their functions in generating specific neuronal

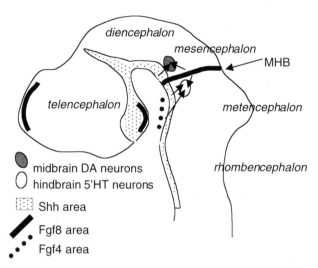

FIGURE 1. Schematic representation of the developing mouse CNS. The figure shows a sagittal section of the embryonic mouse CNS where the floor-plate Shh-positive arease and the MHB Fgf8-postitive areas are marked. Note that the figure represents mouse CNS at approximately E11.5; however, several of the described signaling events occur earlier, as described in the text and in FIGURE 2. At the intersection of Shh and Fgf8 in the MHB, these secreted molecules give rise to DA neurons rostrally of the MHB and 5′HT neurons caudally of this boundary. In addition to Shh and Fgf8, 5′HT neurons require signaling by Fgf4, which might be derived from the primitive streak at earlier developmental stages. The intersection of telencephalic Fgf8 with the floor plate Shh is believed to induce forebrain DA neuron progenitor cells (reviewed in Hynes and Rosenthal 1999).[7] The telencephalon and diencephalon are collectively called the *forebrain*, and the terms *rhombencephalon* and *metencephalon* are collectively called the *hindbrain*. (Drawing adapted from Wurst & Bally-Cuif.[6])

identities.[22–24] Thus, an important future goal should be to identify transcription factors involved in specifying DA neuron identity in the developing midbrain.

POSTMITOTIC DIFFERENTIATION

The first postmitotic differentiating DA cells appear at approximately E10–10.5 in the mouse.[25] The cessation of proliferation is followed by upregulation of general neuronal and specific dopaminergic markers such as TH. Newly formed neurons migrate into medial and lateral positions, to form the A8–A10 areas, and they also begin to initiate target innervation. Several transcription factors influencing these developmental processes have recently been characterized. These factors include the nuclear receptor Nurr1 and the homeodomain transcription factors Lmx1b, Pitx3, and En1/En2. FIGURE 2 shows the temporal sequence whereby these and other dopaminergic markers are induced during DA neuron development. In the following, we will review our current understanding of how these factors influence DA neuron development.

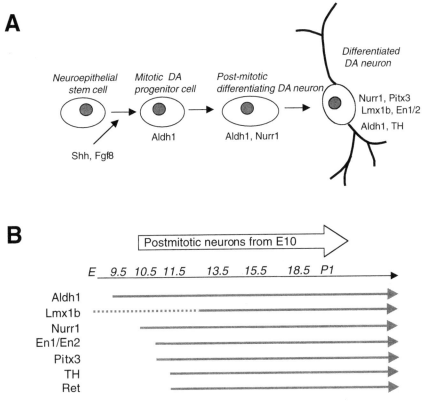

FIGURE 2. (**A**) Midbrain DA cell development in the mouse. Shh and Fgf8 specify a mitotic DA progenitor cell expressing Aldh1. As these cells become postmitotic, *Nurr1* expression is induced, followed by *En1* and *En2*. (**B**) The expression of *Lmx1b* in the ventral midbrain starts at E7.5; however, it is uncertain if the early expression is confined to DA progenitor cells (*broken line*). At later stages, *Lmx1b* is expressed in DA neurons.[24] Representation of the temporal sequence of gene induction in developing DA cells.

Nurr1

Among the transcription factors expressed in postmitotic developing DA cells, Nurr1 has been the most extensively characterized and is therefore the main focus of this review. Nurr1 is a member of the nuclear receptor superfamily of ligand-activated transcription factors.[26] Together with NGFI-B and Nor1, Nurr1 forms a subgroup of three highly homologous receptors. The nuclear receptor family includes receptors for steroid hormones, retinoic acid, thyroid hormone, vitamin D, and several other small, lipophilic signaling molecules (FIG. 3).[27] However, Nurr1, NGFIB, and Nor1, as well as a relatively large number of additional members of this family, lack identified ligands and are therefore referred to as orphan receptors. Nuclear receptors have a common structural organization, with a conserved DNA binding domain and a somewhat less conserved ligand binding domain (FIG. 3). Like other nuclear

A

Nurr1

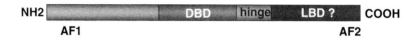

NH2 — AF1 — DBD — hinge — LBD ? — COOH — AF2

B

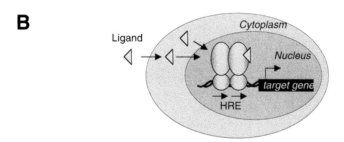

FIGURE 3. The orphan nuclear receptor Nurr1. The nuclear receptor structure with the centrally located DNA binding domain (DBD), flanked by a nonconserved amino-terminal region containing a ligand-independent activatioin function (AF1) and a putative ligand binding domain (LBD), also containing an activation function (AF2). **(B)** Ligand activation of nuclear receptors. Nuclear receptor ligands can be classical endocrine signaling molecules such as steroid hormones and thyroid hormone. They can also act more locally as para- or intracrine signaling molecules. An example of such a paracrine signaling ligand is retinoic acid.

receptors, Nurr1 binds to specific DNA binding sites in the vicinity of regulated genes. Nurr1 can recognize DNA as a monomer, homodimer, or heterodimer with the common heterodimerization partner, the retinoid X receptor (RXR.)[28,29] When binding as a monomer or as a homodimer, Nurr1 can function as a constitutively active transcription factor, apparently in the absence of a ligand. The function of RXR is somewhat enigmatic as it seems to play dual roles. First, RXR is a dimerization partner of many nuclear receptors, including the retinoic acid receptor, the thyroid receptor, and the vitamin D receptor.[30] Second, RXR is a bona fide receptor for 9-cis retinoic acid and fatty acids, such as the brain-enriched docosahexaenoic acid (DHA).[31,32]

Apart from a few scattered *Nurr1*-expressing cells in developing limbs, adult testis, adrenal gland, and thymus, Nurr1 is exclusively localized in the CNS under normal conditions.[26,33–35] Within the CNS, Nurr1 is detected already at E10.5 in developing newly born DA neurons of the ventral mesencephalon.[36] *Nurr1* expression in these cells continues throughout development into adulthood.[33,37] *Nurr1* is expressed in a number of other developing CNS areas in addition to the mesencephalon, including the cortex, hippocampus, thalamus, and spinal cord. Expression continues to be high in several of these brain areas also in adult animals. A unique, interesting feature of Nurr1/NGFI-B/Nor1 is that they are encoded by immediate early response genes, and their expression is highly and transiently upregulated by various stimuli such as growth factors, ischemia, or kainic acid.[38–42] Such induction events are not solely confined to the CNS. For example, *Nurr1* has been shown to be expressed in regenerating liver and in activated T lymphocytes.[43,44]

Mouse knock-out studies from three laboratories have shown that *Nurr1* is essential for the generation of midbrain DA neurons.[35,36,45] In these animals, DA neuron markers such as TH cannot be detected at birth. In contrast, all other catecholaminergic cell groups are intact in *Nurr1* knock-out mice. Even nonmesencephalic DA neurons—in the olfactory bulb and the hypothalamus, for example—develop normally in *Nurr1* knock-out animals, demonstrating that Nurr1 is specifically promoting midbrain DA cell development. *Nurr1* expression is induced as progenitor cells stop proliferating (at approximately E10.5) and migrate from the ventricular neuroepithelial zone into the mantle layer. Although Nurr1 can induce cell cycle arrest when expressed in certain cell lines,[21] analyses of proliferation in wild-type and *Nurr1* knock-out embryos indicate that Nurr1 is not inducing cell cycle exit *in vivo* (our unpublished observation). In knock-out mice, several midbrain DA cell markers—for instance, Pitx3, En1, En2, GFRα1, and Lmx1b—are normally induced even in the absence of Nurr1.[19,20,24,35] However, both TH and the receptor tyrosine kinase signaling subunit *Ret* are absent even from early stages of development in mutant embryos.[20,36] It has subsequently been demonstrated that the TH gene promoter is directly regulated by Nurr1.[46,47] Similarly, the dopamine transporter gene promoter is also regulated by Nurr1 *in vitro*,[48] a finding that has not yet been confirmed *in vivo* in knock-out mice. A corresponding direct regulation of the *Ret* gene promoter has not been reported. However, *Nurr1* and *Ret* are also coexpressed in the dorsal motor nucleus of the vagus nerve in the brain stem. These cells are generated even in the absence of Nurr1, but *Ret* expression is diminished, supporting the idea that Nurr1 is somehow regulating *Ret* gene expression *in vivo*.[20]

Several dopaminergic markers remain in a medial position in the developing *Nurr1* mutant midbrain, indicative of an early migration defect. Moreover, Nurr1-deficient neurons seem unable to innervate their normal forebrain target areas, as demonstrated by retrograde fluorogold tracing in newborn mutant pups.[19] It should be noted that one research group has reported preserved innervation and cellularity in newborn *Nurr1* knock-out mice.[49] One explanation for this discrepancy might be their use of the DiI tracing method, which does not distinguish between ascending and decending pathways. Thus, adjacent nondopaminergic pathways might have been detected. Finally, increased cell death is detected at late gestation in *Nurr1* knock-out mice.[19,35] At this stage, essentially no dopaminergic markers are expressed, cells have not migrated to their final destinations, and target innervation is undetectable. Thus, increased cell death is most likely an indirect consequence of these severe cellular deficiencies, and it remains unclear if Nurr1 is required for long-term survival of DA neurons (also, see below).

Which are the target genes of Nurr1 that can explain the disrupted DA neuron differentiation? Gene targeting of neither *TH* nor *Ret*, both of which are absent in the *Nurr1* mutant midbrain, have resulted in abnormal DA cell development.[50,51] Thus, additional Nurr1 target genes must exist that can explain the drastic developmental phenotype, and identification of such genes should prove instrumental for our understanding of DA neuron generation. However, it remains possible that Nurr1 regulation of *Ret* might be of significance in postnatal DA neuron development. The glial cell line–derived neurotrophic factor (GDNF), which signals via Ret and an associated coreceptor, has recently been implicated in postnatal DA neuron development. Both *GDNF* and *Ret* knock-out mice die shortly after birth, possibly due to their inability to develop kidneys.[52–54] At birth, both types of knock-out mice have developed apparently normal DA neurons and striatal innervation. Due to the early perinatal death of these knock-out animals, it has not been possible to determine the role of these genes in postnatal DA cell development and survival. To circumvent these limitations, Granholm and coworkers grafted embryonic midbrain tissue from *GDNF* knock-out donor embryos into wild-type 6-hydroxy DA–denervated adult rats and showed that GDNF influences the ability of grafts to survive and innervate the host striatal tissue.[55] Thus, the results point to a role for Ret in postnatal development and survival. Whether or not Nurr1, via regulation of *Ret*, influences these processes is unclear. Interestingly, however, Nurr1 may be important for postnatal DA cell survival. Thus, heterozygous *Nurr1* mice, while otherwise apparently normal, are significantly more sensitive than their wild-type littermates to the toxic effects of 1-methyl-4-phenyl-1,2,3,6-tetrahydropyridine (MPTP).[56] As mentioned above, *Nurr1* is strongly induced by various stressful stimuli such as ischemia and kainic acid. An intriguing possibility is thus that Nurr1 is an essential component in a neuroprotective regulatory mechanism, possibly influenced by GDNF or other factors stimulating Ret signal transduction.

Does Nurr1 have an as-yet-unidentified endogenous ligand influencing the development and function of midbrain DA neurons? Such a possibility is intriguing, but it remains possible that Nurr1 is not a "classical" liganded signaling receptor. Ligands for nuclear receptors are often spatially or temporally restricted and bind to receptors whose expression is not highly regulated. It could be argued that the tight spatial distribution of Nurr1 and its regulation as an immediate early gene would indicate that there is no need for a ligand. On the other hand, Nurr1 has a conserved domain that is structurally homologous to ligand binding domains of other nuclear receptors. It can only be concluded that the question remains open. Another realistic and equally interesting possbility is that Nurr1 participates in signaling as a dimerizing partner of RXR. Indeed, Nurr1-RXR heterodimers are very efficiently activated by RXR ligands.[28,29] However, it should be noted that RXR is not required for Nurr1's ability to activate transcription as a monomer, and at least some functions of Nurr1 in developing DA cells are apparently not dependent on Nurr1's ability to dimerize with RXR, as indicated from experiments in a dopaminergic differentiating cell line.[21] Nonetheless, it seems likely that Nurr1-RXR ligand-induced signaling might have functions *in vivo*, perhaps in mature DA neurons or in other unrelated cell types.

Lmx1b, Pitx3, and En1/En2

Homeodomain transcription factors have been identified in developing DA cells. *Lmx1b* is detected from E7.5 in the mouse CNS including the ventral mesencephalon,[24] whereas *Pitx3* is specifically expressed in midbrain TH-positive cells from E11.5 (see FIG. 2).[57] Gene targeting of the *Lmx1b* gene results in loss of embryonic *Pitx3* expression, whereas *Nurr1* and TH were still detected at E12.5. Conversely, *Pitx3* is initially expressed in *Nurr1* knock-out embryos, suggesting the existence of

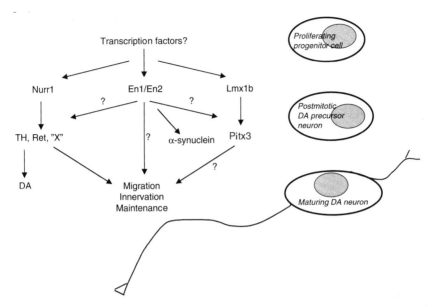

FIGURE 4. Transcriptional control of DA neuron development. Our understanding of genetic interactions remains fragmented, but a few relationships have been described. The transcription factors involved in specification of a DA progenitor cell have not been identified. In newly born postmitotic DA neurons, Nurr1, En1/2, and Lmx1b are involved in the developmental process. Nurr1 and Lmx1b are components in two distinct regulatory cascades and are both induced independently of each other. In addition, Nurr1 is required for normal migration, innervation, and maintenance (survival, sustained innervation, and gene expression) of DA cells. Thus, it is concluded that Nurr1 must regulate additional genes ("X") responsible for the severe phenotype. Lmx1b is required for the induction of Pitx3, although the role of this transcription factor in DA neuron development remains unknown. Lmx1b promotes the maintenance of DA neurons, possibly via upregulation of Pitx3. The role of En1/2 in DA cell maintenance (sustained TH expression) has been described. α-*Synuclein* seem to be a regulated downstream target of En1/2.[63]

at least two independent pathways in developing DA neuron differentiation (see FIG. 4). From E16.5, no TH positive midbrain DA neurons can be detected in *Lmx1b* knock-out mice, demonstrating that Lmx1b is required to sustain the dopaminergic cell fate.[24] The role of Pitx3 has remained elusive as no knockout mice have yet been reported. However, two recent reports have elucidated a phenotype by studying the mouse mutant (*aphakia*), most likely a *Pitx3* null mutation. These reports show that in these mutants, neurons of the substantia nigra fail to develop, thus defining Pitx3 as an essential factor for a subset of mesencephalic DA neurons.[58,59]

The two mouse homologues of the *Drosophila* engrailed gene, *En1* and *En2*, are expressed during early midbrain morphogenesis (E9) and are important for maintaining the MHB structure.[6,22,60,61] These genes show a second phase of expression confined to developing DA cells from approximately E11—that is, somewhat after

Nurr1 is induced. While single knockouts of these genes display no DA neuron deficiencies, TH is downregulated in compound knock-outs at late gestation and is absent at E14.[62,63] *Nurr1, Lmx1b,* or *Pitx3* expression patterns have not been reported in these animals, and it is not known whether the loss of TH is due to downregulation or an increase in cell death.

In conclusion, while the function of Pitx3 remains poorly investigated, homeobox transcription factors Lmx1b and En1/En2, in addition to Nurr1, are clearly important for the normal differentiation and maintenance of the DA neuron phenotype. It should be noted, however, that the null mutations of *Lmx1b* and the *En* genes result in quite severe malformation of mid/hindbrain structures.[24,63] Thus, it remains possible that the dopaminergic phenotypes could be indirect consequences of mid/hindbrain structural abnormalities.

ENGINEERING DA NEURONS FROM STEM CELLS

The elucidation of regulatory cascades influencing the specification and development of neuronal types is of relevance in stem cell research. This is a field attracting considerable interest, not least because of recent breakthroughs illustrating the increasingly realistic perspective of using stem cells and cell replacement strategies in treatment of neurodegenerative diseases.[64–66] However, elucidating the relevant mechanisms involved in development of specific neuronal cell types will prove critical in order to achieve such goals. Indeed, although our current understanding of factors influencing DA neuron development is quite limited, new knowledge has already proved useful in attempts to engineer DA cells *in vitro*. In one recent study expression of Nurr1 in an immortalized neural stem cell line derived from the embryonic cerebellum was shown to result in robust differentiation of TH-expressing neurons when these cells were cocultured with type I astrocytes from the ventral midbrain.[67] Cultures of parental cells did not generate TH-positive neurons under these conditions, indicating an active instructive role of Nurr1. Other DA neuron markers were also expressed, and the cells were shown to synthesize DA. However, their ability to integrate in host brains and restore dopaminergic functions after grafting in rodent Parkinson's disease models remains to be demonstrated. The identity of the astroglial factor is unknown but is evidently produced specifically by astrocytes in the developing ventral midbrain, since glial cells from other regions of the developing CNS were unable to promote DA cell differentiation.[67]

A second striking example of *in vitro*–engineered DA neurons derives from work by McKay and coworkers on embryonic stem cells transfected with a *Nurr1* expression vector.[68] By modifying a protocol previously developed by the same group, a large number of DA neurons could be generated *in vitro*. These neurons expressed several markers specific for midbrain DA neurons, including TH, *Ret, Pitx3,* and *En1*. Impressively, grafting of these neurons into 6-hydroxy-DA–denervated host rat brains resulted in functional integration and restoration of parkinsonian symptoms. Although an ideal scenario would be to avoid the need of gene transfer and depend exclusively on extrinsic signals to manipulate embryonic stem cells in culture, both of these studies illustrate the importance of identifying the appropriate signals and factors that influence normal development of DA cells.

CONCLUSIONS

A great deal of information on transcriptional control of DA neuron development has been acquired during recent years. However, our understanding is still somewhat fragmented, and several areas will require attention in the years to come. For example, most of the current knowledge stems from studies of transcription factors expressed in postmitotic maturing DA neurons. Similarly, a great deal is understood about the general patterning and morphogenetic events shaping the mid/hindbrain region.[6,22] Signaling and the transcriptional events occuring in dividing progenitors leading to the generation of postmitotic DA neurons are much more poorly described. It will also be critical to define mechanisms generating diversity within the dopaminergic system and to define how functionally distinct dopaminergic cell groups are generated. It can be anticipated that characterization of these mechanisms will ultimately allow a complete description of genetic and epigenetic interactions required for generating these clinically important cells. As already shown in previous work, defining such mechanisms will be important in attempts to engineer DA neurons for transplantation and will likely identify mechanisms influencing the behavior and survival of not only developing, but also mature DA neurons. Thus, the strong focus in this area holds excellent prospects of generating data of significance in the treatment of disorders such as Parkinson's disease.

ACKNOWLEDGMENTS

We thank Dr. Bertrand Joseph for critical comments on this manuscript and Dr. Alex Mata for additional help and comments.

REFERENCES

1. FALCK, B., *et al.* 1962. Fluorescence of catechol amines and related compounds condensed with formaldehyde. J. Histochem. Cytochem. **10:** 348–354.
2. DAHLSTRÖM, A. & K. FUXE. 1964. Evidence for the existence of monoamine-containing neurones in the central nervous system. I. Demonstration of monoamines in the cell bodies of brain stem neurones. Acta Physiol. Scand. **62:** 1–55.
3. BJÖRKLUND, A. & O. LINDVALL. 1984. Dopamine-containing systems in the CNS, *In* Handbook of Chemical Neuroanatomy, Vol 2. Classical Transmitters in the CNS, Part I. Björklund, A. & T. Hökfelt, Eds. Elsevier Science Publishers.
4. ARTS, M.P.M., *et al.* 1996. Efferent projections of the retrorubral nucleus to the substantia nigra and ventral tegmental area in cats as shown by anterograde tracing. Brain Res. Bull. **40:** 219–228.
5. UNGERSTEDT, U. 1971. Stereotaxic mapping of the monoamine pathways in the rat brain. Acta Physiol. Scand. Suppl. **367:** 1–48.
6. WURST, W. & L. BALLY-CUIF. 2001. Neural plate patterning: upstream and downstream of the isthmic organizer. Nat. Rev. Neurosci. **2:** 99–108.
7. HYNES, M. & A. ROSENTHAL. 1999. Specification of dopaminergic and serotonergic neurons in the vertebrate CNS. Curr. Opin. Neurobiol. **9:** 26–36.
8. ROSENTHAL, A. 1998. Specification and survival of the dopaminergic neurons in the mammalian midbrain. Adv. Pharmacol. **42:** 908–911.
9. HYNES, M., *et al.* 1995. Control of neuronal diversity by the floor plate: contact-mediated induction of midbrain dopaminergic neurons. Cell **80:** 95–101.
10. HYNES, M., *et al.* 1995. Induction of midbrain dopaminergic neurons by sonic hedgehog. Neuron **15:** 33–44.

11. ERICSON, J., *et al.* 1995. Sonic hedgehog: a common signal for ventral patterning along the rostrocaudal axis of the neural tube. Int. J. Dev. Biol. **39:** 809–816.
12. ERICSON, J., *et al.* 1997. Graded sonic hedgehog signaling and the specification of cell fate in the ventral neural tube. Cold Spring Harb. Symp. Quant. Biol. **62:** 451–466.
13. ERICSON, J., *et al.* 1996. Two critical periods of sonic hedgehog signaling required for the specification of motor neuron identity. Cell **87:** 661–673.
14. ERICSON, J., *et al.* 1995. Sonic hedgehog induces the differentiation of ventral forebrain neurons: a common signal for ventral patterning within the neural tube. Cell **81:** 747–756.
15. CROSSLEY, P.H., S. MARTINEZ & G.R. MARTIN. 1996. Midbrain development induced by FGF8 in the chick embryo. Nature **380:** 66–68.
16. LEE, S.M.K., *et al.* 1997. Evidence that FGF8 signalling from the midbrain-hindbrain junction regulates growth and polarity in the developing midbrain. Development **124:** 959–969.
17. YE, W., *et al.* 1998. FGF and Shh signals control dopaminergic and serotonergic cell fate in the anterior neural tube. Cell **93:** 755–766.
18. LINDAHL, R. & S. EVCES. 1984. Rat liver aldehyde dehydrogenase. II. Isolation and characterization of four inducible isozymes. J. Biol. Chem. **259:** 11991–11996.
19. WALLÉN, Å., *et al.* 1999. Fate of mesencephalic AHD2-expressing dopamine progenitor cells in NURR1 mutant mice. Exp. Cell Res. **253:** 737–746.
20. WALLÉN, Å., *et al.* 2001. Orphan nuclear receptor Nurr1 is essential for Ret expression in the midbrain dopamine neurons and in the brain stem. Mol. Cell. Neurosci. **18:** 649–663.
21. CASTRO, D.S., *et al.* 2001. Induction of cell cycle arrest and morphological differentiation by Nurr1 and retinoids in dopamine MN9D cells. J. Biol. Chem. **276:** 43277–43284.
22. JOYNER, A.L. 1996. Engrailed, Wnt and Pax genes regulate midbrain-hindbrain development. TIG **12:** 15–20.
23. ADAMS, K.A., *et al.* 2000. The transcription factor Lmx1b maintains Wnt1 expression within the isthmic organizer. Development **127:** 1857–1867.
24. SMIDT, M.P., *et al.* 2000. A second independent pathway for development of mesencephalic dopaminergic neurons requires Lmx1b. Nat. Neurosci. **3:** 337–341.
25. LAUDER, J.M. & F.E. BLOOM. 1974. Ontogeny of monoamine neurons in the locus coeruleus, raphe nuclei and substantia nigra of the rat. I. Cell differentiation. J. Comp. Neurol. **155:** 469–481.
26. LAW, S.W., *et al.* 1992. Identification of a new brain-specific transcription factor, NURR1. Mol. Endocrinol. **6:** 2129–2135.
27. MANGELSDORF, D.J., *et al.* 1995. The nuclear receptor superfamily: the second decade. Cell **83:** 835–839.
28. PERLMANN, T. & L. JANSSON. 1995. A novel pathway for vitamin A signaling mediated by RXR heterodimerization with NGFI-B and NURR1. Genes Dev. **9:** 769–782.
29. FORMAN, B.M., *et al.* 1995. Unique response pathways are established by allosteric interactions among nuclear hormone receptors. Cell **81:** 541–550.
30. MANGELSDORF, D.J. & R.M. EVANS. 1995. The RXR heterodimers and orphan receptors. Cell **83:** 841–850.
31. HEYMAN, R.A., *et al.* 1992. 9-cis retinoic acid is a high affinity ligand for the retinoid X receptor. Cell **68:** 397–406.
32. MATA DE URQUIZA, A., *et al.* 2000. Docosahexaenoic acid: a ligand for the retinoid X receptor in the mouse brain. Science **290:** 2140–2144.
33. ZETTERSTRÖM, R.H., *et al.* 1996. Retinoid X receptor heterodimerization and developmental expression distinguish the orphan nuclear receptors NGFI-B, Nurr1 and Nor1. Mol. Endocrinol. **10:** 1656–1666.
34. SAUCEDO-CARDENAS, O. & O.M. CONNEELY. 1996. Comparative distribution of nurr1 and nur77 nuclear receptors in the mouse central nervous system. J. Mol. Neurosci. **7:** 51–63.
35. SAUCEDO-CARDENAS, O., *et al.* 1998. Nurr1 is essential for the induction of the dopaminergic phenotype and the survival of ventral mesencephalic late dopaminergic precursor neurons. Proc. Natl. Acad. Sci. USA **95:** 4013–4018.

36. ZETTERSTRÖM, R.H., et al. 1997. Dopamine neuron agenesis in Nurr1-deficient mice. Science **276:** 248–250.
37. ZETTERSTRÖM, R.H., et al. 1996. Cellular expression of the immediate early transcription factors Nurr1 and NGFI-B suggests a gene regulatory role in several brain regions including the nigrostriatal dopamine system. Mol. Brain Res. **41:** 111–120.
38. HONKANIEMI, J., et al. 1997. Expression of zinc finger immediate early genes in rat brain after permanent middle cerebral artery occlusion. J. Cereb. Blood Flow Metab. **17:** 636–646.
39. HONKANIEMI, J. & F.R. SHARP. 1996. Global ischemia induces immediate-early genes encoding zinc finger transcription factors. J. Cereb. Blood Flow Metab. **16:** 557–565.
40. JOHANSSON, I.M., et al. 2000. Early and delayed induction of immediate early gene expression in a novel focal cerebral ischemia model in the rat. Eur. J. Neurosci. **12:** 3615–3625.
41. LIN, T.N., et al. 1996. Expression of NGFI-B mRNA in a rat focal cerebral ischemia-reperfusion model. Mol. Brain Res. **43:** 149–156.
42. CRISPINO, M., et al. 1998. Nurr1 mRNA expression in neonatal and adult rat brain following kainic acid-induced seizure activity. Mol. Brain Res. **59:** 178–188.
43. SCEARCE, L.M., et al. 1993. RNR-1, a nuclear receptor in the NGFI-B/Nur77 family that is rapidly induced in regenerating liver. J. Biol. Chem. **268:** 8855–8861.
44. MAGES, H.W., et al. 1994. NOT, A human immediate-early response gene closely related to the steroid/thyroid hormone receptor NAK1/TR3. Mol. Endocrinol. **8:** 1583–1591.
45. CASTILLO, S.O., et al. 1998. Dopamine biosynthesis is selectively abolished in substantia nigra/ventral tegmental area but not in hypothalamic neurons in mice with targeted disruption of the Nurr1 gene. Mol. Cell. Neurosci. **11:** 36–46.
46. SAKURADA, K., et al. 1999. Nurr1, an orphan nuclear receptor, is a transcriptional activator of endogenous tyrosine hydroxylase in neural progenitor cells derived from the adult brain. Development **126:** 4017–4026.
47. IWAWAKI, T., K. KOHNO & K. KOBAYASHI. 2000. Identification of a potential nurr1 response element that activates the tyrosine hydroxylase gene promoter in cultured cells. Biochem. Biophys. Res. Commun. **274:** 590–595.
48. SACCHETTI, P., et al. 2001. Nurr1 enhances transcription of the human dopamine transporter gene through a novel mechanism. J. Neurochem. **76:** 1565–1572.
49. WITTA, J., et al. 2000. Nigrostriatal innervation is preserved in Nurr1-null mice, although dopaminergic neuron precursors are arrested from terminal differentiation. Mol. Brain Res. **84:** 67–78.
50. ZHOU, Q.Y. & R.D. PALMITER. 1995. Dopamine-deficient mice are severely hypoactive, adipsic, and aphagic. Cell **83:** 1197–1209.
51. MARCOS, C. & V. PACHNIS. 1996. The effect of the ret- mutation on the normal development of the central and parasympathetic nervous systems. Int. J. Dev. Biol. Suppl **1:** 137S–138S.
52. MOORE, M.W., et al. 1996. Renal and neuronal abnormalities in mice lacking GDNF. Nature **382:** 76–79.
53. SANCHEZ, M.P., et al. 1996. Renal agenesis and the absence of enteric neurons in mice lacking GDNF. Nature **382:** 70–73.
54. SCHUCHARDT, A., et al. 1994. Defects in the kidney and enteric nervous system of mice lacking the tyrosine kinase receptor Ret [see comments]. Nature **367:** 380–383.
55. GRANHOLM, A.C., et al. 2000. Glial cell line-derived neurotrophic factor is essential for postnatal survival of midbrain dopamine neurons. J. Neurosci. **20:** 3182–3190.
56. LE, W.-D., et al. 1999. Reduced Nurr1 expression increases the vulnerability of mesencephalic dopamine neurons to MPTP-induced injury. J. Neurochem. **73:** 2218–2221.
57. SMIDT, M.P., et al. 1997. A homeodomain gene Ptx3 has highly restricted brain expression in mesencephalic dopaminergic neurons. Proc. Natl. Acad. Sci. USA **94:** 13305–13310.
58. NUNES, I., L.T. TOVAMASIAN, R.M. SILVA, et al. 2003. Pitx is required for development of substantia nigra dopaminergic neurons. Proc. Natl. Acad. Sci. USA **100:** 4245–4250.
59. VAN DEN MUNCKHOF, P. K.C. LUK, L. STE.-MARIE, et al. 2003. Pitx is required for motor activity and for survival of a subset of midbrain dopaminergic neurons. Development **130:** 2535–2542.

60. DANIELIAN, P.D. & A.P. MCMAHON. 1996. Engrailed-1 as a target of the wnt-1 signaling pathway in vertebrate midbrain development. Nature **383:** 332–334.
61. JOYNER, A.L. & G.R. MARTIN. 1987. En-1 and En-2, two mouse genes with sequence homology to the Drosophila engrailed gene: expression during embryogenesis. Genes Dev. **1:** 29–38.
62. SIMON, H.H., *et al.* 1998. En-1 and En-2 control the fate of the dopaminergic neurons in the substantia nigra and ventral tegmentum. Eur. J. Neurosci. **10:** 389.
63. SIMON, H.H., *et al.* 2001. Fate of midbrain dopaminergic neurons controlled by the engrailed genes. J. Neurosci. **21:** 3126–3134.
64. GAGE, F.H. 2000. Mammalian neural stem cells. Science **287:** 1433–1438.
65. ANDERSON, D.J. 2001. Stem cells and pattern formation in the nervous system: the possible versus the actual. Neuron **30:** 19–35.
66. MOMMA, S., C.B. JOHANSSON & J. FRISEN. 2000. Get to know your stem cells. Curr Opin. Neurobiol. **10:** 45–49.
67. WAGNER, J., *et al.* 1999. Induction of a midbrain dopaminergic phenotype in Nurr1-overexpressing neural stem cells by type 1 astrocytes. Nat. Biotechnol. **17:** 653–659.
68. KIM, J.H., *et al.* 2002. Dopamine neurons derived from embryonic stem cells function in an animal model of Parkinson's disease. Nature **418:** 50–56.

Transcription Factors in the Development of Midbrain Dopamine Neurons

J. PETER H. BURBACH, SIMONE SMITS, AND MARTEN P. SMIDT

Rudolf Magnus Institute of Neuroscience, Department of Pharmacology and Anatomy, University Medical Center Utrecht, Utrecht, the Netherlands

ABSTRACT: The development of midbrain dopamine (DA) neurons follows a number of stages marked by distinct events. After preparation of the region by signals that provide induction and patterning, at least two cascades of transcription factors contribute to the fully matured midbrain DA systems. One cascade involving the nuclear receptor Nurr1 is required to synthesize the neurotransmitter DA; the enzyme tyrosine hydroxylase (TH) depends on it. The other cascade involves homeobox genes. Lmx1b and engrailed genes are expressed before the genesis of DA neurons and maintain their expression in these neurons. Lmx1b drives Ptx3, which is the latest transcription factor known to be induced. Its induction coincides with that of TH. Disruption of the function of Ptx3 affects the formation of the substantia nigra (SN) and alters the anatomical organization of the midbrain DA systems. While each cascade contributes to a specific aspect of DA neurons, both cascades are required for survival during development, indicating that the maintenance of DA neurons is delicately dependent on the appropriate activity of multiple transcriptional cascades.

KEYWORDS: transcription factors; midbrain; dopamine neurons

INTRODUCTION: MULTIPLICITY OF MIDBRAIN DOPAMINE NEURONS

Midbrain dopamine (DA) neurons comprise a heterogenous group of neurons that control elementary brain functions. First, they are involved in the control of movement; hence their prime role in Parkinson's disease. Second, they are part of circuits controling mood and reward, and thereby behavior. These two functions of midbrain DA systems are partly distinguished anatomically in the nigrostriatal system (movement) and the mesolimbic system (behavior).

Despite differentiation in anatomy and functions, all midbrain DA systems share the dopaminergic transmission machinery to communicate with postsynaptic elements of the networks they are part of. Dopaminergic transmission requires coordinated expression of specific gene products in order to synthesize and recycle the transmitter, to receive and control the chemical signal, and to transduce this into rel-

Address for correspondence: J.P.H. Burbach, Ph.D., Rudolf Magnus Institute of Neuroscience, Department of Pharmacology and Anatomy, University Medical Center Utrecht, Utrecht, the Netherlands. Voice: +31 (0)30 2538848; fax +31 (0)30 2539032.

j.p.h.burbach@med.uu.nl

Ann. N.Y. Acad. Sci. 991: 61–68 (2003). © 2003 New York Academy of Sciences.

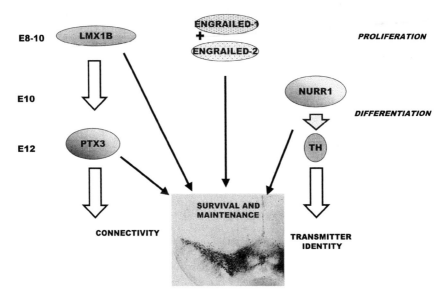

FIGURE 1. Cascades of transcription factors enrolling in the development of midbrain DA neurons. Relationships are based on loss-of-function studies in mice. All transcription factors affect the survival of developing DA neurons (see text).

evant cellular responses. Thus, midbrain neurons, despite their heterogeneous functions, have in common the transcriptional control to activate the gene sets necessary for dopaminergic transmission.

The distinction between functionally different groups of midbrain DA neurons is made at the level of the anatomy of cell bodies and the connectivity of axonal efferents with postsynaptic structures. DA signaling by substantia nigra (SN) neurons innervating the striatum modifies brain circuits controlling movement, while behavioral responses are triggered by ventral tegmental (VTA) DA neurons in the nucleus accumbens and other limbic areas. Thus, transcriptional control of genes involved in migration and axonal guidance is likely different from those involved in determination of the DA identity and is possibly variable between populations of midbrain DA neurons.

In this chapter we present our current view on how transcription factor cascades that unfold during development of midbrain DA neurons are linked to neurotransmission, connectivity, and survival. This view is illustrated in FIGURE 1.

THE FOREPLAY: PREPARATION OF THE EARLY MIDBRAIN

The development of midbrain dopamine neurons is largely dependent on the proper development of the ventral midbrain and the midbrain-hindbrain border that precedes the induction of midbrain dopamine neurons. Genes involved in boundary formation will have effects on the emergence of midbrain DA neurons. The first midbrain DA neurons arise at the most ventral rim of the neuroepithelium, lining up along the mesencephalic flexure of the ventral midbrain, where the expression of the growth factors Fgf8 and Shh interact.[1] Before the expression of DA-specific markers, ventral midbrain markers are present in these cells. Among the earliest markers of the region are the homeobox genes engrailed-1 (En1), engrailed-2 (En2), Pax2 and Pax5, and the growth factor Wnt1. The expression of En1 and En2 is maintained by the expression of the signaling molecule Wnt1.[2] Another homeobox gene implicated in the early specification of the ventral midbrain is Lmx1b. This gene is expressed at E7.5 in the ventral midbrain and diencephalon, and remains expressed in the adult in brain structures derived from these areas, including midbrain DA neurons.[3]

The first specific signs of the birth of midbrain DA neurons is the expression of the key enzyme in DA synthesis, tyrosine hydroxylase (TH), at E11. This moment follows the induction of the nuclear receptor Nurr1 (E10.5) and coincides with the expression of the midbrain DA–specific homeobox gene Ptx3.[4]

THE HOMEOBOX PATHWAY: SPECIFICATION OF ARCHITECTURE AND CONNECTIVITY

As yet, four homeobox genes have been shown to be expressed in DA neurons: En1, En2, Lmx1b, and Ptx3. Ptx3 differs from the others in both timing and space: Ptx3 is induced late, and its brain expression is confined to DA neurons. En1, En2, and Lmx1b are expressed in the ventral midbrain, well before induction of TH; their expression extends largely beyond DA progenitors.[3,5]

In situ hybridization on mouse embryos from E8.5 to E16.5 showed the induction of Ptx3 expression with appearance of midbrain DA neurons. At E11.5, a small layer at the ventral surface of the mesencephalic flexure expresses Ptx3. At E12.5 a complete field of TH-positive, Ptx3-positive neurons has been obtained. These Ptx3-positive cells are restricted to the marginal layer of the mesencephalic tegmentum. This group of about 50 cells corresponds to the first TH-expressing cells in the developing rodent brain. At later stages, the expression remains restricted to the midbrain DA system, and this association is conserved in adult rat brain and human SN tissue. This has also been demonstrated by 6-hydroxy DA lesions that take away all Ptx3-positive neurons.[4] Extraneural Ptx3 expression is found in the developing skeletal muscle, in the tongue and in the developing eye lens.[4,6]

Lmx1b is a member of the LIM homeodomain family and is an essential regulator of dorsoventral patterning of the developing limbs. Lmx1b mutations evoke the nail-patella syndrome.[7,8] Neural Lmx1b expression starts already at E7.5 (Johnson and Chen, personal communication). Early embryonic expression is extending anterior to the midbrain DA region into the ventral hypothalamic area, and posterior in the dorsal hindbrain and the dorsal spinal cord. In the ventral midbrain, Lmx1b is expressed in midbrain DA neurons. Lmx1b expression is maintained in the adult SN and VTA of rodents and in the melanin-containing SN neurons of man.[3] *Engrailed* genes also have an early (E8 onwards), regionally broad expression field in the midbrain and hindbrain.[5] Interesting, like Lmx1b, their expression is maintained in adult midbrain DA neurons.[9] En1 is highly expressed in all adult midbrain DA neurons, and En2 in only a subset[9] or is not detectable (unpublished).

The intrinsic potential of the Lmx1b and En1/En2 genes as developmental regulators, together with the fact that these homeobox genes are expressed earlier than Nurr1, TH, and Ptx3, initially raised the hypothesis that Lmx1b and En genes may act genetically as upstream activators of these genes, in addition to preparing the ventral midbrain for genesis and differentiation of the midbrain DA system. To validate this hypothesis we analyzed expression of TH, Ptx3, and Nurr1 in brain sections of homozygous Lmx1b knock-out mice[8] of stage E12.5, when the field of expression of TH and Ptx3 is first complete. Lmx1b$^{-/-}$ embryos contained TH-positive cells in the ventral tegmentum, but these cells did not express Ptx3, indicating that Ptx3 is not necessary for TH expression. En1-null mutants are indistinguishable from wild-type mice, except for a high expression of En2 in all midbrain DA neurons.[9] In En1/En2–double-null mutants TH-positive neurons are initially generated, but soon lost.[9] A similar observation has been made in Lmx1b-null mutants. Apparently, Lmx1b and En1/En2 genes are each required for survival of midbrain DA neurons.

AN END STATION OF THE HOMEOBOX PATHWAY

To test the contribution of Ptx3 to the development of midbrain neurons, mice homozygous for a defective Ptx3 allele were analyzed. These mice are blind, due to the function of Ptx3 in eye development, but grow and breed normally. These mice contain TH-positive neurons in the midbrain, but the anatomical organization is altered in two ways. First, TH-positive neurons are absent in the SN, and second, a central cell group exists frontal to the VTA. The organization of TH neurons in the VTA appears normal. Correlating with this phenotype is the lack of innervation of the dorsal striatum, which receives input from the SN DA neurons in wild-type mice. The innervation of the nucleus accumbens and olfactory tubercle exists as in wild-type mice. This phenotype suggests that Ptx3 disrupts processes required for expansion of DA neurons from E11.5 onwards. These processes significantly affect neurons that will form the SN—that is, neurons that need to migrate laterally from the mesencephalic flexure. Whether or not Ptx3 drives the survival, migration, or axonal pathfinding of this subset of neurons still needs to be established.

THE NURR1 PATHWAY: INDUCTION OF THE DOPAMINERGIC TRANSMITTER PHENOTYPE AND SURVIVAL

Nurr1 is an orphan member of the nuclear hormone receptor superfamily of transcription factors.[10] Nurr1 has a relatively wide field of expression in the embryonic midbrain, covering the entire ventral region.[3] Only a small proportion of Nurr1-expressing neurons overlap with the midbrain DA progenitor neurons (FIG. 2). Thus, brain expression of Nurr1 is not uniquely linked to midbrain DA neurons, in contrast to the homeobox gene Ptx3. The onset of Nurr1 expression in midbrain DA neurons is at E10.5 in the mouse, just before the induction of TH and Ptx3 atE11.5.[4,11,12] The expression of Nurr1 is maintained in the adult stage, albeit in a more limited pattern, but including the midbrain DA system (FIG. 2). Multiple regions of the adult brain

EMBRYO E12.5

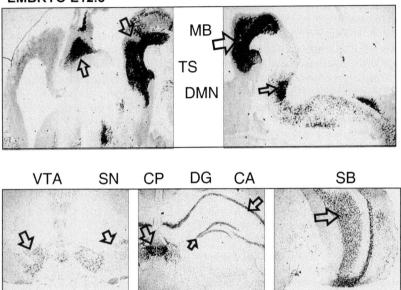

ADULT BRAIN

FIGURE 2. Expression of Nurr1 in the embryonic and adult mouse brain. MB: midbrain; TS: thalamic subfield; DMN: dorsal motor nucleus; VTA: ventral tegmental area; SN: substantia nigra; CP: choroid plexus; CA: CA1, 2, and 3 field of the hippocampus; DG: dentate gyrus; SB: subiculum.

express Nurr1.[13–15] The Nurr1 protein may therefore serve developmental and regulatory functions that are not restricted to DA neurons.

The function of Nurr1 in the brain has been addressed by the creation of null-mutant mice by three groups.[12,16,17] Mice with a targeted deletion of the Nurr1 gene die soon after birth. Analysis of the brain of these animals using such markers as Adh2, cRet, and TH showed that in the newborn animals no midbrain DA neurons are present. Although it was initially concluded that this is due to "agenesis" of midbrain DA neurons,[12] several additional studies demonstrated a more refined role of Nurr1 in midbrain DA neurons. At E12.5 Nurr1-null mutants express other markers associated with midbrain DA neurons, including HNF 3β, Ptx3, and Lmx1b, but fail to induce TH.[11,18] CRet expression was also found to be absent in the ventral midbrain of Nurr1-null mutants.[18] These findings link Nurr1 to the growth factor glia-derived neurotrophic factor (GDNF), which promotes the survival of DA neurons.[20]

The role of Nurr1 as the key factor in the determination of the dopaminergic phenotype of midbrain DA neurons has been extended by two significant findings. First, it was shown that Nurr1[+/−] mice display diminished DA levels, suggesting that TH activity, which is rate limiting in neurotransmitter synthesis, is strictly regulated by Nurr1.[11] Second, in humans a correlation between Nurr1 and TH has been found in the age-related decrease of Nurr1 in the SN.[21] In cocain addicts Nurr1 expression levels were decreased,[22] but this finding has not been compared to levels of TH.

The mechanism by which Nurr1 induces TH has not been elucidated. Although Nurr1 has a weak transacting potential on 5'-flanking regulatory regions of the TH gene in heterologous cell lines,[23,24] this cannot explain a total dependence of TH expression on Nurr1. Therefore, Nurr1 may engage unique cofactors in DA neurons. Moreover, differentiation of embryonic stem cells into DA-expressing neurons is enhanced by survival-promoting factors that upregulate Nurr1 and TH in parallel.[25] Also, stable expression of Nurr1 in embryonic stem cells enhances the differentiation in a TH-expressing neuronal phenotype.[26]

Recent data suggest that the function of Nurr1 in DA neurons is not cell autonomous. In contrast to observations *in vivo*, it has been observed that TH can be induced in cultured ventral midbrain tissue of Nurr1$^{-/-}$ mice. Cultured ventral midbrain of these animals contains normal numbers of TH neurons when dissected at E10.5 or E15.5. These displayed a failure to develop nerve fiber bundles.[27]

The developmental program of midbrain DA neurons in the Nurr1$^{-/-}$ animals does proceed, as illustrated by the proper induction of the midbrain DA-specific homeobox gene Ptx3[16] and maintenance of Lmx1b.[3] The perinatal survival of these Nurr1$^{-/-}$ midbrain DA neurons is not entirely clear, since there have been conflicting findings.[16,28,29] Whether these cells are lost gradually or maintained postnatally may depend on secondary influences, such as, perhaps, genetic background of Nurr1-null mutants.

We speculate that the degeneration of the midbrain DA neurons in Nurr1$^{-/-}$ is not only due to the fact that there is no DA synthesis because of the lack of TH, but that other cellular functions of Nurr1 in survival mechanisms are involved. The absence of TH alone is probably not sufficient for the severe neuronal loss that is found in Nurr1$^{-/-}$ mice, since DA-deficient mice still form projections to the striatum.[30] This degeneration may be indirect. Possibly, the Nurr1$^{-/-}$ midbrain DA neurons cannot form or maintain the connections to their targets, and therefore the neurons degenerate, as is found after transection of the projecting axons. Alternatively, Nurr1 drives other downstream targets that are required for survival. The dependence of cRet, a component of the GDNF receptor, on Nurr1 may link Nurr1 to survival.

Humans heterozygous for a mutation in the Ptx3 suffer from cataract and anterior segment mesenchymal dysgenesis (ASMDS), in line with early eye expression of Ptx3,[7] but have no reported neurological abnormalities. Interestingly, human subjects with nail-patella syndrome, an autosomal-dominant disorder resulting from loss-of-function mutations in Lmx1b,[31] seem to display a behavioral phenotype.[32]

INTERRELATIONSHIPS BETWEEN PATHWAYS

The data obtained from Nurr1- and Lmx1b-null mutants lead to the differentiation of two genetic pathways that operate in parallel in developing midbrain DA neurons (FIG. 1). One pathway links Nurr1 to the induction of TH. The function of this pathway is to specify the identity of the neurotransmitter that will be employed by these neurons. The other pathway positions Lmx1b upstream of Ptx3. It is not yet clear whether the En genes operate fully independently of this pathway or are part of it. Disruption of this pathway by deletion of Lmx1b leads to rapid loss of TH-positive neurons after E12.5. Since this is not the case when Ptx3 is inactivated, Lmx1b must attribute additional survival properties to developing midbrain DA neurons. It is remarkable to note that disruption of transcription factors in separate pathways— Nurr1, En1/En2, and Lmx1b—affects the survival of developing DA neurons. Perhaps, also the phenotype of Ptx3-null mutants will turn out to be caused by compromised survival. This suggests that the maintenance of DA neurons is delicately dependent on the appropriate activity of multiple transcriptional cascades. This may render the midbrain DA neuron a cell prone to degenerate if transcriptional pathways are affected.

ACKNOWLEDGMENTS

Research from our lab was supported by grants from the Korczak Foundation for Autism and Related Disorders, and the Netherlands Organizaton for Scientific Research, NWO. We thank members from our lab for contributing data to this paper, and Ms. Ria van Vlaardingen-Priester for her help in preparing the manuscript.

REFERENCES

1. YE, W., K. SHIMAMURA, J.L. RUBENSTEIN, *et al.* 1998. FGF and Shh signals control dopaminergic and serotonergic cell fate in the anterior neural plate. Cell **93**: 755–766.
2. DANIELIAN, P.S. & A.P. MCMAHON. 1996. Engrailed-1 as a target of the Wnt-1 signalling pathway in vertebrate midbrain development. Nature **383**: 332–334.
3. SMIDT, M.P., C.H. ASBREUK, J.J. COX, *et al.* 2000. A second independent pathway for development of mesencephalic dopaminergic neurons requires Lmx1b. Nat. Neurosci. **3**: 337–341.
4. SMIDT, M.P., H.S. VAN SCHAICK, C. LANCTOT, *et al.* 1997. A homeodomain gene Ptx3 has highly restricted brain expression in mesencephalic dopaminergic neurons. Proc. Natl. Acad. Sci. USA **94**: 13305–13310.
5. JOYNER, A.L. 1996. Engrailed, Wnt, and Pax genes regulate midbrain-hindbrain development. Trends Genet. **12**: 15–20.
6. SEMINA, E.V., R.S. REITER & J.C. MURRAY. 1997. Isolation of a new homeobox gene belonging to the Pitx/Rieg family: expression during lens development and mapping to the aphakia region on mouse chromosome 19. Hum. Mol. Genet. **6**: 2109–2116.
7. DREYER, S.D., G. ZHOU, A. BALDINI, *et al.* 1998. Mutations in LMX1B cause abnormal skeletal patterning and renal dysplasia in nail patella syndrome. Nat. Genet. **19**: 47–50.
8. CHEN, H., Y. LUN, D. OVCHINNIKOV, *et al.* 1998. Limb and kidney defects in Lmx1b mutant mice suggest an involvement of LMX1B in human nail patella syndrome. Nat. Genet. **19**: 51–55.
9. SIMON, H.H., H. SAUERESSIG, W. WURST, *et al.* 2001. Fate of midbrain dopaminergic neurons controlled by the engrailed genes. J. Neurosci. **21**: 3126–3134.
10. LAW, S.W., O.M. CONNEELY, F.J. DEMAYO & B.W. O'MALLEY. 1992. Identification of a new brain-specific transcription factor, NURR1. Mol. Endocrinol. **6**: 2129–2135.
11. ZETTERSTROM, R.H., R. WILLIAMS, T. PERLMANN & L. OLSON. 1996. Cellular expression of the immediate early transcription factors Nurr1 and NGFI-B suggests a gene regulatory role in several brain regions including the nigrostriatal dopamine system. Brain Res. Mol. Brain Res. **41**: 111–120.
12. ZETTERSTROM, R.H., L. SOLOMIN, L. JANSSON, *et al.* 1997. Dopamine neuron agenesis in Nurr1-deficient mice. Science **276**: 248–250.
13. SAUCEDO-CARDENAS, O. & O.M. CONNEELY. 1996. Comparative distribution of NURR1 and NUR77 nuclear receptors in the mouse central nervous system. J. Mol. Neurosci. **7**: 51–63.
14. XIAO, Q., S.O. CASTILLO & V.M. NIKODEM. 1996. Distribution of messenger RNAs for the orphan nuclear receptors Nurr1 and Nur77 (NGFI-B) in adult rat brain using in situ hybridization. Neuroscience **75**: 221–230.

15. BACKMAN, C., T. PERLMANN, A. WALLEN, et al. 1999. A selective group of dopaminergic neurons express Nurr1 in the adult mouse brain. Brain Res. **851:** 125–132.
16. SAUCEDO-CARDENAS, O., J.D. QUINTANA-HAU, W.D. LE, et al. 1998. Nurr1 is essential for the induction of the dopaminergic phenotype and the survival of ventral mesencephalic late dopaminergic precursor neurons. Proc. Natl. Acad. Sci. USA **95:** 4013–4018.
17. CASTILLO, S.O., J.S. BAFFI, M. PALKOVITS, et al. 1998. Dopamine biosynthesis is selectively abolished in substantia nigra/ventral tegmental area but not in hypothalamic neurons in mice with targeted disruption of the Nurr1 gene. Mol. Cell Neurosci. **11:** 36–46.
18. SAUCEDO-CARDENAS, O., R. KARDON, T.R. EDIGER, et al. 1997. Cloning and structural organization of the gene encoding the murine nuclear receptor transcription factor, NURR1. Gene **187:** 135–139.
19. WALLEN, A.A., D.S. CASTRO, R.H. ZETTERSTROM, et al. 2001. Orphan nuclear receptor Nurr1 is essential for Ret expression in midbrain dopamine neurons and in the brain stem. Mol. Cell Neurosci. **18:** 649–663.
20. BECK, K.D., J. VALVERDE, T. ALEXI, et al. 1995. Mesencephalic dopaminergic neurons protected by GDNF from axotomy-induced degeneration in the adult brain. Nature **373:** 339–341.
21. CHU, Y., K. KOMPOLITI, E.J. COCHRAN, et al. 2002. Age-related decreases in Nurr1 immunoreactivity in the human substantia nigra. J. Comp. Neurol. **450:** 203–214.
22. BANNON, M.J., B. PRUETZ, A.B. MANNING-BOG, et al. 2002. Decreased expression of the transcription factor NURR1 in dopamine neurons of cocaine abusers. Proc. Natl. Acad. Sci. USA **99:** 6382–6385.
23. SAKURADA, K., M. OHSHIMA-SAKURADA, T.D. PALMER & F.H. GAGE. 1999. Nurr1, an orphan nuclear receptor, is a transcriptional activator of endogenous tyrosine hydroxylase in neural progenitor cells derived from the adult brain. Development **126:** 4017–4026.
24. CAZORLA, P., M.P. SMIDT, K.L. O'MALLEY & J.P. BURBACH. 2000. A response element for the homeodomain transcription factor Ptx3 in the tyrosine hydroxylase gene promoter. J. Neurochem. **74:** 1829–1837.
25. ROLLETSCHEK, A., H. CHANG, K. GUAN, et al. 2001. Differentiation of embryonic stem cell-derived dopaminergic neurons is enhanced by survival-promoting factors. Mech. Dev. **105:** 93–104.
26. KIM, J.H., J.M. AUERBACH, J.A. RODRIGUEZ-GOMEZ, et al. 2002. Dopamine neurons derived from embryonic stem cells function in an animal model of Parkinson's disease. Nature **418:** 50–56.
27. TORNQVIST, N., E. HERMANSON, T. PERLMANN & I. STROMBERG. 2002. Generation of tyrosine hydroxylase-immunoreactive neurons in ventral mesencephalic tissue of Nurr1 deficient mice. Dev. Brain Res. **133:** 37–47.
28. LE, W., O.M. CONNEELY, L. ZOU, et al. 1999. Selective agenesis of mesencephalic dopaminergic neurons in Nurr1-deficient mice. Exp. Neurol. **159:** 451–458.
29. WALLEN, A., R.H. ZETTERSTROM, L. SOLOMIN, et al. 1999. Fate of mesencephalic AHD2-expressing dopamine progenitor cells in NURR1 mutant mice. Exp. Cell Res. **253:** 737–746.
30. ZHOU, Q.Y. & R.D. PALMITER. 1995. Dopamine-deficient mice are severely hypoactive, adipsic, and aphagic. Cell **83:** 1197–1209.
31. BONGERS, E.M., M.C. GUBLER & N.V. KNOERS. 2002. Nail-patella syndrome. Overview on clinical and molecular findings. Pediatr. Nephrol. **17:** 703–712.
32. MCINTOSH, I., E. TIERNEY, I. BUKELIS & L. MARSH. 2001. Behavioral phenotype of nail-patella syndrome. Presented at the 51st Annual Meeting of the American Association of Human Genetics, San Diego, CA, October 13–16, 2001. Abstr. 571/S.

Postnatal Developmental Programmed Cell Death in Dopamine Neurons

ROBERT E. BURKE

Departments of Neurology and Pathology, The College of Physicians and Surgeons, Columbia University, New York, New York 10032, USA

ABSTRACT: The prenatal development of dopamine (DA) neurons of the substantia nigra (SN) is characterized by their birth, specification, and migration to their final positions. Their postnatal development is characterized by the establishment of contact and interactions between the SN and other neural nuclei, particularly the striatal target, by extension of axons, terminal differentiation, and synapse formation. In this postnatal context there is a natural cell death event, which is apoptotic in nature and biphasic in time course, with an initial peak on postnatal day (PND) 2, and a second on PND14. By PND20 the event has largely subsided. This natural cell death event is regulated *in vivo* by interaction with striatal target: it is augmented by axon-sparing target lesion, DA terminal destruction, and medial forebrain bundle axotomy. This target dependence is present largely within only the first two postnatal weeks. The striatal target–derived neurotrophic factor(s) that regulate this death event are unknown. We have shown, in a postnatal primary culture model of mesencephalic DA neurons, that glia-derived neurotrophic factor (GDNF) is unique in its ability to support their viability by suppressing apoptosis. We have also recently found that intrastriatal injection of GDNF *in vivo* suppresses apoptosis, and injection of neutralizing antibodies augments it. Thus, GDNF is a leading candidate for a striatum-derived neurotrophic factor for DA neurons during development.

KEYWORDS: apoptosis; programmed cell death; neurotrophic factors; Parkinson's disease; striatum; substantia nigra

In evaluating research approaches to Parkinson's disease (PD), it is certainly reasonable to ask, how valuable is it to study developmental processes affecting dopamine (DA) neurons in relation to an adult-onset (and age-related) neurodegenerative disease? There are several important reasons, related both to developing therapies for the treatment of patients today, and to furthering our understanding of pathogenesis for the development of prevention and cure. In relation to the treatment of patients today, some of the most promising approaches are based on cell replacement therapies. For all of these approaches, but especially for those based on the utilization of stem cells, critical issues in the developmental biology of dopamine neurons must be

Address for correspondence: Robert E. Burke, M.D., Department of Neurology, Room 308, Black Building, Columbia University, 650 West 168th Street, New York, NY 10032. Voice: +1-212-305-7374; fax: +1-212-305-5450.
rb43@columbia.edu

Ann. N.Y. Acad. Sci. 991: 69–79 (2003). © 2003 New York Academy of Sciences.

addressed in order to succeed: How is the mesencephalic dopamine neuron phenotype specified? What extrinsic molecules and intrinsic signaling systems do the neurons depend upon to differentiate? At different stages in their development, what
trophic factors and signaling pathways do they depend upon for viability? How do
their axons find their way to appropriate targets and establish functional synaptic
contacts?

In relation to the pathogenesis of PD, it is likely that the developmental neurobiology of dopamine neurons holds clues. Synuclein has been clearly implicated in the
pathogenesis of familial and sporadic PD, and yet we do not know its normal func-

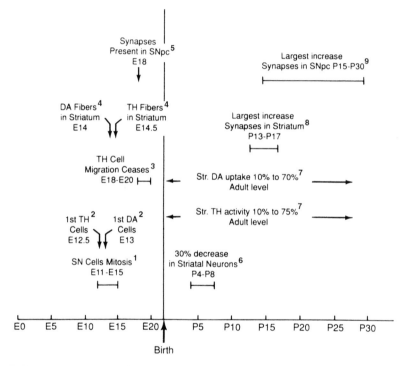

FIGURE 1. Important milestones in the development of the nigrostriatal dopaminergic
system in rat. (1) SN dopamine neurons are born between E11 and E15, with a peak on
E13.[66,67] (2) Immunoreactivity for TH is first observed on E12.5;[68] for dopamine on E13.[9]
(3) Prior to E18, dopaminergic neurons can be observed from the aqueduct to the ventral pial
surface of the mesencephalon, in association with radial glia; they are likely to be migrating
from their locus of origin to their final positions in the mesencephalon.[69] By E20, dopamine
neurons assume a topography similar to that of the adult brain,[69] so it is likely that extra-
nigral migration has ceased. (4) Dopaminergic fibers are first observed in the striatum by
TH immunohistochemistry at E14.5;[68] by dopamine immunohistochemistry at E14.[9] (5)
Synapses are first observed in SNpc at E18.[70] (6) In the postnatal period, a natural cell death
event occurs in striatum between PND4 and 8.[71] (7) Differentiation of dopamine terminals
takes place postnatally, indicated by large increases in TH activity and dopamine uptake between birth and PND30.[10] (8) Synapses form in the striatum postnatally, with the most rapid
increase occurring between PNDs13 and 17.[11] (9) The largest increase in synapses in SNpc
occurs between P15 and 30.[70]

tion. One of our few clues is that it is highly upregulated during normal development.[1,2] The proteasome complex has been proposed to play a role in the pathogenesis of PD and other neurodegenerative disorders.[3] What are the principal roles of this complex in the normal physiology of dopamine neurons? Again, development may hold clues: mRNAs for several components of the proteasome are highly upregulated.[4] There is a growing consensus that programmed cell death (PCD) may play a role in the pathogenesis of neurodegenerative diseases. The concept of PCD derived in large part from developmental studies in neurobiology demonstrating the universal occurrence of natural cell death.[5] Many of the major classes of molecules known today that regulate PCD, including the Bcl-2 family and the caspase family, were first identified by molecular studies of developmental cell death in *C. elegans*.[6] Of all the features of development, the cell cycle would seem the least likely to play a role in adult-onset neurodegenerative diseases affecting postmitotic neurons, and yet components of the cell cycle have been implicated as PCD mediators[7] and identified in Alzheimer brains.[8] Surely we have much to learn about potential mechanisms of neurodegeneration by the study of developmental processes.

The development of dopamine neurons of the substantia nigra (SN) in rat can be thought of as proceeding in two broad phases (FIG. 1). In the prenatal phase, the population of dopamine neurons is established, and the architecture of the SN as a nucleus is formed, by the processes of mitosis, phenotype specification, and neuronal migration. In this volume Drs. Simon, Perlmann, and Burbach address important advances in the molecular basis of dopamine neuron phenotype specification. In the second phase of development, which begins in the perinatal period and extends into the postnatal period, the DA neurons of the SN establish interactions with other neural groups by extending axons, forming synapses, and receiving afferents (FIG. 1). The first dopaminergic projections to reach the striatum do so by E14,[9] but most of the innervation takes place between E18 and postnatal day (PND) 4.[9] During the postnatal period, dopaminergic terminals in the striatum undergo extensive differentiation, indicated by major increases in tyrosine hydroxylase (TH) activity and dopamine reuptake.[10] During the postnatal period synapses form in the striatum, with most of the rapid rate of increase observed between PNDs13 and 17.[11] It is in this context of developing target interactions with the striatum that a natural cell death (NCD) event takes place among dopamine neurons of the SN.

NATURAL CELL DEATH IN DOPAMINE NEURONS OF THE SN

NCD in dopamine neurons of the SN begins shortly before birth in rat and achieves an initial peak on PND2[12,13] (FIG. 2). There is a second, smaller peak of NCD on PND14, and by PND20 the event has largely abated. Qualitatively, the morphology of this NCD event is exclusively apoptotic. While other morphologies of cell death have been identified in the setting of developmental cell death,[14] we have observed only classic apoptotic morphology using a suppressed silver stain technique.[12] We have previously shown that this technique will detect nonapoptotic, variant morphologies of programmed cell death,[15,16] and yet none are observed in the SN during normal development.

We believe that this NCD event is likely to be a universal feature of nigral development in mammals. Based on counts of TH-immunostained neurons in SN, it had been claimed that there is no evidence for NCD in mice.[17] However, interpretation of such data is complicated by the fact that increasing expression of levels of TH during development add to the numbers of counted TH neurons; thus, loss of some of them could be masked.[5] Indeed, Jackson-Lewis *et al.* have shown that a NCD event does occur in mice; classic nuclear apoptotic chromatin clumps are observed in TH-positive neurons.[18] This morphology was confirmed to be apoptotic at the light microscope level by TUNEL labeling and immunostaining for the activated form of caspase-3. It was confirmed at the ultrastructural level by the appearance of electron-dense nuclear chromatin clumps and preservation of intracellular organelles as classically described.[19]

Our approach to quantifying the NCD event in SN warrants a brief methodological point. It will be noted in FIGURE 2 that two sets of counts are presented. Apoptotic nuclei meeting *cellular* criteria are surrounded by TH-positive cytoplasm, and are therefore defined as dopaminergic at the cellular level. It can be seen that only a small number of profiles meet this criterion. We had previously observed at an ultrastructural level that apoptotic neurons are stripped of their cytoplasm as they die,[20] and it had previously been shown that neuronal cytoplasmic markers are diminished in their expression as cells die by apoptosis.[21] It is therefore to be expected that only a small portion of dopamine neurons dying by apoptosis would be identifiable as such at the cellular level. In order to obtain an estimate of profiles derived from dopamine neurons, which otherwise would not be counted, we developed a *regional* criterion: any apoptotic profile in the SNpc, within 15 μm of two TH-positive neurons, is counted. It can be seen in FIGURE 2 that the time courses of counts obtained by the cellular and regional criteria are identical.

Relatively little is known about the specific programmed cell death mechanisms in NCD in SN dopamine neurons. Of the three general pathways that mediate programmed cell death, the extrinsic, the intrinsic, and the endoplasmic reticulum stress-mediated pathways,[22] it is the intrinsic that is likely to be operative, given that NCD in SN appears to be regulated by the availability of trophic support (see below). In the intrinsic pathway, members of the Bcl-2 family of proteins act upstream to mitochondria to regulate release of cytochrome c and the resulting activation of

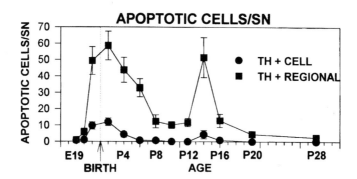

FIGURE 2. The time course of natural cell death in dopamine neurons in the SN. Counts for apoptotic profiles meeting cellular and regional criteria, as discussed in the text, are presented. Natural cell death in dopamine neurons has a biphasic time course, with an initial peak at PND2 and a second at PND14.

caspases.[23] In transgenic mice overexpressing the antiapoptotic protein Bcl-2 under the control of the TH promoter, there is a reduction in the level of NCD in dopamine neurons and an increase in the number of SN TH-positive neurons surviving into adulthood.[18] These animals are also resistant to the induction of developmental cell death due to striatal target lesion (see below). On the other hand, the proapoptotic protein Bax appears to be important for this induction, because it is reduced in Bax-null mice.[24] While Bax-null mice show a trend for diminished levels of NCD, the effect does not reach significance, suggesting that mechanisms independent of Bax must also be operative.

Within the intrinsic pathway, mitochondrial release of cytochrome c, and its association with Apaf and pro-caspase-9 in the presence of ATP, results in the activation of caspase-9, with the subsequent proteolytic cleavage, and activation of caspase-3 and other effector caspases.[25,26] Activated caspase-3 is observed in apoptotic profiles in SN in a nuclear distribution during NCD,[27] as are caspase protein cleavage products.[18] However, whether caspase-3 is an essential mediator of NCD in dopamine neurons is unknown. In many postmitotic neurons, it is not; caspase-3–null animals show diminished apoptotic nuclear chromatin changes, but no alteration in the levels of NCD.[28]

REGULATION OF NCD IN DOPAMINE NEURONS BY STRIATAL TARGET INTERACTIONS

According to classic neurotrophic theory, the magnitude of the NCD event within a projecting nucleus is regulated by interactions with its target.[29,30] The target provides a necessary trophic factor in limiting quantities by retrograde transport, such that only projecting neurons that successfully make target contact will survive. It is important to realize, however, that most of the experimental data upon which classic theory rests was developed from systems with peripheral projections; far less is known about systems with central projections. For dopamine neurons of the SN, it would appear likely that target interactions would regulate the NCD event, given that it occurs within the developmental period most characterized by elaboration of target contact and synapse formation (FIG. 1). In support of this concept, we have previously shown that axon-sparing lesions of the target striatum during development result in a reduction in the ultimate number of dopamine neurons at maturity.[31] Furthermore, numerous investigations in tissue culture have demonstrated the ability of various striatal preparations to support the viability and differentiation of dopamine neurons.[32–35]

Based on these considerations, it would be predicted that disruption of striatal target, or access to target, would result in an augmentation of NCD in dopamine neurons, and we have shown in a number of studies that this is indeed the case: developmental axon-sparing lesion of the striatum[20] or selective disruption of dopamine terminals by 6-hydroxydopamine (6OHDA)[36] or axotomy[37] lead to an induction of apoptotic death in dopamine neurons (FIG. 3).

For the striatal target lesion model and the 6OHDA model, there is a developmental window for this effect. In both models the effect is largely achieved within the first two postnatal weeks, corresponding, interestingly, to the period of NCD. Thereafter, the models differ; in the striatal lesion model, there is very little induction of death in SN pars compacta (pc) after PND14[38] and none in adult.[16,39] Thus, there is

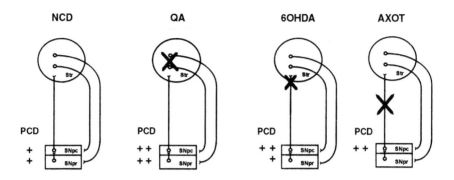

FIGURE 3. The NCD event in SNpc is augmented during development by disruption of target interactions by axon-sparing striatal target lesion with quinolinate (QA),[20] dopamine terminal destruction with 6OHDA,[36] or axotomy (Axot).[37] PCD: programmed cell death.

no evidence that adult SN dopamine neurons depend on target support for viability. In the 6OHDA model, although the levels of death are reduced, it remains possible, even in adult animals, to induce apoptosis in SN dopamine neurons.[40] Thus, in the 6OHDA model, induction of death probably occurs not only on the basis of disrupted target support, in the developmental context, by destruction of terminals, but also on the basis of a direct toxic effect as well. In the axotomy model, induction of apoptosis is also developmentally dependent; it can be induced at PNDs 3, 7, and 14,[37] but not in adults.[41]

EVALUATION OF GDNF AS A STRIATAL TARGET–DERIVED NEUROTROPHIC FACTOR FOR DOPAMINE NEURONS OF THE SN

While there is therefore much evidence that developmental cell death in dopamine neurons is regulated by target interaction, as envisioned by classic neurotrophic theory, the factor(s) that mediate this regulation are unknown. One candidate has been glial cell line–derived neurotrophic factor (GDNF), based on its original identification as a protein capable of supporting the development of embryonic mesencephalic dopamine neurons in tissue culture.[42] In keeping with such a possible role for GDNF, its mRNA is present in striatum and is expressed at highest levels during early postnatal development.[43–47] GDNF protein is expressed in striatum and is most abundant after birth.[48] The GDNF receptor GFRα1 and the tyrosine kinase Ret are both expressed in SNpc.[49–51] GDNF can be specifically transported retrograde from striatum to SNpc.[52] The strongest evidence against a possible role for GDNF in this capacity has been that homozygous null mice for GDNF[53–55] and for GFRα1[56,57] show no reduction in the number of SN dopamine neurons at birth. These results have led some authorities to conclude that GDNF is not a physiologic neurotrophic factor for developing dopamine neurons.[58]

However, mice homozygous for GDNF- and GFRα1-null mutations die shortly after birth, due to abnormalities in the development of the kidneys and enteric nervous system. Thus, they die quite early in the course of the NCD event in these neurons, and it is possible that they die before an effect on NCD can become apparent. Furthermore, none of these null mutations were regionally or temporally regulated; it is possible that compensatory changes occurred, masking a phenotype.

To reassess the possible role of GDNF as a physiologic trophic factor for dopamine neurons, we examined its ability to support their viability in a unique postnatal primary culture model,[59] established during the period of NCD for these neurons. It is important to realize that all prior *in vitro* work on trophic factors for dopamine neurons, including that on GDNF itself, had been performed on early embryonic cultures, often derived at E14–E16. This is not a developmental period when dopamine neurons are making significant target contact (FIG. 1), so there is little reason to expect that they should at this time be responsive to target-derived factors. The postnatal culture model provides an opportunity to examine putative neurotrophic factors for dopamine neurons in a context in which target support is more likely to be operative. In the postnatal cultures, we assessed GDNF in comparison to other factors that had previously been reported to support embryonic dopamine neurons, including brain-derived neurotrophic factor (BDNF),[60] transforming growth factors (TGF) β2 and β3,[61] TGFα,[62] epidermal growth factor,[63] and basic fibroblast growth factor.[63] We found that GDNF alone was able to support the viability of postnatal dopamine neurons *in vitro*, and it did so by suppressing apoptosis.[64] This effect of GDNF was specific at the cellular level for dopamine neurons and at the regional level for dopamine neurons derived from the SN.

We have recently evaluated effects of GDNF on levels of NCD in dopamine neurons *in vivo*. We have found that 1.0 µg GDNF administered into the striatum of rats on PND2 is able to suppress levels of NCD, quantified using either cellular or regional criteria for apoptosis among dopamine neurons.[65] In support of a possible physiologic role for endogenous GDNF, we have also found, using a passive immunization approach, that acute intrastriatal neutralization of GDNF augments NCD among dopamine neurons.[65] This effect is developmentally dependent; it is observed on PNDs 2 and 6, but not PNDs 14 or 21. Thus, striatal GDNF appears to play a role primarily in the regulation of the first phase of NCD in dopamine neurons. This observation is in keeping with our assessment of the time course of GDNF mRNA expression in striatum during development. It is most abundant during the first postnatal week, and it declines thereafter (see Cho, Kholodilov, and Burke; this volume).

In order to be certain that endogenous striatal GDNF plays a physiologic role in regulating the NCD event and long-term survival of dopamine neurons, regional and temporally regulated knockout mice must be developed. To determine if GDNF alone is sufficient to regulate the NCD events in dopamine neurons, long-term overexpression in target areas must be achieved, and effects on the ultimate number of dopamine neurons in adult animals determined. We must also determine whether GDNF plays a role selectively in the early phase of NCD.

SUMMARY AND CONCLUSIONS

In summary, it is clear that a NCD event occurs during the normal development of dopamine neurons and that the magnitude of this event is regulated by early target interactions. It remains unknown what factor(s) derived from the striatal target regulate the NCD event, but in spite of observations in homozygous null mice, GDNF remains an important candidate.

Certainly this hypothesis does not exclude the possibility that there may be other equally important neurotrophic factors. To develop therapeutic approaches, and to better understand the pathogenesis of PD, the identification of physiologic trophic factors for dopamine neurons should be a foremost priority.

ACKNOWLEDGMENTS

The author is supported by NIH NS26836, NS38370, the Parkinson's Disease Foundation, and the Lowenstein Foundation.

REFERENCES

1. KHOLODILOV, N.G., M. NEYSTAT, T.F. OO, et al. 1999. Increased expression of rat synuclein1 in the substantia nigra pars compacta identified by differential display in a model of developmental target injury. J. Neurochem. **73:** 2586–2599.
2. PETERSEN, K., O.F. OLESEN & J.D. MIKKELSEN. 1999. Developmental expression of alpha-synuclein in rat hippocampus and cerebral cortex [in-process citation]. Neuroscience **91:** 651–659.
3. II, K., H. ITO, K. TANAKA & A. HIRANO. 1997. Immunocytochemical co-localization of the proteasome in ubiquitinated structures in neurodegenerative diseases and the elderly. J. Neuropathol. Exp. Neurol. **56:** 125–131.
4. EL-KHODOR, B.F., N.G. KHOLODILOV, O. YARYGINA & R.E. BURKE. 2001. The expression of mRNAs for the proteasome complex is developmentally regulated in the rat mesencephalon. Dev. Brain Res. **129:** 47–56.
5. OPPENHEIM, R.W. 1991. Cell death during development of the nervous system. Ann. Rev. Neurosci. **14:** 453–501.
6. ELLIS, R.E., J. YUAN & H.R. HORVITZ. 1991. Mechanisms and functions of cell death. Annu. Rev. Cell Biol. **7:** 663–698.
7. PARK, D.S., E.J. MORRIS, R. BREMNER, et al. 2000. Involvement of retinoblastoma family members and E2F/DP complexes in the death of neurons evoked by DNA damage. J. Neurosci. **20:** 3104–3114.
8. HUSSEMAN, J.W., D. NOCHLIN & I. VINCENT. 2000. Mitotic activation: a convergent mechanism for a cohort of neurodegenerative diseases. Neurobiol. Aging **21:** 815–828.
9. VOORN, P., A. KALSBEEK, B. JORRITSMA-BYHAM & H.J. GROENEWEGEN. 1988. The pre- and postnatal development of the dopaminergic cell groups in the ventral mesencephalon and the dopaminergic innervation of the striatum of the rat. Neuroscience **25:** 857–887.
10. COYLE, J.T. 1977. Biochemical aspects of neurotransmission in the developing brain. Int. Rev. Neurobiol. **20:** 65–102.
11. HATTORI, T. & P.L. MCGEER. 1973. Synaptogenesis in the corpus striatum of infant rat. Exp. Neurol. **38:** 70–79.
12. JANEC, E. & R.E. BURKE. 1993. Naturally occurring cell death during postnatal development of the substantia nigra of the rat. Mol. Cell Neurosci. **4:** 30–35.
13. OO, T.F. & R.E. BURKE. 1997. The time course of developmental cell death in phenotypically defined dopaminergic neurons of the substantia nigra. Dev. Brain Res. **98:** 191–196.
14. CLARKE, P.G.H. 1990. Developmental cell death: morphological diversity and multiple mechanisms. Anat. Embryol. **181:** 195–213.
15. OO, T.F., R. BLAZESKI, S.M.W. HARRISON, et al. 1996. Neuron death in the substantia nigra of weaver mouse occurs late in development and is not apoptotic. J. Neurosci. **16:** 6134–6145.

16. STEFANIS, L. & R.E. BURKE. 1996. Transneuronal degeneration in substantia nigra pars reticulata following striatal excitotoxic injury in adult rat: time course, distribution, and morphology of cell death. Neuroscience **74:** 997–1008.
17. BLUM, M. 1998. A null mutation in TGF-alpha leads to a reduction in midbrain dopaminergic neurons in the substantia nigra. Nat. Neurosci. **1:** 374–377.
18. JACKSON-LEWIS, V., M. VILA, R. DJALDETTI, *et al.* 2000. Developmental cell death in dopaminergic neurons of the substantia nigra of mice. J. Comp. Neurol. **424:** 476–488.
19. KERR, J.F.R., G.C. GOBE, C.M. WINTERFORD & B.V. HARMON. 1995. Anatomical methods in cell death. *In* Methods in Cell Biology: Cell Death. L.M. Schwartz & B.A. Osborne, Eds.: 1–27. Academic Press. New York.
20. MACAYA, A., F. MUNELL, R.M. GUBITS & R.E. BURKE. 1994. Apoptosis in substantia nigra following developmental striatal excitotoxic injury. Proc. Natl. Acad. Sci. USA **91:** 8117–8121.
21. FREEMAN, R.S., S. ESTUS & E.M. JOHNSON. 1994. Analysis of cell cycle related gene expression in postmitotic neurons selective induction of cyclin D1 during programmed cell death. Neuron **12:** 343–355.
22. MEHMET, H. 2000. Caspases find a new place to hide [news]. Nature **403:** 29–30.
23. ADAMS, J.M. & S. CORY. 1998. The Bcl-2 protein family: arbiters of cell survival. Science **281:** 1322–1326.
24. VILA, M., V. JACKSON-LEWIS, S. VUKOSAVIC, *et al.* 2001. Bax ablation prevents dopaminergic neurodegeneration in the 1-methyl-4-phenyl-1,2,3,6-tetrahydropyridine mouse model of Parkinson's disease. Proc. Natl. Acad. Sci. USA **98:** 2837–2842.
25. BUDIHARDJO, I., H. OLIVER, M. LUTTER, *et al.* 1999. Biochemical pathways of caspase activation during apoptosis. Annu. Rev. Cell Dev. Biol. **15:** 269–290.
26. GREEN, D.R. & J.C. REED. 1998. Mitochondria and apoptosis. Science **281:** 1309–1312.
27. JEON, B.S., N.G. KHOLODILOV, T.F. OO, *et al.* 1999. Activation of caspase-3 in developmental models of programmed cell death in neurons of the substantia nigra. J. Neurochem. **73:** 322–333.
28. OPPENHEIM, R.W., R.A. FLAVELL, S. VINSANT, *et al.* 2001. Programmed cell death of developing mammalian neurons after genetic deletion of caspases. J. Neurosci. **21:** 4752–4760.
29. CLARKE, P.G.H. 1985. Neuronal death in the development of the vertebrate nervous system. Trends Neurosci. **8:** 345–349.
30. BARDE, Y.A. 1989. Trophic factors and neuronal survival. Neuron **2:** 1525–1534.
31. BURKE, R.E., A. MACAYA, D. DEVIVO, *et al.* 1992. Neonatal hypoxic-ischemic or excitotoxic striatal injury results in a decreased adult number of substantia nigra neurons. Neuroscience **50:** 559–569.
32. PROCHIANTZ, A., U. DI PORZIO, A. KATO, *et al.* 1979. *In vitro* maturation of mesencephalic dopaminergic neurons from mouse embryos is enhanced in presence of their striatal target cells. Proc. Natl. Acad. Sci. USA **76:** 5387–5391.
33. HEMMENDINGER, L.M., B.B. GARBER, P.C. HOFFMANN & A. HELLER. 1981. Target neuron-specific process formation by embryonic mesencephalic dopamine neurons *in vitro*. Proc. Natl. Acad. Sci. USA **78:** 1264–1268.
34. HOFFMANN, P.C., L.M. HEMMENDINGER, C. KOTAKE & A. HELLER. 1983. Enhanced dopamine cell survival in reaggregates containing target cells. Brain Res. **274:** 275–281.
35. TOMOZAWA, Y. & S.H. APPEL. 1986. Soluble striatal extracts enhance development of mesencephalic dopaminergic neurons *in vitro*. Brain Res. **399:** 111–124.
36. MARTI, M.J., C.J. JAMES, T.F. OO, *et al.* 1997. Early developmental destruction of terminals in the striatal target induces apoptosis in dopamine neurons of the substantia nigra. J. Neurosci. **17:** 2030–2039.
37. EL-KHODOR, B.F. & R.E. BURKE. 2002. Medial forebrain bundle axotomy during development induces apoptosis in dopamine neurons of the substantia nigra and activation of caspases in their degenerating axons. J. Comp. Neurol. **452:** 65–79.
38. KELLY, W.J. & R.E. BURKE. 1996. Apoptotic neuron death in rat substantia nigra induced by striatal excitotoxic injury is developmentally dependent. Neurosci. Lett. **220:** 85–88.

39. LUNDBERG, C., K. WICTORIN & A. BJORKLUND. 1994. Retrograde degenerative changes in the substantia nigra pars compacta following an excitotoxic lesion of the striatum. Brain Res. **644:** 205–212.
40. MARTI, M.J., J. SAURA, R.E. BURKE, et al. 2002. Striatal 6–hydroxydopamine induces apoptosis of nigral neurons in the adult rat. Brain Res. **958:** 185–191.
41. CROCKER, S.J., N. WIGLE, P. LISTON, et al. 2001. NAIP protects the nigrostriatal dopamine pathway in an intrastriatal 6-OHDA rat model of Parkinson's disease. Eur. J. Neurosci. **14:** 391–400.
42. LIN, L.-F.H., D.H. DOHERTY, J.D. LILE, et al. 1993. GDNF: a glial cell line-derived neurotrophic factor for midbrain dopaminergic neurons. Science **260:** 1130–1132.
43. SCHAAR, D.G., B.A. SIEBER, C.F. DREYFUS & I.B. BLACK. 1993. Regional and cell specific expression of GDNF in rat brain. Exp. Neurol. **124:** 368–371.
44. STROMBERG, I., L. BJORKLUND, M. JOHANSSON, et al. 1993. Glial cell line derived neurotrophic factor is expressed in the developing but not adult striatum and stimulates developing dopamine neurons in vivo. Exp. Neurol. **124:** 401–412.
45. BLUM, M. & C.S. WEICKERT. 1995. GDNF mRNA expression in normal postnatal development, aging, and in weaver mutant mice. Neurobiol. Aging **16:** 925–929.
46. CHOI-LUNDBERG, D.L. & M.C. BOHN. 1995. Ontogeny and distribution of glial cell line-derived neurotrophic factor (GDNF) mRNA in rat. Dev. Brain Res. **85:** 80–88.
47. GOLDEN, J.P., J.A. DEMARO, P.A. OSBORNE, et al. 1999. Expression of neurturin, GDNF, and GDNF family-receptor mRNA in the developing and mature mouse. Exp. Neurol. **158:** 504–528.
48. LOPEZ-MARTIN, E., H.J. CARUNCHO, J. RODRIGUEZ-PALLARES, et al. 1999. Striatal dopaminergic afferents concentrate in GDNF-positive patches during development and in developing intrastriatal striatal grafts. J. Comp. Neurol. **406:** 199–206.
49. TREANOR, J.J., L. GOODMAN, F. DE SAUVAGE, et al. 1996. Characterization of a multicomponent receptor for GDNF. Nature **382:** 80–83.
50. YU, T., S. SCULLY, Y. YU, et al. 1998. Expression of GDNF family receptor components during development: implications in the mechanisms of interaction. J. Neurosci. **18:** 4684–4696.
51. GLAZNER, G.W., X. MU & J.E. SPRINGER. 1998. Localization of glial cell line-derived neurotrophic factor receptor alpha and c-ret mRNA in rat central nervous system. J. Comp. Neurol. **391:** 42–49.
52. TOMAC, A., J. WIDENFALK, L.H. LIN, et al. 1995. Retrograde axonal transport of glial cell line-derived neurotrophic factor in the adult nigrostriatal system suggests a trophic role in the adult. Proc. Natl. Acad. Sci. USA **92:** 8274–8278.
53. MOORE, M.W., R.D. KLEIN, I. FARINAS, et al. 1996. Renal and neuronal abnormalities in mice lacking GDNF. Nature **382:** 76–79.
54. PICHEL, J.G., L. SHEN, H.Z. SHENG, et al. 1996. Defects in enteric innervation and kidney development in mice lacking GDNF. Nature **382:** 73–76.
55. SANCHEZ, M.P., I. SILOS-SANTIAGO, J. FRISEN, et al. 1996. Renal agenesis and the absence of enteric neurons in mice lacking GDNF. Nature **382:** 70–73.
56. CACALANO, G., I. FARINAS, L.C. WANG, et al. 1998. GFRalpha1 is an essential receptor component for GDNF in the developing nervous system and kidney. Neuron **21:** 53–62.
57. ENOMOTO, H., T. ARAKI, A. SACKMAN, et al. 1998. GFRalpha-1 deficient mice have deficits in the enteric nervous system and kidneys. Neuron **21:** 317–324.
58. ROSENTHAL, A. 1999. The GDNF protein family: gene ablation studies reveal what they really do and how. Neuron **22:** 201–203.
59. RAYPORT, S., D. SULZER, W.X. SHI, et al. 1992. Identified postnatal mesolimbic dopamine neurons in culture morphology and electrophysiology. J. Neurosci. **12:** 4264–4280.
60. HYMAN, C., M. HOFER, Y.A. BARDE, et al. 1991. BDNF is a neurotrophic factor for dopaminergic neurons of the substantia nigra. Nature **350:** 230–232.
61. POULSEN, K.T., M.P. ARMANINI, R.D. KLEIN, et al. 1994. TGFβ2 and TGF β3 are potent survival factors for midbrain dopaminergic neurons. Neuron **13:** 1245–1252.
62. ALEXI, T. & F. HEFTI. 1993. Trophic actions of transforming growth factor α on mesencephalic dopaminergic neurons developing in culture. Neuroscience **55:** 903–918.

63. KNUSEL, B., P.P. MICHEL, J.S. SCHWABER & F. HEFTI. 1990. Selective and nonselective stimulation of central cholinergic and dopaminergic development *in vitro* by nerve growth factor, basic fibroblast growth factor, epidermal growth factor, insulin and the insulin-like growth factors I and II. J. Neurosci. **10:** 558–570.

64. BURKE, R.E., M. ANTONELLI & D. SULZER. 1998. Glial cell line-derived neurotrophic growth factor inhibits apoptotic death of postnatal substantia nigra dopamine neurons in primary culture. J. Neurochem. **71:** 517–525.

65. OO, T.F., N. KHOLODILOV & R.E. BURKE. 2003. Regulation of natural cell death in dopaminergic neurons of the substantia nigra by striatal glial cell line-derived neurotrophic factor in vivo. J. Neurosci. **23:** in press.

66. MARCHAND, R. & L.J. POIRER. 1983. Isthmic origin of neurons of the rat substantia nigra. Neuroscience **9:** 373–381.

67. LAUDER, J.M. & F.E. BLOOM. 1974. Ontogeny of monoamine neurons in the locus coeruleus, raphe nuclei and substantia nigra of the rat. J. Comp. Neurol. **155:** 469–482.

68. SPECHT, L.A., V.M. PICKEL, T.H. JOH & D.J. REIS. 1981. Light-microscopic immunocytochemical localization of tyrosine hydroxylase in prenatal brain. I. Early ontogeny. J. Comp. Neurol. **199:** 233–253.

69. SHULTS, C.W., R. HASIMOTO, R.M. BRADY & F.H. GAGE. 1990. Dopaminergic cells align along radial glia in the developing mesencephalon of the rat. Neuroscience **38:** 427–436.

70. LAUDER, J.M. & F.E. BLOOM. 1975. Ontogeny of monoamine neurons in the locus coeruleus, raphe nuclei and substantia nigra of the rat. J. Comp. Neurol. **163:** 251–264.

71. FENTRESS, J.C., B.B. STANFIELD & W.M. COWAN. 1981. Observations on the development of the striatum in mice and rats. Anat. Embryol. **163:** 275–298.

The Cast of Molecular Characters in Parkinson's Disease

Felons, Conspirators, and Suspects

KAH LEONG LIM,[a] VALINA L. DAWSON,[b,c,d,e] AND TED M. DAWSON[b,c,d]

[a]*Neurodegeneration Research Laboratory, National Neuroscience Institute, 11 Jalan Tan Tock Seng, Singapore 308433*

[b]*Institute for Cell Engineering and Departments of [c]Neurology, [d]Neuroscience, and [e]Physiology, Johns Hopkins University School of Medicine, Baltimore, Maryland 21287, USA*

ABSTRACT: Parkinson's Disease (PD) is a common neurodegenerative disorder characterized by the progressive loss of dopamine neurons and the accumulation of Lewy bodies and neurites. Recent advances indicate that PD is due in some individuals to genetic mutations in α-synuclein, parkin, and ubiquitin C-terminal hydrolase L1 (UCHL1). All three PD-linked gene products are related directly or indirectly to the functioning of the cellular ubiquitin proteasomal system (UPS), suggesting that UPS dysfunction may be important in PD pathogenesis. Indeed, emerging evidence indicates that derangements of the UPS may be one of the underlying mechanisms of PD pathogenesis. The function of parkin as an ubiquitin protein ligase positions it as an important player in both familial and idiopathic PD. We recently demonstrated that parkin mediates a nondegradative form of ubiquitination on synphilin-1 that could contribute to synphilin-1's aggregation in PD. Our results implicate parkin involvement in the formation of Lewy bodies associated with sporadic PD. This review discusses the role of the UPS, as well as the modus operandi of the three PD candidate felons (α-synuclein, parkin, and UCHL1) along with their conspirators in bringing about dopaminergic cell death in PD.

KEYWORDS: Parkinson's disease; α-synuclein; parkin; UCHL1; ubiquitin-proteasome system; ubiquitination

INTRODUCTION

Parkinson's disease (PD) is a progressive neurodegenerative disorder affecting 1–2% of the population above the age of 65.[1,2] Pathologically, the disease is characterized by the relatively selective loss of midbrain dopaminergic neurons in the substantia nigra pars compacta (SNpc) and the presence of Lewy bodies, eosinophilic

Address for correspondence: Ted M. Dawson, M.D., Ph.D., Institute for Cell Engineering, Departments of Neurology and Neuroscience, Johns Hopkins University School of Medicine, 600 N. Wolfe St., Carnegie 214, Baltimore, MD 21287. Voice: 410-614-3359; fax: 410-614-9568.

tdawson@jhmi.edu

Ann. N.Y. Acad. Sci. 991: 80–92 (2003). © 2003 New York Academy of Sciences.

intracytoplasmic inclusions that are abundantly enriched in ubiquitin. The loss of nigral dopaminergic neurons results in a severe depletion of striatal dopamine and gives rise to a constellation of motoric deficits that include bradykinesia, rest tremor, rigidity, and postural instability. Although the etiology of PD remains unknown, the recent identification of several genetic mutations that cause familial PD has contributed significantly to our understanding of the molecular pathogenesis of idiopathic PD. Mutations in α-synuclein, one of the major components of Lewy bodies, is linked to autosomal-dominant familial PD, and mutations in parkin cause autosomal recessive PD. Mutation in a third gene, encoding ubiquitin C-terminal hydrolase L1 (UCHL1), may cause a rare autosomal-dominant form of PD.[3] Interestingly, all the three PD-linked gene products are functionally associated directly or indirectly with the cellular ubiquitin proteasomal system (UPS).

The UPS plays an important role in maintaining cell homeostasis through the clearance of unwanted proteins. In this system, proteins destined for proteasomal degradation are covalently tagged with ubiquitin, a 76–amino acid residue protein, by the sequential actions of ubiquitin-activating (E1), -conjugating (E2) and -ligating (E3) enzymes. The ligation process is usually repeated many times to form a polyubiquitin chain in which the C terminal glycine residue of each ubiquitin unit is linked to a specific lysine (K) residue (most commonly K-48) of the previous ubiquitin.[4] We and others have shown that parkin functions as an E2 dependent-E3 ligase.[5–7] Thus, one can envisage that a loss of parkin function would lead to aberrations in the UPS and contribute to the pathogenesis of PD. Indeed, dysfunction of the UPS is emerging as a popular hypothesis to explain nigral degeneration in both familial and idiopathic PD.[8] The formation of α-synuclein aggregates that are evident in brain lesions in many neurodegenerative diseases including PD also suggests a derangement in intracellular protein handling. Finally, the function of UCHL1 in the hydrolysis of polyubiquitin further implicates an involvement of the UPS machinery in PD. We review here our current understanding of the various felons, conspirators, and suspects involved in the molecular pathogenesis of PD.

α-SYNUCLEIN

The association of two missense mutations in α-synuclein (A30P and A53T) in a small subset of familial PD patients generated an intense and widespread interest among PD researchers.[9,10] Fueling this excitement was the discovery that Lewy bodies, the pathologic hallmark of sporadic PD, were strongly immunoreactive for α-synuclein.[11] These findings made α-synuclein a compelling candidate felon in PD. Although the physiological function of α-synuclein remains to be elucidated, we now have a wealth of knowledge regarding its role in PD pathogenesis.

The α-synuclein protein belongs to a family of structurally related proteins that are expressed abundantly in the central nervous system. In humans, the synuclein family includes two other members, β- and γ-synuclein. Structurally, synucleins have a highly conserved aminoterminal region containing repetitive imperfect repeats that bear the consensus sequence KTKEGV, a hydrophobic middle section, and a less well conserved acidic carboxyl terminal. While α- and β-synucleins are concentrated in close proximity to synaptic vesicles in nerve terminals, γ-synuclein is more ubiquitously expressed throughout nerve cells.[12]

TABLE 1. Rodent models of Parkinson's disease based on α-synuclein ablation or overespression

Animal	α-Synuclein	Transgene promoter	Protein inclusions	Nigral pathology	Motor impairment	Reference
Mouse	knockout	NA	−	−	−	13
Mouse	WT	PDGF-β	+	−	+	56
Mouse	WT	TH	−	−	−	57
Mouse	WT	TH	−	−	−	58
Mouse	WT	Prp	−	−	−	19
Mouse	WT	Prp	−	−	−	20
Mouse	A53T	Thy-1	+	−	+	59
Mouse	A53T	TH	−	−	−	57
Mouse	A53T	Prp	+	−	+	19
Mouse	A53T	Prp	+	−	+	20
Mouse	A30P	TH	−	−	−	57
Mouse	A30P	Prp	−	−	−	20
Rat	WT	PGK	+	+	nd	16
Rat	WT	CBA	+	+	+	17
Rat	A53T	PGK	+	+	nd	16
Rat	A53T	CBA	+	+	+	17
Rat	A30P	PGK	+	+	nd	16

ABBREVIATIONS: NA, not applicable; PDGF, platelet-derived growth factor; TH, tyrosine hydroxylase; Prp, prion; CBA, chicken beta-actin; PGK, phosphoglycerate kinase; nd, not described.

To elucidate the physiological function of α-synuclein and its role in PD, several animal models based on the manipulation of α-synuclein expression were generated (TABLE 1). Targeted ablation of α-synuclein expression in mice, however, did not offer many clues to its endogenous function. α-Synuclein knockout mice developed normally without an overt neurological phenotype, showing only mild electrophysiological and behavioral alterations.[13] It thus would appear that loss of α-synuclein function is unlikely a direct contributor to PD pathogenesis. This is consistent with the dominant transmission of familial PD–linked α-synuclein mutations, which indicates a gain of function in α-synuclein. Transgenic rodents and flies overexpressing either wild-type or mutant α-synuclein do recapitulate some of the behavioral and pathologic features of human PD, including developing Lewy body-like intracytoplasmic inclusions[14] (TABLE 1). However, the mammalian animal models generally mirror synucleinopathies better than PD, as the substantia nigra is not the most severely affected brain area. Interestingly, in the Contursi kindred with α-synuclein A53T substitution, α-synuclein pathology was not isolated to the substantia nigra but were also found throughout other brain regions including the limbic system, striatum, and locus coeruleus.[15] Thus, the pathogenicity arising from derangements in α-synuclein function is not localized to a particular subset of neurons per se. It is likely that in PD, exogenous or other endogenous factors participate to predispose the nigral dopaminergic neurons to α-synuclein–mediated toxicity. To achieve a more localized effect of α-synuclein overexpression, direct intranigral injections of viral vectors expressing α-synuclein in rats induces Parkinson-like neurodegeneration including selective dopaminergic neuron loss and formation of α-synuclein positive inclusions[16,17] (TABLE 1).

How do derangements in α-synuclein lead to neuronal death? Several lines of evidence seem to converge on a common theme: dysfunction in protein handling. The propensity of α-synuclein to aggregate and fibrillize into structures that are resistant to cellular degradation may be central to its neurotoxicity. The transformation of α-synuclein from a soluble state to a disease-associated fibrillar state involves a progressive oligomerization of β-folded proteins known as protofibrils. Giasson and colleagues showed that the A53T α-synuclein has an increased tendency to polymerize into fibrils *in vitro* and that the polymerization is concentration dependent.[18] They proposed that α-synuclein fibrillization eventually leads to the formation of neuronal inclusions that would disrupt cellular function and result in cell death. The same group recently confirmed their hypothesis in mice overexpressing A53T α-synuclein (TABLE 1), as mice overexpressing A53T α-synuclein develop a progressive neurodegenerative disorder characterized by the presence of insoluble aggregates of α-synuclein and fibrillar inclusions composed of α-synuclein.[19] In contrast, mice overexpressing wild-type α-synuclein lack Lewy body-like inclusions, and they do not develop a disease phenotype.[19] Lee and colleagues also recently observed that the A53T mutant α-synuclein is significantly more pathogenic than either wild-type α-synuclein or A30P mutant α-synuclein in transgenic mice.[20] A53T mutant α-synuclein–mediated neurodegeneration is associated with abnormal accumulation of detergent-insoluble α-synuclein that undergoes unique proteolytic processing.[20] Thus, proteolytic processing may in part drive the transformation of α-synuclein from a soluble state to a disease-associated fibrillar state through progressive oligomerization. Clearly, additional conspirators are required to induce the formation of similar lesions from wild-type α-synuclein. Experimental cell culture models based on the ectopic expression of α-synuclein or its mutants have given us many clues to the nature of these conspirators. Agents that cause oxidative or nitrative damage can alter the solubility of α-synuclein and result in the formation of α-synuclein aggregates.[21–23] Posttranslational modifications such as phosphorylation may also play a role in synuclein aggregation.[24] Phosphorylation of synuclein at Ser-129 promoted fibril formation *in vitro*, and this residue is selectively and extensively phosphorylated in synucleinopathy lesions.[25] Interestingly, some evidence indicates the protofibril, rather than the fibril, to be the pathogenic species.[26] Biophysical studies conducted by Conway and colleagues showed that the two PD-linked α-synuclein mutations accelerated the rate of protofibril formation.[27] Furthermore, cytosolic dopamine seems to interact with α-synuclein to produce adducts that inhibit the conversion of protofibrils to fibrils.[28] The stabilization of α-synuclein protofibrils by the dopamine–α-synuclein adducts might explain the specific neurodegeneration of nigral neurons in PD. Provoking further suspicion that dopamine may be an accomplice in PD pathogenesis is the observation that accumulation of α-synuclein is toxic to cultured dopaminergic neurons, but not to nondopaminergic neurons.[29] However, dopamine–α-synuclein adducts did not account for the selective degeneration of dopamine neurons; instead they showed that α-synuclein and 14-3-3 coexist in a 36–83-kDa protein complex and that the levels of this complex are selectively increased in the substantia nigra, but not in the cerebellum or cortex. The 14-3-3 family of protein chaperones fulfill diverse roles in the cell, including the sequestration and inhibition of proapoptotic proteins.[30] Complex formation between α-synuclein and 14-3-3 is likely to decrease the free pool of cellular 14-3-3 to counteract apoptosis and to result in increased cellular susceptibility to stress.[31] The involvement of dopamine in α-synuclein–mediated toxicity is a very appealing explanation on the selectivity of dopaminergic cell death in PD. It also highlights potential mechanistic differences in α-synuclein–mediated cell death among different subsets of the neuronal populations in synucleinopathies.

PARKIN

Mutations in the parkin gene cause autosomal-recessive juvenile parkinsonism (ARJP). Pathologically, ARJP is characterized by a severe loss of nigral dopaminergic neurons and the absence of classic Lewy bodies. Affected individuals also tend to have an earlier mean age of onset (typically before 40 years of age). Following the discovery of parkin mutations in Japanese ARJP patients, several families with recessively inherited PD throughout the world were also found to carry parkin mutations. These findings are in stark contrast to the restricted occurrence of α-synuclein mutations. Indeed, mutations in parkin have become the main contributor not only to autosomal-recessive PD, but also to familial PD. It is thus important to understand how parkin acts as a felon in PD.

Parkin is a 465–amino acid ubiquitin protein ligase with a molecular mass of 52 kDa. The parkin protein has a modular structure consisting of an ubiquitin-like (UBL) domain at its N terminus, a RING (*really interesting new gene*) box domain at its C terminus, and a unique middle segment that links the two domains. The RING box contains two RING finger motifs (termed RING 1 and RING 2) flanking a Cys-rich in-between RING (IBR). The RING box is important for the recruitment of E2s and represents the catalytic moiety of parkin.[5–7] Not surprisingly, the majority of familial point mutations in parkin reside in this region. The function of the UBL is currently unknown, although this domain shares 32% identity and 62% similarity with ubiquitin. Interestingly, the highly conserved lysine-48 (K-48) on the ubiquitin molecule is also conserved among UBL domains from different parkin orthologues (Lim *et al.*, unpublished observations). During the synthesis of polyubiquitin chains, individual ubiquitin molecules are usually linked to one another through K-48–G76 isopeptide bonds.[4] We have shown that parkin promotes its own degradation through self-ubiquitination.[7] Potentially, K-48 on the UBL domain of parkin could represent a putative site on which the polyubiquitin chain is formed and, as such, may be important in the regulation of cellular parkin levels.

We and others have shown that familial associated mutations in parkin impair its catalytic function. These mutations disrupt parkin binding either to its cognate E2s or to its substrates. As a result, parkin-targeted substrates could not be ubiquitinated.[5–7] Our findings suggest that a loss of parkin function would lead to the toxic accumulation of its substrates, eventually killing the cell. However, it is not clear why dopaminergic neurons are preferentially susceptible. Undoubtedly, the identification of the spectrum of parkin substrates, together with the characterization of the biochemical pathways involved, will shed some light on the selective death of dopaminergic neurons in PD. To date, six parkin substrate have been described: (1) CDCrel-1;[7] (2) CDCrel2A (Choi *et al.*, submitted); (3) an O-glycosylated form of α-synuclein;[32] (4) synphilin-1;[33] (5) tau (Petrucelli *et al.*, submitted); and (6) Pael-R (*P*arkin-*a*ssociated *e*ndothelin receptor-*l*ike *r*eceptor).[34]

The synaptic vesicle–associated protein, CDCrel-1, was the first parkin substrate identified.[7] Parkin interacts with and promotes the ubiquitination and degradation of CDCrel-1. Conversely, the familial parkin mutants Q311stop and T415N fail to affect CDCrel-1 turnover. Relatively little is known about CDCrel-1 function, but recent work from Trimble's group has suggested that it regulates synaptic vesicle release in the nervous system.[35] More recently, the same group generated CDCrel-1– null mice and showed that CDCrel-1 is not essential for neuronal development or function.[36] This observation is reminiscent of the mild neurological phenotype in α-synuclein knockout mice. Perhaps neuronal dysregulation results from CDCrel-1 accumulation rather than from its absence. Potentially, the elevation of CDCrel-1 in the absence of parkin-mediated degradation could disrupt dopamine release and eventually lead to PD. Although this possibility remains to be evaluated, CDCrel 1 and a close homologue, CDCrel 2A, were recently found to accumulate in the brain of patients with ARJP (Choi *et al.*, submitted). CDCrel 2A is a newly described parkin-binding protein that was identified using a yeast–two-hydrid screen (Choi *et al.*, submitted). Structurally, CDCrel 2A and CDCrel 1 share extensive homology except for their N terminal regions. Parkin interacts with and regulates the degradation of CDCrel 2A. Parkin also colocalizes with CDCrel 2A in neuronal cell bodies and synapses (Choi *et al.*, submitted). The association of both CDCrel members with parkin suggests an important functional relationship between parkin and the septins.

Since mutations in α-synuclein are associated with PD, it is tempting to link derangements in parkin and α-synuclein in a common pathogenic pathway. Naturally, this presynaptic protein became a much sought-after candidate substrate of parkin. However, in our coimmunoprecipitation studies we found that parkin neither interacts with nor ubiquitinates α-synuclein.[33] It turned out that α-synuclein needs to undergo a complex modification before it becomes a substrate of parkin. Shimura and colleagues described an O-glycosylated form of α-synuclein (αSP22) that could interact with and be ubiquitinated by parkin. They further showed that the level of αSP22 is elevated in ARJP brains and proposed that ubiquitination of αSP22 may be a prerequisite in the formation of Lewy bodies, which are generally absent in ARJP patients.[32] Parkin interaction with the glycosylated form of α-synuclein is highly selective, as the major nonglycosylated form of α-synuclein is totally inert to parkin.[32] This result is consistent with our inability to demonstrate an interaction between parkin and the normal form of α-synuclein. Curiously, most laboratories have not been able to detect the glycosylated form of α-synuclein. Indeed, this type of complex glycosylation is more commonly found in extracellular proteins and is highly unusual for a cytoplasmic protein. Additionally, αSP22 to date has not been described in the several transgenic mouse models overexpressing α-synuclein. The relevance of αSP22 in the pathogenesis of PD thus awaits further characterization.

Synphilin-1, an interactor with α-synuclein, is a synaptic vesicle–enriched protein that has previously been shown to form Lewy body-like inclusions when coexpressed with α-synuclein.[37] Synphilin-1 is found in Lewy bodies, and abnormal accumulation of synphilin-1 is specific for brain lesions in which α-synuclein is a major component.[38] We recently identified synphilin-1 as a direct target for parkin-mediated ubiquitination and further showed that parkin ubiquitinates proteins within cytosolic inclusions formed by coexpression of synphilin-1 and α-synuclein.[33] Our results suggest a molecular link between the formation of Lewy bodies, the UPS, parkin, and synphilin-1 and support the speculation that functional parkin is required for Lewy body formation. Our results also linked the major nonglycosylated form of α-synuclein and parkin in a common biochemical pathway through their interactions with synphilin-1. Although the function of synphilin-1 is currently unknown, its ability to generate inclusions in the presence of α-synuclein indicates that it may play a role in Lewy body formation. We recently observed that parkin could mediate both K-48– and K-63–linked polyubiquitination of synphilin-1.[39] Unlike K-48– linked polyubiquitination, K-63–linked polyubiquitination of proteins is not associated with proteasomal degradation.[4] Indeed, while K-48–linked ubiquitination of synphilin-1 leads to a reduction in its steady state levels, the K-63–linked ubiquitination of synphilin-1 did not affect its turnover rate. It is therefore conceivable that aberrant K-63–linked ubiquitination of synphilin-1 could lead to the intracytoplasmic accumulation of protein. Interestingly, parkin-mediated ubiquitination of proteins present in cytoplasmic inclusions formed by coexpression of α-synuclein and synphilin-1 occurs via K-63 but not K-48 linkage.[39] Our results suggest that K-63– linked ubiquitination of synphilin-1 by parkin may be involved in Lewy body pathology associated with idiopathic PD.

The microtubule-associated protein tau is another protein present in Lewy bodies that is a parkin substrate (Petrucelli *et al.*, submitted). While tauopathies and synucleinopathies are quite distinct phenomena, several recent genetic studies implicate tau in PD.[40,41] Furthermore, tau pathology was found in a case of autosomal-recessive early-onset PD caused by parkin mutations.[42] Petrucelli *et al.* demonstrated physical and functional interactions between tau and parkin and, further, showed that tau accumulates in the brain of ARJP patients (Petrucelli *et al.*, submitted). These findings indicate that tau pathology may contribute to the demise of nigral neurons in PD caused by parkin mutations.

A more general role for parkin in the ubiquitin degradation pathway is suggested by the observation that parkin is upregulated in response to cellular unfolded protein stress.[6] Elevation of parkin relieves unfolded protein-mediated toxicity through ubiquitinating and targeting improperly folded protein to the proteasome for clearance. For this purpose, parkin recruits a different set of E2s, UBC6 and UBC7. Both UBC6 and UBC7 are resident to the endoplasmic recticulum (ER). Indeed, recent evidence showed that parkin ubiquitinates the putative G protein–coupled transmembrane receptor Pael-R when it becomes unfolded.[34] When overexpressed in cells, Pael-R has a propensity to become unfolded and insoluble. The accumulation of unfolded Pael-R can be toxic to cells. Parkin protects against unfolded Pael-R–mediated cytotoxicity by facilitating unfolded Pael-R removal in the proteasome through ubiquitination.[34] Consistent with this notion is the observation that there is an elevation of insoluble Pael-R in the brain of ARJP patients lacking functional parkin.

While more substrates of parkin undoubtedly will be identified with time, the current spectrum of parkin substrates is already indicative of the involvement of parkin in both familial and sporadic PD (FIG. 1). Under normal circumstances, parkin acts as an E3 ligase that will control the fate of the target proteins it ubiquitinates. Parkin-mediated K-48–linked ubiquitination will target its substrates for proteasomal clearance, while parkin-mediated K-63–linked ubiquitination is likely to modulate its tar-

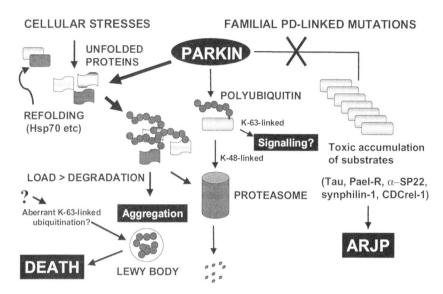

FIGURE 1. Depiction of the cast of molecular characters, felons, conspirators and suspects in PD.

get substrate's function—for example, in cell signaling. In ARJP patients lacking functional parkin, parkin substrates destined for degradation accumulate instead. The accumulation of these parkin substrates, such as αSP22, tau, and Pael-R, would be toxic to cells. It is likely that these cells fail to sequester the accumulated toxic proteins as inclusion bodies due to a loss in parkin-mediated ubiquitination.[43,44] However, Farrer and colleagues recently described the presence of Lewy bodies and Lewy neurites in an ARJP patient with compound heterozygous parkin mutations.[45] This patient contains a null mutation in one parkin allele and a R275W substitution in the other. We have shown that the R275W mutation in parkin substantially reduces, but does not abolish, its catalytic competency.[33] Hence, the Lewy bodies and neuritic inclusions described by Farrer and colleagues could be related to the activity of parkin. This would be consistent with the speculation that functional parkin is required for Lewy body formation and the finding that ARJP patients with homologous null mutations in parkin lack Lewy body pathology. It is not known at this moment whether failure of parkin-mediated K-63–linked ubiquitination of proteins would contribute to ARJP. However, this mode of ubiquitination could potentially be linked to Lewy body formation in sporadic PD. The etiology of sporadic PD is likely complex, with environmental factors possibly playing an integral part, through the potential modulation of susceptibility genes for PD. Environmental insults that cause oxidative damage and other cellular stresses would, among other effects, increase the number of misfolded or unfolded proteins. The latter would trigger the unfolded protein response (UPR) that would initially involve the upregulation of chaperone proteins such as members of the Hsp70 family. These chaperones would be instrumental in alleviating stresses due to unfolded proteins through the refolding of these proteins. Indeed, overexpression of Hsp70 rescues the motoric and neuropathologic features of transgenic flies expressing normal and mutant forms of α-synuclein.[46] In the presence of continuous or more intense insults, the unfolded protein load is likely to overwhelm chaperones. The UPS, whose response would include the elevation of parkin expression to aid ER-associated degradation, would then fulfill the second line of cellular defence against unfolded proteins. The recruitment of an alternative set of E2s resident in the ER by parkin may be dedicated to degradation-linked ubiquitination of proteins. Another collaborator of parkin function is a protein called CHIP. Recent evidence from Takahashi's group showed that CHIP is a mammalian E4-like molecule that positively regulates parkin activity.[47] CHIP and Hsp70 are both binding partners of parkin, and all three proteins exist as a complex with Pael-R. However, the amount of CHIP in the complex increases during ER stress. Apparently, CHIP facilitates parkin-mediated ubiquitination of Pael-R by promoting the dissociation of Hsp70 from parkin and Pael-R. Interestingly, the association of Hsp70 with Pael-R inhibits the E3 ligase activity of parkin.[47] This observation supports our model that Hsp70 chaperone activity represents the first line of defence against unfolded proteins. When Hsp70 activity becomes insufficient to cope with the unfolded protein stress, E3 ligases such as parkin would take over. We envisaged that if unfolded proteins accumulate beyond a certain threshold, leading to proteasomal impairment, the cell would sequester the ubiquitinated unfolded proteins in the form of Lewy body inclusions in an attempt to prolong its survival. Our model thus supports the general hypothesis that functional parkin is required for Lewy body formation and the notion that the formation of Lewy body-like inclusions is a cellular mechanism to sequester toxic products that would otherwise be an immediate threat to the cell. Although Lewy bodies may be beneficial initially, they are space-filling entities that would ultimately disrupt cellular function, leading to cell death. Additionally, the sequestration of parkin in such inclusions would also deplete the cell of functional parkin and further contribute to neuronal death. In this light, the operating level of parkin in the cell is therefore crucial. Supporting this view is the increasing evidence that parkin haploinsufficiency may be sufficient for disease in some cases.[48] As ubiquitination and proteasomal degradation are both ATP-dependent processes, it is conceivable that events depleting the cell of its ATP could tax the UPS function. Blockage of UPS activity would, in turn, lead to increased oxidative stress. Thus, mitochondrion dysfunction and reduction of complex 1 activity in sporadic PD may be intimately linked with UPS derangements.

UCHL1 AND OTHER SUSPECTS

UCHL1 is a member of a gene family whose products hydrolyze small C terminal adducts of ubiquitin to generate the ubiquitin monomer. Expression of UCHL1 is highly specific to neurons and to cells of neuroendocrine lineage. An I93M missense mutation in the UCHL1 gene has been linked to PD in a sibling pair from a small German pedigree.[49] The I93M mutation causes a partial loss of its ubiquitin hydrolase activity *in vitro*.[49] Since hydrolysis of ubiquitin adducts is important in the proper functioning of the UPS, impairment of UCHL1 activity could lead to aberrations in the proteolytic pathway and aggregation of proteins, including the UCHL1 protein itself. Indeed, UCHL1 is present in Lewy bodies. The occurrence of UCHL1 in Lewy bodies and its function in the proteasome pathway thus make it a persuasive candidate gene in PD. However, subsequent sequence analyses of UCHL1 performed by others in several dominantly inherited PD cases have failed to detect the I93M substitution.[50,51] Currently, the general view of this mutation is that it represents either a rare cause of PD or a benign substitution occurring in a single family. We speculate that an alternative way in which UCHL1 could potentially act as a felon in PD is when its activity becomes overpromoted. Rapid and aberrant deubiquitination of polyubiquitinated proteins could stabilize proteins intended for degradation and contribute to their accumulation. A novel p53-interacting protein, herpesvirus-associated ubiquitin-specific protease (HAUSP), has recently been shown to stabilize the levels of p53 by direct deubiquitination.[52] HAUSP has intrinsic enzymatic activity that specifically deubiquitinates p53, leading to increased p53 levels both *in vitro* and *in vivo*. In contrast, expression of a catalytically inactive point mutant of HAUSP in cells increases the level of p53 ubiquitination and destabilizes p53. It is not known at this moment whether genetic mutations or environmental factors could modulate UCHL1 activity or expression level. But aberrant UCHL1 deubiquitination could be a mechanism contributing to protein aggregation.

There are many other suspects abetting PD pathogenesis, including (1) cytochrome P450 enzymes, which are involved in the detoxification of xenobiotics; (2) N-acetyltransferase 2, whose activity governs the rate of aromatic amine detoxification; and (3) apolipoprotein E (APOE), an extracellular ligand for receptors that clears remnants of chylomicrons and very-low-density lipoproteins.[53] Due to the lack of strong evidence for roles in PD, interest in these suspects has dissipated. Some newer suspects whose dysfunction may contribute to PD include transcription factors such as Nurr 1, Ptx-3, and Lmx1b, which regulate dopaminergic cell neurogenesis, and the protein kinase PKCγ. Comprehensive reviews of these newer PD candidates have appeared elsewhere.[3,54]

CONCLUSIONS

It is tempting to try to unify the multiple genes and sporadic causes of PD into one pathogenic biochemical pathway. The identification and characterization of the three PD gene products, α-synuclein, parkin, and UCHL1, has certainly helped us to conceive a general molecular pathway leading to PD. While we await the identity of the genes in other PD loci to be elucidated, the evolving picture of PD pathogenesis is one that converges onto cellular protein mishandling linked to UPS dysfunction. The firm establishment of UPS derangements as a major pathogenic biochemical pathway for PD would be instrumental in the design of rational therapeutic targets for PD patients. Potential druggable targets for PD could then include components of the protein handling squad, such as the chaperones, cochaperones, E3 ligases, and collaborators of E3 ligases. Other cellular components that help police the dopaminergic activities would also be potential targets for PD therapy. For example, β-synuclein has recently been suggested to be a natural negative regulator of α-synuclein aggregation.[55] Thus, the antiamyloidogenic property of β-synuclein might also provide a novel strategy for the treatment of neurodegenerative disorders such as PD. Undoubtedly, with better understanding of the molecular mechanisms underlying PD, new and useful therapeutic targets will emerge. As we move into the postgenomic era, we certainly hope to move towards novel and effective treatment strategies for PD that go beyond L-DOPA.

ACKNOWLEDGMENTS

This work was supported by USPHS Grant NS38377 and the Edward D. and Anna Mitchell Family Foundation. K. L. Lim is a recipient of the National Science Scholarship International Fellowship awarded by A*STAR (Singapore).

REFERENCES

1. LANG, A.E. & A.M. LOZANO. 1998. Parkinson's disease. First of two parts. N. Engl. J. Med. **339:** 1044–1053.
2. LANG, A.E. & A.M. LOZANO. 1998. Parkinson's disease. Second of two parts. N. Engl. J. Med. **339:** 1130–1143.
3. LIM, K.L., V.L. DAWSON & T.M. DAWSON. 2002. The genetics of Parkinson's disease. Curr. Neurol. Neurosci. Rep. **2:** 439–446.
4. PICKART, C.M. 2001. Mechanisms underlying ubiquitination. Annu. Rev. Biochem. **70:** 503–533.
5. SHIMURA, H., N. HATTORI, S. KUBO, et al. 2000. Familial Parkinson disease gene product, parkin, is a ubiquitin-protein ligase. Nat. Genet. **25:** 302–305.
6. IMAI, Y., M. SODA & R. TAKAHASHI. 2000. Parkin suppresses unfolded protein stress-induced cell death through its E3 ubiquitin-protein ligase activity. J. Biol. Chem. **275:** 35661–35664.
7. ZHANG, Y., J. GAO, K.K. CHUNG, et al. 2000. Parkin functions as an E2-dependent ubiquitin- protein ligase and promotes the degradation of the synaptic vesicle-associated protein, CDCrel-1. Proc. Natl. Acad. Sci. USA **97:** 13354–13359.
8. KRUGER, R., O. EBERHARDT, O. RIESS, et al. 2002. Parkinson's disease: one biochemical pathway to fit all genes? Trends Mol. Med. **8:** 236–240.
9. POLYMEROPOULOS, M.H., C. LAVEDAN, E. LEROY, et al. 1997. Mutation in the alpha-synuclein gene identified in families with Parkinson's disease. Science **276:** 2045–2047.
10. KRUGER, R., W. KUHN, T. MULLER, et al. 1998. Ala30Pro mutation in the gene encoding alpha-synuclein in Parkinson's disease. Nat. Genet. **18:** 106–108.
11. SPILLANTINI, M.G., M.L. SCHMIDT, V.M. LEE, et al. 1997. Alpha-synuclein in Lewy bodies. Nature **388:** 839–840.
12. GOEDERT, M. 2001. Alpha-synuclein and neurodegenerative diseases. Nat. Rev. Neurosci. **2:** 492–501.
13. ABELIOVICH, A., Y. SCHMITZ, I. FARINAS, et al. 2000. Mice lacking alpha-synuclein display functional deficits in the nigrostriatal dopamine system. Neuron **25:** 239–252
14. DAWSON, T., A. MANDIR & M. LEE. 2002. Animal models of PD: pieces of the same puzzle? Neuron **35:** 219–222.
15. SPIRA, P.J., D.M. SHARPE, G. HALLIDAY, et al. 2001. Clinical and pathological features of a Parkinsonian syndrome in a family with an Ala53Thr alpha-synuclein mutation. Ann. Neurol. **49:** 313–319.
16. LO BIANCO, C., J.L. RIDET, B.L. SCHNEIDER, et al. 2002. alpha-Synucleinopathy and selective dopaminergic neuron loss in a rat lentiviral-based model of Parkinson's disease. Proc. Natl. Acad. Sci. USA **99:** 10813–10818.
17. KIRIK, D., C. ROSENBLAD, C. BURGER, et al. 2002. Parkinson-like neurodegeneration induced by targeted overexpression of alpha-synuclein in the nigrostriatal system. J. Neurosci. **22:** 2780–2791.
18. GIASSON, B.I., K. URYU, J.Q. TROJANOWSKI, et al. 1999. Mutant and wild type human alpha-synucleins assemble into elongated filaments with distinct morphologies in vitro. J. Biol. Chem. **274:** 7619–7622.

19. GIASSON, B.I., J.E. DUDA, S.M. QUINN, *et al.* 2002. Neuronal alpha-synucleinopathy with severe movement disorder in mice expressing A53T human alpha-synuclein. Neuron **34**: 521–533.

20. LEE, M.K., W. STIRLING, Y. XU, *et al.* 2002. Human alpha-synuclein-harboring familial Parkinson's disease-linked Ala-53 → Thr mutation causes neurodegenerative disease with alpha-synuclein aggregation in transgenic mice. Proc. Natl. Acad. Sci. USA **99**: 8968–8973.

21. PAXINOU, E., Q. CHEN, M. WEISSE, *et al.* 2001. Induction of alpha-synuclein aggregation by intracellular nitrative insult. J. Neurosci. **21**: 8053–8061.

22. SHERER, T.B., R. BETARBET, A.K. STOUT, *et al.* 2002. An in vitro model of Parkinson's disease: linking mitochondrial impairment to altered alpha-synuclein metabolism and oxidative damage. J. Neurosci. **22**: 7006–7015.

23. LEE, H.J., S.Y. SHIN, C. CHOI, *et al.* 2002. Formation and removal of alpha-synuclein aggregates in cells exposed to mitochondrial inhibitors. J. Biol. Chem. **277**: 5411–5417.

24. OKOCHI, M., WALTER, J., KOYAMA, A., *et al.* 2000. Constitutive phosphorylation of the Parkinson's disease associated alpha-synuclein. J. Biol. Chem. **275**: 390–397.

25. FUJIWARA, H., M. HASEGAWA, N. DOHMAE, *et al.* 2002. alpha-Synuclein is phosphorylated in synucleinopathy lesions. Nat. Cell Biol. **4**: 160–164.

26. GOLDBERG, M.S. & P.T. LANSBURY, JR. 2000. Is there a cause-and-effect relationship between alpha-synuclein fibrillization and Parkinson's disease? Nat. Cell Biol. **2**: E115–119.

27. CONWAY, K.A., S.J. LEE, J.C. ROCHET, *et al.* 2000. Acceleration of oligomerization, not fibrillization, is a shared property of both alpha-synuclein mutations linked to early-onset Parkinson's disease: implications for pathogenesis and therapy. Proc. Natl. Acad. Sci. USA **97**: 571–576.

28. CONWAY, K.A., J.C. ROCHET, R.M. BIEGANSKI, *et al.* 2001. Kinetic stabilization of the alpha-synuclein protofibril by a dopamine-alpha-synuclein adduct. Science **294**: 1346–1349.

29. XU, J., S.Y. KAO, F.J. LEE, *et al.* 2002. Dopamine-dependent neurotoxicity of alpha-synuclein: a mechanism for selective neurodegeneration in Parkinson disease. Nat. Med. **8**: 600–606.

30. VAN HEMERT, M.J., H.Y. STEENSMA & G.P. VAN HEUSDEN. 2001. 14-3-3 proteins: key regulators of cell division, signalling, and apoptosis. Bioessays **23**: 936–946.

31. WELCH, K. & J. YUAN. 2002. Releasing the nerve cell killers. Nat. Med. **8**: 564–565.

32. SHIMURA, H., M.G. SCHLOSSMACHER, N. HATTORI, *et al.* 2001. Ubiquitination of a new form of alpha-synuclein by parkin from human brain: implications for Parkinson's disease. Science **293**: 263–269.

33. CHUNG, K.K., Y. ZHANG, K.L. LIM, *et al.* 2001. Parkin ubiquitinates the alpha-synuclein-interacting protein, synphilin-1: implications for Lewy-body formation in Parkinson disease. Nat. Med. **7**: 1144–1150.

34. IMAI, Y., M. SODA, H. INOUE, *et al.* 2001. An unfolded putative transmembrane polypeptide, which can lead to endoplasmic reticulum stress, is a substrate of Parkin. Cell **105**: 891–902.

35. BEITES, C.L., H. XIE, R. BOWSER, *et al.* 1999. The septin CDCrel-1 binds syntaxin and inhibits exocytosis. Nat. Neurosci. **2**: 434–439.

36. PENG, X.R., Z. JIA, Y. ZHANG, *et al.* 2002. The septin CDCrel-1 is dispensable for normal development and neurotransmitter release. Mol. Cell Biol. **22**: 378–387.

37. ENGELENDER, S., Z. KAMINSKY, X. GUO, *et al.* 1999. Synphilin-1 associates with alpha-synuclein and promotes the formation of cytosolic inclusions. Nat. Genet. **22**: 110–114.

38. WAKABAYASHI, K., S. ENGELENDER, M. YOSHIMOTO, *et al.* 2000. Synphilin-1 is present in Lewy bodies in Parkinson's disease. Ann. Neurol. **47**: 521–523.

39. LIM, K.L., Y. TANAKA & Y. ZHANG. 2002. Parkin mediates lysine-63 (K-63)-linked ubiquitination of synphilin-1: Implications for Lewy Body formation. Soc. Neurosci. Abst.

40. SCOTT, W.K., M.A. NANCE, R.L. WATTS, *et al.* 2001. Complete genomic screen in Parkinson disease: evidence for multiple genes. JAMA **286**: 2239–2244.

41. MARTIN, E.R., W.K. SCOTT, M.A. NANCE, *et al.* 2001. Association of single-nucleotide polymorphisms of the tau gene with late-onset Parkinson disease. JAMA **286:** 2245–2250.
42. VAN DE WARRENBURG, B.P., M. LAMMENS, C.B. LUCKING, *et al.* 2001. Clinical and pathologic abnormalities in a family with parkinsonism and parkin gene mutations. Neurology **56:** 555–557.
43. DAWSON, T.M. 2000. New animal models for Parkinson's disease. Cell **101:** 115–118.
44. CHUNG, K.K., V.L. DAWSON & T.M. DAWSON. 2001. The role of the ubiquitin-proteasomal pathway in Parkinson's disease and other neurodegenerative disorders. Trends Neurosci. **24:** S7–14.
45. FARRER, M., P. CHAN, R. CHEN, *et al.* 2001. Lewy bodies and parkinsonism in families with parkin mutations. Ann. Neurol. **50:** 293–300.
46. AULUCK, P.K., H.Y. CHAN, J.Q. TROJANOWSKI, *et al.* 2002. Chaperone suppression of alpha-synuclein toxicity in a Drosophila model for Parkinson's disease. Science **295:** 865–868.
47. IMAI, Y., M. SODA, S. HATAKEYAMA, *et al.* 2002. CHIP is associated with Parkin, a gene responsible for familial Parkinson's disease, and enhances its ubiquitin ligase activity. Mol. Cell **10:** 55–67.
48. WEST, A.M. 2002. Complex relationship between Parkin mutations and Parkinson disease. Am. J. Med. Genet. **114:** 584–591.
49. LEROY, E., R. BOYER, G. AUBURGER, *et al.* 1998. The ubiquitin pathway in Parkinson's disease. Nature **395:** 451–452.
50. LINCOLN, S., J. VAUGHAN, N. WOOD, *et al.* 1999. Low frequency of pathogenic mutations in the ubiquitin carboxy-terminal hydrolase gene in familial Parkinson's disease. Neuroreport **10:** 427–429.
51. MARAGANORE, D.M., M.J. FARRER, J.A. HARDY, *et al.* 1999. Case-control study of the ubiquitin carboxy-terminal hydrolase L1 gene in Parkinson's disease. Neurology **53:** 1858–1860.
52. LI, M., D. CHEN, A. SHILOH, *et al.* 2002. Deubiquitination of p53 by HAUSP is an important pathway for p53 stabilization. Nature **416:** 648–653.
53. VAUGHAN, J.R., M.B. DAVIS & N.W. WOOD. 2001. Genetics of Parkinsonism: a review. Ann. Hum. Genet. **65:** 111–126.
54. RAMSDEN, D.B., R.B. PARSONS, S.L. HO, *et al.* 2001. The aetiology of idiopathic Parkinson's disease. Mol. Pathol. **54:** 369–380.
55. HASHIMOTO, M., E. ROCKENSTEIN & M. MANTE. 2001. beta-Synuclein inhibits alpha-synuclein aggregation: a possible role as an anti-parkinsonian factor. Neuron **32:** 213–223
56. MASLIAH, E., E. ROCKENSTEIN, I. VEINBERGS, *et al.* 2000. Dopaminergic loss and inclusion body formation in alpha-synuclein mice: implications for neurodegenerative disorders. Science **287:** 1265–1269.
57. MATSUOKA, Y., M. VILA, S. LINCOLN, *et al.* 2001. Lack of nigral pathology in transgenic mice expressing human alpha-synuclein driven by the tyrosine hydroxylase promoter. Neurobiol. Dis. **8:** 535–539.
58. RICHFIELD, E.K., M.J. THIRUCHELVAM, D.A. CORY-SLECHTA, *et al.* 2002. Behavioral and neurochemical effects of wild-type and mutated human alpha-synuclein in transgenic mice. Exp. Neurol. **175:** 35–48.
59. VAN DER PUTTEN, H., K.H. WIEDERHOLD, A. PROBST, *et al.* 2000. Neuropathology in mice expressing human alpha-synuclein. J. Neurosci. **20:** 6021–6029.

Oxidative Modifications of α-Synuclein

HARRY ISCHIROPOULOS

Stokes Research Institute, Department of Biochemistry and Biophysics,
Children's Hospital of Philadelphia and the University of Pennsylvania,
Philadelphia, Pennsylvania 19104, USA

ABSTRACT: Hallmark lesions of neurodegenerative synucleinopathies contain α-synuclein (α-syn) that is modified by nitration of tyrosine residues and possibly by dityrosine cross-linking to generated stable oligomers. Data gathered from *in vitro* experiments and from model systems of cells transfected with wild-type and mutant α-syn revealed that conditions resulting in α-syn nitration also induce formation of α-syn inclusions with similar biochemical characteristics to protein extracted from human lesions. The detection of tyrosine-nitrated α-syn signifies the formation of reactive nitrogen species capable of both radical and electrophilic attack on aromatic residues as well as nucleophilic additions and oxidations. The cellular sources and biochemical reactivity of reactive nitrogen species in the central nervous system remain largely unknown, but kinetically fast reactions of nitric oxide with superoxide to form peroxynitrite as well as enzymatic one-electron oxidation of nitrite are two important sources of reactive nitrogen species. Based on these findings a model is proposed where the process of fibrilization can be differentially affected by oxidants and nitrating species. Posttranslational modifications of α-syn by reactive nitrogen species inhibits fibril formation and results in urea- and SDS-insoluble, protease-resistant α-syn aggregates that maybe responsible for cellular toxicity.

KEYWORDS: oxidative stress; tyrosine nitration; dityrosine; α-synuclein; protein aggregation

OXIDATIVE AND NITRATIVE STRESSES IN NEURODEGENERATIVE DISORDERS

Partial reduction of oxygen by one electron produces superoxide, whereas two-electron reduction produces hydrogen peroxide. Enzymatic and other scavenging pathways rapidly remove superoxide and hydrogen peroxide to avoid formation of secondary strong oxidants. Under pathological conditions the overproduction of oxidants may overwhelm the cellular antioxidant capacity, resulting in undesired oxidation of cellular molecules and ultimately cell death. Augmentation of intracellular defenses in humans as well as in model systems of neurodegenerative disorders has

Address for correspondence: Harry Ischiropoulos, Ph.D., Stokes Research Institute, Children's Hospital of Philadelphia, 416D Abramson Research Center, 34th St. and Civic Center Blvd., Philadelphia, PA 19104-4318. Voice: 215-590-5320; fax: 215-590-4267.
ischirop@mail.med.upenn.edu

Ann. N.Y. Acad. Sci. 991: 93–100 (2003). © 2003 New York Academy of Sciences.

provided support for the generally held hypothesis that oxidative stress is a critical component in the pathogenesis of neurodegeneration.[1-3] A major obstacle in determining the oxidative burden in human subjects and in animal models is the inability to measure reactive species directly. Due to their highly reactive and evanescent biochemical and biophysical nature, reactive species cannot be quantified directly; and evidence for their existence in disease comes from the detection of relatively stable products derived by the oxidation of cellular macromolecules. During aging or under low but continuous production of oxidants during pathological states the frequency of oxidation of biological targets increases; and possibly as repair processes slow, detection of oxidized proteins, lipids, and even DNA becomes apparent.[4]

The production of reactive oxygen species during oxidative stress could also alter the biological targets affected by nitric oxide, a versatile signaling molecule in the central nervous system (CNS) and vascular compartments.[5] Nitric oxide has been implicated in both neuroprotective and neurodestructive mechanisms and in the presence of reactive oxygen intermediates forms reactive nitrogen species capable of modifying tyrosine residues in proteins to 3-nitrotyrosine.[6] Support for the role of nitric oxide in neuronal injury, in the presence or absence of oxidative stress, comes from animals models utilizing inhibitors of nitric oxide synthesis as well as mice deficient either in the neuronal or the inducible form of nitric oxide synthase. These mice were found to be resistant to stroke and ischemia,[7,8] NMDA neurotoxicity,[9] 1-methyl-4-phenyl-1,2,3,6 tetrahydropyridine (MPTP) toxicity,[10,11] and various mitochondrial neurotoxins.[12,13] In all the model systems where nitric oxide appears to contribute to neurotoxicity, nitration of specific proteins has been detected by a variety of immunological and analytical approaches[12,14,15] only within the cells affected by the insult. Among human pathologies nitrated proteins have been detected in postmortem brain lesions associated with multiple sclerosis, amyotrophic lateral sclerosis, and Alzheimer's and Parkinson's diseases.[13,16-20] Therefore, nitration of proteins may serve as another index of stress (nitrative) associated with oxidative stress, since the nitrating agents are derived from the biochemical interaction of nitric oxide with reactive oxygen species.

ACCUMULATIONS OF ABNORMAL PROTEIN FILAMENTS ARE HALLMARKS OF SYNUCLEINOPATHIES AND OTHER NEURODEGENERATIVE DISORDERS

Accumulation of proteinacious fibrils are a common neuropathological feature of several different sporadic and hereditary neurodegenerative diseases.[21] Wild-type α–synuclein (α-syn) is a major component of Lewy bodies (LBs) in sporadic Parkinson's diseae, dementia with LBs, a subtype of Alzheimer's disease known as the LB variant of Alzheimer's disease, as well as of glial cytoplasmic inclusions in multiple system atrophy.[22-27] Wild-type α-syn as well as aggregated and truncated α-syn have been recovered from purified LBs, and α-syn solubility is reduced in affected regions of Lewy body disease and multiple system atrophy brains.[22] These findings and in vitro evidence[28-30] that wild-type as well as mutant α-syn aggregate and assemble into filaments suggest that alterations in α-syn may lead to the formation of filamentous α-syn inclusions in vivo.

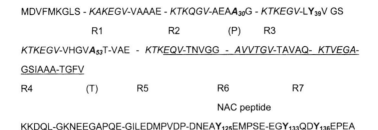

MDVFMKGLS - *KAKEGV*-VAAAE - *KTKQGV*-AEA**A**$_{30}$G - *KTKEGV*-L**Y**$_{39}$V GS

R1   R2   (P)   R3

KTKEGV-VHGV**A**$_{53}$T-VAE - *KTKEQV*-TNVGG - *AVVTGV*-TAVAQ- *KTVEGA*-

GSIAAA-TGFV

R4   (T)   R5   R6   R7

NAC peptide

KKDQL-GKNEEGAPQE-GILEDMPVDP-DNEA**Y**$_{125}$EMPSE-EG**Y**$_{133}$QD**Y**$_{136}$EPEA

FIGURE 1. Amino acid sequence of α-synuclein. A unique feature of the peptide sequence is the presence of 6 or possibly 7 imperfect 11-residue repeats of *KTKEGV* (R) in the conserved core in the N terminal (residues 10–86). The repeating domains consist of residues with a high tendency for helical conformation (A, L, K, and E). The first five repeats are hydrophilic and are predicted to form amphipathic α-helices that would promote lipid association.[33] The last two repeats are part of the hydrophobic core of the protein, residues 61–95. This peptide sequence (*underlined*) has been identified as the non-Aβ component of amyloid (NAC peptide).[46] The minimal peptide required for fibril formation is residues 71–82.[29] Mutations responsible for familial forms of PD are A30P and A53T.[47,48] In human brain inclusions α-syn is modified by tyrosine nitration in all four residues, and all four residue are capable of cross-linking via dityrosine formation.

α-SUNUCLEIN: RANDOM STRUCTURE AND NO APPARENT FUNCTION

α-Synuclein is a soluble protein consisting of 140 amino acids (sequence in Fig. 1) with a predicated molecular mass of 14,460.16 and an isoelectric point of 4.67. Spectroscopic techniques revealed that the wild-type α-syn contains as little as 3% α-helices and 23% β-sheets, whereas the rest of the protein assumes a random conformation. The function of α-syn remains uncertain, although the preferential localization to presynaptic nerve terminals and its interaction with lipids and proteins suggest some regulatory function associated with dopamine production and lipid vesicle trafficking.[31,32] Of interest are the numerous interactions of α-syn with proteins, suggesting that the abundance of this relatively unstructured protein may be important in allowing stochiometric protein–protein interactions that may regulate the function of the interactive proteins.[33–38] A focus of our investigations has been the C terminus, which is rich in negatively charged residues and three tyrosine residues. Sequence alignment of a ([either E or D]-X-X-[ED]-X-X-[ED]) motif revealed possible similarities with proteins such as tubulin, neurofilament, and the mitochondrial chaperonin CNP60 protein; and published data indicated that α-syn, but not β-synuclein—another member of the synclein family, can associate with proteins in a manner consistent with a chaperone-like activity.[39] The chaperone-like function of α-syn requires stochiometric amounts of protein, suggesting that this putative function would require sufficiently high concentrations of α-syn. Interactions with synphilin-1,[40] parkin,[41] tyrosine hydroxylase,[38] dopamine transporter,[32] phospholipase D,[35] and β-synuclein[34] may be critical in understanding both the physiological and pathological function of this protein. In addition posttranslation modification such

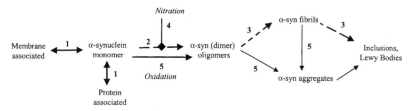

FIGURE 2. Working model for the role of oxidative/nitrative modifications on α-synuclein aggregation. The relative slow turnover rate of α-syn allows the protein to establish reversible associations with lipid membranes and proteins. **(1)** Monomeric α-synuclein exists in equilibrium with vesicle lipids as well as in association with proteins. **(2)** Although the *in vivo* conditions that induce α-syn to dimerize have not been identified, dimerization of monomeric synuclein leads to the formation of oligomers that initiate the cascade of fibril formation **(3)** that ultimately leads to formation of inclusions and Lewy bodies.[28,30] **(4)** The process of fibril formation can be disrupted by tyrosine nitration of α-syn or by oxidative formation of dopamine adduct(s) but not by oxidation of the protein.[44,49] However, oxidative cross-linking via dityrosine formation may initiate the cascade of fibril production.[44] **(5)** Moreover, oxidants and nitrating species can covalently cross-link either α-syn-oligomers or fibers forming urea- and SDS-insoluble, protease-resistant α-syn aggregates.[39,50] If the oxidants and nitrating agents encounter α-syn in fibril form, then the aggregated synuclein can be incorporated in the inclusions or Lewy bodies. It remains unknown if protofibril oligomers, fibrils, or insoluble aggregates (or even all three) cause cellular toxicity. Possibly toxicity is derived by multiple pathways: (a) loss of monomeric α-syn to fibrils may disturb the equilibrium and thus the association with lipids and proteins, resulting in disturbances of normal cellular functions; (b) the oligomers, fibrils, and covalently cross-linked post-translationally modified synuclein exhibit a cytotoxic gain of function; and finally (c) the cell becomes metabolically stressed by the energetic demand to repair oligomers, fibrils, and covalently cross-linked α-syn. This metabolic demand, coupled with the presence of oxidative/nitrative stresses in part derived from mitochondria or dopamine-mediated production of reactive intermediates,[32,50–53] results in cellular dysfunction. Alternatively the cell consumes considerable energy attempting to remove the modified synuclein, and as a result normal turnover of cellular proteins is impaired or ignored, resulting in inappropriate signaling and dysfunction.

as glycosylation[41] and serine phosphorylation[23,42,43] have been detected, and their potential role in the pathogenesis of synucleipathies is under investigation.

α-SYNUCLEIN IS POSTTRANSLATIONALLY MODIFIED BY NITRATION AND OXIDATION *IN VIVO*

Based on data gathered to understand the molecular basis of the selectivity of protein tyrosine nitration *in vivo* we uncovered that tyrosine residues in the vicinity of charged amino acids (mostly acidic residues) are primary targets for nitration.[14,44] Within the α-syn sequence the carboxyl terminus contains there tyrosine residues in an aspartate- and glutamate-rich environment, suggesting a reasonable site for modification. Indeed, *in vitro* exposure of the protein to nitrating agents resulted in nitration of these three tyrosine residues; and, moreover, in oxidation of tyrosine to form dityrosine that cross-linked the protein to form SDS and urea-stable dimer and multi-oligomeric forms.[44] A series of monoclonal antibodies were then raised and characterized by mutational analysis that recognizes only nitrated α-syn or only nitrated and oxidized α-syn.[20,22] These antibodies revealed a highly selective labeling of α-syn not only in LBs but also in dystrophic neurites, indicating a wide-spread but highly selective modification of α-syn in PD and other related synucleopathies.[20,22] Selective nitration of α-syn but not of other presynaptic proteins has also been detected in MPTP-challenged mice.[45] This selective targeting of α-syn for oxidative and nitrative modification clearly implies the formation of nitrating agents and is derived in part, as alluded to before, from the protein structure and not the biochemical nature of the nitrating agent, the abundance of the protein, or even the number of tyrosine residues in the protein. This selective targeting may provide some clues regarding the molecular and biochemical events that lead to the pathogenesis of PD, as an important determinant in the selection of protein(s) for nitration is the site of formation of the nitrating agent. Based on these observations a model is proposed that implicates oxidative/nitrative stress in the formation of α-syn inclusions and cellular death in PD.

ACKNOWLEDGMENTS

I am grateful to all members of my laboratory, the members of the synuclein group at the Center for Neurodegenerative Disorders (Virginia M-Y. Lee, John Q. Trojanowski, codirectors), for their support and stimulating discussions; and to Dr. Akiva Cohen for comments and critical reading of the manuscript. Major contributions in this project have been made by Dr. Jose "Pepe" Souza, Dr. Qiping Chen, and Jenny Paxinou, with support from National Institute on Aging, National Institutes of Health.

REFERENCES

1. DESNUELLE, C., M. DIB, C. GARREL & A. FAVIER. 2001. A double-blind, placebo-controlled randomized clinical trial of alpha-tocopherol (vitamin E) in the treatment of amyotrophic lateral sclerosis. ALS Riluzole-Tocopherol Study Group. Amyotroph. Lateral Scler. Other Motor Neuron Disord. **2:** 9–18.
2. SANO, M., C. ERNESTO, R.G. THOMAS, et al. 1997. A controlled trial of selegiline, alpha-tocopherol, or both as treatment for Alzheimer's disease. The Alzheimer's Disease Cooperative Study. N. Eng. J. Med. **336:** 1216–1222.
3. PRZEDBORSKI, S., Q. CHEN, M. VILA, et al. 2001. Oxidative post-translational modifications of α-synuclein in the MPTP mouse model of Parkinson's disease. J. Neurochem. **76:** 637–640.
4. STADTMAN, E.R. 1992. Protein oxidation and aging. Science **257:** 1220–1224.
5. LIPTON, S.A, Y-B. CHOI, Z-H. PAN, et al. 1993. A redox-based mechanism for the neuroprotective and neurodestructive effects of nitric oxide and related compounds. Nature **364:** 626–631.
6. ISCHIROPOULOS, H. 1998. Biological tyrosine nitration: a pathophysiological function of nitric oxide and reactive oxygen species. Arch. Biochem. Biophys. **356:** 1–11.
7. HUANG, Z., P.L. HUANG, N. PANAHIAN, et al. 1994. Effects of cerebral ischemia in mice deficient in neuronal nitric oxide synthase. Science **265:** 1883–1885.
8. ELIASSON, M.J., Z. HUANG, R.J. FERRANTE, et al. 1999. Neuronal nitric oxide synthase activation and peroxynitrite formation in ischemic stroke linked to neural damage. J. Neurosci. **19:** 5910–5918.

9. AYATA, C., G. AYATAM, H. HARA, et al. 1997. Mechanisms of reduced striatal NMDA excitotoxicity in type 1 nitric oxide synthase knock-out mice. J. Neurosci. **17:** 6908–6917.

10. PRZEDBORSKI, S., V. JACKSON-LEWIS, R. YOKOYAMA, et al. 1996. Role of neuronal nitric oxide in MPTP (1-methyl-4-phenyl-1,2,3,6-tetrahydropyridine)-induced dopaminergic neurotoxicity. Proc. Natl. Acad. Sci. USA **93:** 4565–4571.

11. LIBERATORE, G.T., V. JACKSON-LEWIS, S. VUKOSAVIC, et al. 1999. Inducible nitric oxide synthase stimulates dopaminergic neurodegeneration in the MPTP model of Parkinson disease. Nat. Med. **5:** 1403–1409.

12. SCHULZ, J.B., P.L. HUANG, R.T. MATTHEWS, et al. 1996. Striatal malonate lesions are attenuated in nitric oxide oxide synthase knockout mice. J. Neurochem. **67:** 430–433.

13. SMITH, M.A., P.L. RICHEY HARRIS, L.M. SAYRE, et al. 1997. Widespread peroxynitrite-mediated damage in Alzheimer's disease. J. Neurosci. **17:** 2653–2657.

14. ARA, J., S. PRZEDBORSKI, A.B. NAINI, et al. 1998. Inactivation of tyrosine hydroxylase following exposure to peroxynitrite and MPTP. Proc. Natl. Acad. Sci. USA **95:** 7659–7663.

15. PENNATHUR S., V. JAKSON-LEWIS, S. PRZEDBORSKI & J.W. HEINECKE. 1999. Mass spectrometric quantification of 3-nitrotyrosine, ortho-tyrosine, and o,o'-dityrosine in brain tissue of 1-methyl-4-phenyl-1,2,3, 6-tetrahydropyridine-treated mice, a model of oxidative stress in Parkinson's disease. J. Biol. Chem. **274:** 34621–34628.

16. BASARGA, O., F.H. MICHAELS, Y.M. ZHENG, et al. 1995. Activation of the inducible form of nitric oxide synthase in the brains of patients with multiple sclerosis. Proc. Natl. Acad. Sci. USA **92:** 12041–12045.

17. BEAL, M.F., R.J. FERRANTE, S.E. BROWNE, et al. 1997. Increased 3-nitrotyrosine in both sporadic and familial amyotrophic lateral sclerosis. Ann. Neurol. **42:** 644–654.

18. HENSLEY, K., M.L. MAIDT, Z.Q. YU, et al. 1998. Electrochemical analysis of protein nitrotyrosine and dityrosine in the Alzheimer brain indicates region-specific accumulation. J. Neurosci. **18:** 8126–8132.

19. DUDA, J.E., B.I. GIASSON, Q. CHEN, et al. 2000. Widespread nitration of pathological inclusions in neurodegenerative synucleinopathies. Am. J. Pathol. **157:** 1439–1445.

20. GIASSON, B.I., J.E. DUDA, I.V. MURRAY, et al. 2000. Oxidative damage linked to neurodegeneration by selective alpha-synuclein nitration in synucleinopathy lesions. Science **290:** 985–989.

21. TROJANOWSKI, J.Q., M. GOEDERT, T. IWATSUBO & V.M-Y. LEE. 1998. Fatal attractions: abnormal protein aggregation and neuron death in Parkinson's disease and Lewy body dementia. Cell Death Differ. **5:** 832–837.

22. DUDA. J.E., B.I. GIASSON, M.E. MABON, et al. 2002. Novel antibodies to synuclein show abundant striatal pathology in Lewy body diseases. Ann. Neurol. **52:** 205–210.

23. FUJIWARA, H., M. HASEGAWA, N. DOHMAE, et al. 2002. Alpha-synuclein is phosphorylated in synucleinopathy lesions. Nat. Cell Biol. **4:** 160–164.

24. IRIZARRY, M.C., W. GROWDON, T. GOMEZ-ISLA, et al. 1998. Nigral and cortical Lewy bodies and dystrophic nigral neurites in Parkinson's disease and cortical Lewy body disease contain α-synuclein. J. Neuropath. Exp. Neurol. **57:** 334–337.

25. LANGSTON, J.W., S. SASTRY, P. CHAN, et al. 1998. Novel alpha-synuclein-immunoreactive proteins in brain samples from the Contursi kindred, Parkinson's, and Alzheimer's disease. Exp. Neurol. **154:** 684–690.

26. SPILLANTINI, M.G, M.L. SCHMIDT, V.M-Y. LEE, et al. 1997. α-Synuclein in Lewy bodies. Nature **388:** 839–840.

27. WAKABAYASHI, K., M. YOSHIMOTO, S. TSUJI & H. TAKAHASHI. 1998. Alpha-synuclein immunoreactivity in glial cytoplasmic inclusions in multiple system atrophy. Neurosci. Lett. **249:** 180–182.

28. CONWAY, K.A., J.D. HARPER & P.T. LANSBURY. 1998. Accelerated in vitro fibril formation by a mutant alpha-synuclein linked to early-onset Parkinson disease. Nature Med. **4:** 1318–1320.

29. GIASSON, B.I, I.V. MURRAY, J.Q. TROJANOWSKI & V.M. LEE. 2001. A hydrophobic stretch of 12 amino acid residues in the middle of alpha-synuclein is essential for filament assembly. J. Biol. Chem. **276:** 2380–2386.

30. UVERSKY, V.N., J. LI & A.L. FINK. 2001. Metal-triggered structural transformations, aggregation, and fibrillation of human alpha-synuclein. A possible molecular link between Parkinson's disease and heavy metal exposure. J. Biol. Chem. **276:** 44284–44296.

31. DAVIDSON, W.S., A. JONAS, D.F. CLAYTON & J.M. GEORGES. 1998. Stabilization of alpha-synuclein secondary structure upon binding to synthetic membranes. J. Biol. Chem. **273:** 9443–9449.

32. LEE, F.J.S., F. LIU, Z.B. PRISTUPA & H.B. NIZNIK. 2001. Direct binding and functional coupling of α-synuclein to the dopamine transporters accelerate dopamine-induced apoptosis. FASEB J. **15:** 916–926.

33. HASHIMOTO, M., A. TAKEDA, L.J. HSU, et al. 1999. Role of cytochrome c as a stimulator of α-synuclein aggregation in Lewy Body disease. J. Biol. Chem. **274:** 28849–28852.

34. HASHIMOTO, M., E. ROCKENSTEIN, M. MANTE, et al. 2001. beta-Synuclein inhibits alpha-synuclein aggregation: a possible role as an anti-parkinsonian factor. Neuron **32:** 213–223.

35. JENCO, J.M., A. RAWLINGTON, B. DANIELS & A. J. MORRIS. 1998. Regulation of phosholipase D2: selective inhibition of mammalian phospholipase D isoenzyme by alpha- and beta-synucleins. Biochemistry **37:** 4901–4909.

36. OSTREROVA-GOLTS, N., L. PETRUCELLI, M. FARER, et al. 1999. Alpha-synuclein shares physical and functional homology with 14-3-3 proteins. J. Neurosci. **19:** 5782–5791.

37. PAYTON J.E., R.J. PERRIN, D.F. CLAYTON & J.M. GEORGE. 2001. Protein-protein interactions of alpha-synuclein in brain homogenates and transfected cells. Brain Res. Mol. Brain Res. **95:** 138–145.

38. PEREZ, R.G., J.C. WAYMIRE, E. LIN, et al. 2002. A role for a-synuclein in the regulation of dopamine biosynthesis. J. Neurosci. **22:** 3090–3099.

39. SOUZA, J.M., B.I. GIASSON, V. M-Y. LEE & H. ISCHIROPOULOS. 2000. Chaperone-like activity of synucleins. FEBS Lett. **474:** 116–119.

40. ENGELENDER, S., Z. KAMINSKY, X. GUO, et al. 1999. Synphilin-1 associates with a-synuclein and promotes the formation of cytosolic inclusions. Nat. Genet. **22:** 110–114.

41. SHIMURA, H., M.G. SCHLOSSMACHER, N. HATTORI, et al. 2001. Ubiquitination of a new form of alpha-synuclein by parkin from human brain: implications for Parkinson's disease. Science **293:** 263–269.

42. ELLIS C.E., P.L. SCHWARTZBERG, T.L. GRIDER, et al. 2001. alpha-Synuclein is phosphorylated by members of the Src family of protein-tyrosine kinases. J. Biol. Chem. **276:** 3879–3884.

43. OKOCHI, M., J. WALTER, A. KOYAMA, et al. 2000. Constitutive phosphorylation of the Parkinson's disease associated α-synuclein. J. Biol. Chem. **275:** 390–397.

44. SOUZA, J.M., B.I. GIASSON, Q. CHEN, et al. 2000. Dityrosine cross-linking promotes formation of stable alpha-synuclein polymers. Implication of nitrative and oxidative stress in the pathogenesis of neurodegenerative synucleinopathies. J. Biol. Chem. **275:** 18344–18349.

45. PRZEDBORSKI, S., V. KOSTIC, V. JACKSON-LEWIS, et al. 1992. Transgenic mice with increased Cu/Zn-superoxide dismutase activity are resistant to N-methyl-4-phenyl-1,2,3,6-tetrahydropyridine-induced neurotoxicity. J. Neurosci. **12:** 1658–1667.

46. TAKEDA, A., M. MALLORY, M. SUNDSMO, et al. 1998. Abnormal accumulation of NACP/alpha-synuclein in neurodegenerative disorders. Am. J. Pathol. **152:** 367–372.

47. KRUGER, R., W. KUHN, T. MULLER, et al. 1998. Ala30-to-pro mutation in the gene encoding alpha-synuclein in Parkinson's disease. Nat. Genet. **18:** 106–108.

48. POLYMEROPOULOS, M.H., C. LAVEDANM, E. LEROY, et al. 1997. Mutation in the alpha-synuclein gene identified in families with Parkinson's disease. Science **276:** 2045–2047.

49. CONWAY, K.A., J.C. ROCHET, R.M. BIEGANSKI & P.T. LANSBURY, JR. 2001. Kinetic stabilization of the alpha-synuclein protfibril by a dopamine-alpha-synuclein adduct. Science **294:** 1396–1349.

50. PAXINOU, E., Q. CHEN, M. WEISSE, et al. 2001. Induction of alpha-synuclein aggregation by intracellular nitrative insult. J. Neurosci. **21:** 8053–8061.

51. LEE, H.J., S.Y. SHIN, C. CHOI, *et al.* 2002. Formation and removal of alpha-synuclein aggregates in cells exposesed to mitochondrial inhibitors. J. Biol. Chem. **277:** 5411–5417.
52. TABIRZI, S.J., M. ORTH, J.M. WILKINSON, *et al.* 2000. Expression of mutant alpha-synuclein causes increased susceptibility to dopamine toxicity. Hum. Mol. Genet. **9:** 2683–2689.
53. XU, J., S.Y. KAO, F.J. LEE, *et al.* 2002. Dopamine-dependent neurotoxicity of alpha-synulcein: a mechanism for selective neurodegeneration in Parkinson's disease. Nat. Med. **8:** 600–606.

Parkin and Endoplasmic Reticulum Stress

RYOSUKE TAKAHASHI,[a] YUZURU IMAI,[a] NOBUTAKA HATTORI,[b] AND
YOSHIKUNI MIZUNO[b]

[a]Laboratory for Motor System Neurodegeneration, RIKEN Brain Science Institute (BSI),
Saitama 351-0198, Japan

[b]Department of Neurology, Juntendo University School of Medicine, Bunkyo-ku,
Tokyo, 113-0033, Japan

ABSTRACT: Autosomal-recessive juvenile parkinsonism (AR-JP) is caused by
mutations in the *parkin* gene. Parkin protein is characterized by a ubiquitin-
like domain at its NH_2 terminus and by two RING finger motifs and one IBR
(in *b*etween *R*ING finger) motif at its COOH-terminus (RING-IBR-RING). We
showed that the parkin protein is an E3 ubiquitin ligase, which binds to ubiquitin-conjugating enzymes (E2s) through its RING-IBR-RING motif. The
pathogenesis of AR-JP, therefore, was hypothesized to be accumulation of unidentified neurotoxic protein (a substrate of parkin). On the basis of this hypothesis, the substrate of parkin was sought using a yeast two-hybrid system.
A putative G protein–coupled transmembrane polypeptide, named Pael (*p*ar-
kin-*a*ssociated *e*ndothelin receptor-*l*ike) receptor, was identified as a parkin
binding protein. When overexpressed in cells, this receptor tends to become unfolded, insoluble, and ubiquitinated. The insoluble Pael receptor leads to endoplasmic reticulum (ER) stress-induced cell death. Parkin specifically
ubiquitinates this receptor in the presence of ER-resident E2s and promotes
the degradation of unfolded Pael receptor, resulting in suppression of the cell
death induced by the accumulation of unfolded Pael receptor in the ER. Moreover, the insoluble form of Pael receptor accumulates in the brain of AR-JP patients. This protein is highly expressed in the dopaminergic neurons in the
substantia nigra, which is specifically affected in Parkinson's disease; although
it is also widely expressed in oligodendroglias in the fiber tract. In conclusion,
we showed that the accumulation of unfolded Pael receptor (a substrate of parkin) may cause selective death of dopaminergic neurons in AR-JP.

KEYWORDS: AR-JP; parkin; Pael receptor; ER stress; ERAD

INTRODUCTION

Parkinson's disease (PD) is the second most common neurodegenerative disease
among elderly people. More than 1% of people aged 65 or older are afflicted with
PD. The main clinical feature of PD is progressive motor disturbances (tremor, rigidity, and akinesia). Although the rate of disease progression is variable, wheel
chair or bed confinement usually occurs years after disease onset.

Address for correspondence: Ryosuke Takahashi, M.D., Ph.D., Laboratory for Motor System
Neurodegeneration, RIKEN Brain Science Institute (BSI), 2-1 Hirosawa, Wako, Saitama 351-
0198, Japan. Voice: +81-48-467-6072; fax: +81-48-462-4796.
ryosuke@brain.riken.go.jp

Ann. N.Y. Acad. Sci. 991: 101–106 (2003). © 2003 New York Academy of Sciences.

Most PD cases are sporadic rather than familial (5–10%) and are presumably inherited. Autosomal-recessive juvenile parkinsonism (AR-JP), the most frequent cause of familial PD, is characterized by several unique features including young age at onset (most under age 40) and superb responsiveness to L-dopa. The neuropathological hallmark of AR-JP is selective degeneration of dopaminergic neurons in the substantia nigra, similar to that of the common form of Parkinson's disease. However, the pathology of AR-JP is not usually accompanied by Lewy bodies (cytoplasmic neuronal inclusions), which are the histopathological signature for common PD.[1–3]

In 1998, *parkin* was identified as the gene responsible for AR-JP.[4] Here, the physiological and pathophysiological function of parkin in ER stress is discussed.

RESULTS AND DISCUSSION

The Structure and Function of the Parkin Protein

Parkin is a 465–amino acid protein characterized by a ubiquitin-like domain at its NH_2 terminus and two RING finger motifs and one IBR (*in between RING* fingers) motif at its COOH-terminus (RING-IBR-RING). The RING finger motif is a variant of the zinc finger motif, which has metal binding activity and cysteine and histidine residues present at certain intervals.

Although the RING finger motif is found in a wide variety of proteins, the physiological function of this motif has been unknown until recently. However, recent findings implicate the RING domain in specific ubiquitination events.[5] Protein ubiquitination begins with the formation of a thiol-ester linkage between the COOH terminus of ubiquitin and the active-site cysteine of the ubiquitin-activating enzyme (E1). Ubiquitin then is transferred to a ubiquitin-conjugating enzyme (E2), again through a thiol-ester linkage. Ubiquitin-protein ligases (E3s), which are primarily responsible for providing specificity to ubiquitin conjugation, interact with E2 and the substrate, facilitating the formation of isopeptide bonds between the COOH-terminus of ubiquitin and lysines either on a target protein or on the last ubiquitin of a protein-bound multiubiquitin chain. Multiubiquitin chains are potent targeting signals for protein degradation in proteasomes.[6] A number of RING finger–containing proteins including Mdm2 and Siah are shown to be E3s. In RING-type E3s, RING finger motifs serve as recruiting motifs for specific E2 enzymes. These facts suggest that parkin, which contains the RING-IBR-RING motif, is a new E3 ubiquitin ligase.

Parkin actually turned out to be a RING-type E3 ubiquitin ligase.[7–9] We have shown that wild-type parkin ubiquitinates an unidentified substrate protein. By contrast, disease-related mutated parkin has lost its E3 activity, indicating a close inverse correlation between enzymatic activity and disease phenotype.[8] These results suggest that a genetic defect in parkin causes the substrate of parkin to escape degradation and accumulate, and may lead to PD. This hypothesis implies a key role for the substrate of parkin in the neurodegenerative process.

The Identification of Pael Receptor as a Substrate of Parkin

To identify the substrate of parkin, we carried out a yeast two-hybrid screening of human adult brain cDNA libraries using full-length parkin as bait. One of the isolated clones contained a COOH terminal portion of endothelin receptor-like protein, which is a putative G protein–coupled receptor with its unidentified ligand, very similar to endothelin receptor type B in sequence. We renamed this receptor Pael (*par*kin-*a*ssociated *e*ndothelin receptor-*l*ike) receptor (Pael-R; GenBank accession number: AF502281).[10]

Pael-R was specifically ubiquitinated by parkin in the presence of Ubc6 and Ubc7 in an *in vitro* ubiquitination assay. Moreover, the half-life of Pael-R in cultured neuroblastoma cells transiently transfected with a Pael-R expression vector was dramatically shortened from one hour to less than 30 minutes by parkin coexpression. These results indicate that Pael-R is an *in vivo* substrate of parkin.

Pael-R Is a Substrate of Endoplasmic Reticulum–Associated Degradation

It has been shown that the ubiquitin-proteasome pathway plays an important role in the degradation of membrane or secretory protein at the level of endoplasmic reticulum (ER). The ER is an organelle that carries out the quality control of membrane or secretory protein folding. Newly synthesized secretory proteins enter the ER, where ER chaperones such as BiP bind and help the proper folding of these proteins. Properly folded proteins are then allowed to enter the normal secretory pathway composed of Golgi apparatus, plasma membrane, endosome, lysosome, and various intermediate transport compartments. However, the proteins that do not fold correctly are retrotranslocated to the cytosol, where these "failed" proteins are degraded. This process is called endoplasmic reticulum–associated degradation (ERAD).[11] ERAD substrates (i.e., ER luminal or ER transmembrane proteins) are transported through a channel-like protein complex termed a "translocon" back to the cytosol, where they are subject to ubiquitin-proteasome degradation.

Because parkin binds to Ubc6 and Ubc7 (ER-resident E2s involved in ERAD) and Pael-R was ubiquitinated *in vitro* in the presence of both parkin and Ubc6/7, it has been suggested that parkin is an E3 involved in ERAD and Pael-R is a substrate of ERAD. To test this idea, we caused overexpression of Pael-R in a dopaminergic neuroblastoma cell line, SH-SY5Y. When these cells were lysed with a nonionic detergent such as Triton X-100, properly folded and unfolded proteins substantially partitioned into detergent-soluble and -insoluble fractions, respectively.[12]

Interestingly, a significant amount (up to 50%) of Pael-R was detected in the insoluble fraction when cells transiently transfected with a plasmid containing a Pael-R cDNA were given no additional treatment, suggesting that the proper folding of Pael-R is inherently difficult. Treatment with ER stress–inducing reagents such as tunicamycin and 2-mercaptoethanol increased the level of insoluble Pael-R and decreased the level of soluble Pael-R, indicating that the soluble and insoluble Pael-R correspond to properly folded and unfolded species of Pael-R. Moreover, treatment with lactacystin, a selective proteasomal inhibitor, dramatically increased the level of insoluble Pael-R without affecting the level of soluble Pael-R. This result indicates that inhibition of ERAD by lactacystin resulted in the accumulation of unfolded, insoluble Pael-R and provides strong evidence that Pael-R is a substrate of ERAD.

Abnormal Accumulation of Pael-R and ER Stress–Induced Cell Death

To examine the effect of Pael-R accumulation on cell viability, Pael-R overexpressing cells were treated with lactacystin to induce forced accumulation of Pael-

R. Immunofluorescence analysis revealed the accumulation of Pael-R in the ER 6 h after the addition of lactacystin. Prolonged lactacystin treatment led to Pael-R aggregate formation. As the aggregate formed, the cells became round and shrunken, suggesting apoptotic cell death and that accumulation of Pael-R causes cell death.

Then what is the mechanism underlying Pael-R–induced cell death? Abnormal accumulation of unfolded proteins in the ER constitutes a major threat to cell viability. This situation is called "unfolded protein stress" or ER stress. Cells make attempts to overcome ER stress in various ways including transcriptional upregulation of ER chaperones (such as GRP78/BiP) and components of ERAD (such as Ubc7), and general translational suppression. These cellular responses are collectively called the "unfolded protein response" (UPR). When the amount of accumulated unfolded protein exceeds the threshold level, the cells undergo cell death accompanied by activation of c-Jun N terminal kinase (JNK) and caspase-12.[13,14] At the early stage of Pael-R accumulation, GRP78/BiP was upregulated at the transcriptional level, indicating that accumulation of Pael-R indeed induced ER stress. Moreover, we have already found that parkin mRNA is increased when cells are subjected to tunicamycin- or 2-mercaptoethanol–induced ER stress and that the resulting parkin overexpression suppressed ER stress–induced cell death of the human neuroblastoma cell line SH-SY5Y expressing endogenous Pael-R. Parkin-mediated cell death suppression is at least partially explained by parkin-mediated degradation of Pael-R. Consistent with this idea, Pael-R overexpression–induced cell death is suppressed by coexpression of parkin, which is accompanied by a significant decrease of insoluble, but not soluble, Pael-R.

On the basis of these findings, accumulation of Pael-R is most likely the pathogenetic mechanism underlying AR-JP. Seeking direct evidence to support this idea, we examined brains from AR-JP patients to determined whether they contained accumulated Pael-R. We prepared homogenates of AR-JP as well as control brain samples, separated them into detergent-soluble and -insoluble fractions, and measured the amount of Pael-R in each fraction. The protein level of insoluble, but not soluble, Pael-R was 10–30-fold higher in AR-JP brains than that in non-AR-JP brains. Moreover, in three out of four AR-JP brains examined, an increased level of GRP78/BiP was observed, suggesting that AR-JP brains were also under ER stress caused by the accumulation of unfolded Pael-R. Given that neurodegeneration in AR-JP is caused by ER stress–induced cell death, cytoplasmic inclusions composed of unfolded Pael-R may not be formed before cellular demise, providing reasonable explanation for the absence of Lewy bodies or other types of neuronal inclusion bodies in AR-JP.

Tissue Distribution Pattern of Pael-R

Pael-R mRNA is highly expressed in the central nervous system, especially in the substantia nigra and the corpus callosum, the latter being composed mainly of nerve fibers and not of neuronal cell bodies.[15,16] Immunohistochemical analysis revealed that Pael-R is generally strongly expressed in oligodendrocytes and poorly expressed in neurons except hippocampal neurons and dopaminergic neurons in the substantia nigra. Assuming that postmitotic neurons are more vulnerable to ER stress than renewable oligodendrocytes, selective degeneration of dopaminergic neurons in AR-JP can be partly explained by this unique distribution pattern of Pael-R. On the other hand, dopaminergic neurons are thought to be constitutively exposed to oxidative

Normal:

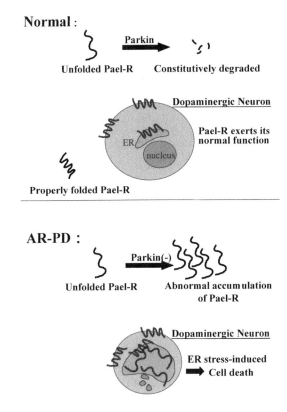

FIGURE 1. Diagram showing **(top)** the normal functioning of Pael-R and **(bottom)** the pathogenic mechanism of AR-JP.

stress and especially sensitive to various stresses, providing another factor contributing to the lesion selectivity in AR-JP.

CONCLUSION

Taken together, our evidence strongly suggests that accumulation of Pael-R is causative in AR-JP (FIG. 1).[10] Recently, the accumulation of misfolded proteins has been implicated in the pathogenesis of many neurodegenerative diseases including amyotrophic lateral sclerosis, Alzheimer's disease, Parkinson's disease, and polyglutamine disease.[17,18] Our study showed that AR-JP is also one of these so-called "conformational diseases." Potentially cytotoxic misfolded protein is usually detoxified either by refolding with molecular chaperones or degradation through the ubiquitin-proteasome pathway. Manipulations of such refolding or degrading machineries may provide opportunities for treatment of currently intractable neurodegenerative diseases.

ACKNOWLEDGMENTS

We would like to thank Ms. Mariko Soda and Dr. Haruhisa Inoue for their kind collaborative efforts. This study was supported by a Grant-in-Aid for Scientific Research from the Ministry of Education, Culture, Sports, Science and Technology, Japan (R.T., N.H., and Y.M.); and a Grant-in-Aid for Encouragement of Young Scientists from the Japan Society for the Promotion of Science (Y.I.).

REFERENCES

1. YAMAMURA, Y., I. SOBUE, K. ANDO, et al. 1973. Paralysis agitans of early onset with marked diurnal fluctuation of symptoms. Neurology **23:** 239–244.
2. ISHIKAWA, A. & S. TSUJI. 1996. Clinical analysis of 17 patients in 12 Japanese families with autosomal-recessive type juvenile parkinsonism. Neurology **47:** 160–166.
3. YOKOCHI, M. 2000. Development of the nosological analysis of juvenile parkinsonism. Brain Dev. **22** Suppl. 1: S81–86.
4. KITADA, T., S. ASAKAWA, N. HATTORI, et al. 1998. Mutations in the parkin gene cause autosomal recessive juvenile parkinsonism. Nature **392:** 605–608.
5. JOAZEIRO, C.A. & A.M. WEISSMAN. 2000. RING finger proteins: mediators of ubiquitin ligase activity. Cell **102:** 549–552.
6. HERSHKO, A. & A. CIECHANOVER. 1998. The ubiquitin system. Annu. Rev. Biochem. **67:** 425–479.
7. SHIMURA, H., N. HATTORI, S. KUBO, et al. 2000. Familial Parkinson disease gene product, parkin, is a ubiquitin-protein ligase. Nat. Genet. **25:** 302–305.
8. IMAI, Y., M. SODA & R. TAKAHASHI. 2000. Parkin suppresses unfolded protein stress-induced cell death through its E3 ubiquitin-protein ligase activity. J. Biol. Chem. **275:** 35661–35664.
9. ZHANG, Y., J. GAO, K.K. CHUNG, et al. 2000. Parkin functions as an E2-dependent ubiquitin-protein ligase and promotes the degradation of the synaptic vesicle-associated protein, CDCrel-1. Proc. Natl. Acad. Sci. USA **97:** 13354–13359.
10. IMAI, Y., M. SODA, H. INOUE, et al. 2001. An unfolded putative transmembrane polypeptide, which can lead to endoplasmic reticulum stress, is a substrate of parkin. Cell **105:** 891–902.
11. PLEMPER, R.K. & D.H. WOLF. 1999. Retrograde protein translocation: ERADication of secretory proteins in health and disease. Trends Biochem. Sci. **24:** 266–270.
12. WARD, C.L., S. OMURA & R.R. KOPITO. 1995. Degradation of CFTR by the ubiquitin-proteasome pathway. Cell **83:** 121–127.
13. URANO, F., X. WANG, A. BERTOLOTTI, et al. 2000. Coupling of stress in the ER to activation of JNK protein kinases by transmembrane protein kinase IRE1. Science **287:** 664–666.
14. NAKAGAWA, T., H. ZHU, N. MORISHIMA, et al. 2000. Caspase-12 mediates endoplasmic-reticulum-specific apoptosis and cytotoxicity by amyloid-beta. Nature **403:** 98–103.
15. ZENG, Z., K. SU, H. KYAW, et al. 1997. A novel endothelin receptor type-B-like gene enriched in the brain. Biochem. Biophys. Res. Commun. **233:** 559–567.
16. DONOHUE, P.J., H. SHAPIRA, S. A. MANTEY, et al. 1998. A human gene encodes a putative G protein-coupled receptor highly expressed in the central nervous system. Brain Res. Mol. Brain Res. **54:** 152–160.
17. SHERMAN, M.Y. & A.L. GOLDBERG. 2001. Cellular defenses against unfolded proteins: a cell biologist thinks about neurodegenerative diseases. Neuron **29:** 15–32.
18. JULIEN, J. 2001. Amyotrophic lateral sclerosis. Unfolding the toxicity of the misfolded. Cell **104:** 581–591.

Parkinson's Disease and Related α-Synucleinopathies Are Brain Amyloidoses

JOHN Q. TROJANOWSKI AND VIRGINIA M-Y. LEE

Center for Neurodegenerative Disease Research, Department of Pathology and Laboratory Medicine, and the Institute on Aging, the University of Pennsylvania School of Medicine, Philadelphia, Pennsylvania 19104, USA

ABSTRACT: A paradigm shift in understanding Parkinson's disease (PD) and related disorders is emerging from studies showing that alpha-synuclein (AS) gene mutations cause familial PD; AS is abnormally nitrated, phosphorylated, and ubiquitinated; AS forms neuronal and glial inclusions; AS fibrillizes *in vitro*; and AS transgenic animals develop neurodegeneration with AS amyloid inclusions. Thus, PD and related synucleinopathies are brain amyloidoses that may share similar mechanisms and targets for drug discovery.

KEYWORDS: Parkinson's disease; alpha-synuclein; synucleinopathies; neurodegenerative brain amyloidoses

Parkinson's disease (PD) is the most common neurodegenerative movement disorder, but because its underlying mechanisms are poorly understood, only symptomatic treatments that partially or transiently ameliorate some of the impairments associated with PD are available (reviewed in Ref. 1). However, recent research breakthroughs implicate α-synuclein (AS) abnormalities in mechanisms of PD (reviewed in Refs. 2–7), and this will hasten development of more effective PD therapies. For example, AS pathologies are now recognized as the defining brain amyloid lesions of diverse neurodegenerative disorders known as α-synucleinopathies (also called synucleinopathies) that appear to share similar disease mechanisms (TABLE 1); and further insights into the role that AS plays in PD and other neurodegenerative brain amyloidoses are likely to provide new targets for the discovery of drugs to treat these diseases (reviewed in Refs. 2–9).

As summarized and discussed in more detail elsewhere,[2–12] a paradigm shift in understanding mechanisms of PD began in 1997, and this is resulting in the convergence of several lines of evidence implicating brain amyloid deposits formed by

Address for correspondence: John Q. Trojanowski, M.D., Ph.D., Center for Neurodegenerative Disease Research, Department of Pathology and Laboratory Medicine, University of Pennsylvania School of Medicine, HUP, Maloney Building, 3rd Floor, Philadelphia, PA 19104. Voice: 215-662-6399/6427; fax: 215-349-5909.
trojanow@mail.med.upenn.edu

Ann. N.Y. Acad. Sci. 991: 107–110 (2003). © 2003 New York Academy of Sciences.

TABLE 1. Neurodegenerative diseases with prominent filamentous AS lesions

Sporadic and familial Parkinson's disease
Sporadic and familial Alzheimer's disease
Dementia with Lewy bodies
Multiple system atrophy
Down's syndrome
Neuronal degeneration with brain iron accumulation type 1 (Hallervorden-Spatz disease)
Pure autonomic failure
REM sleep behavior disorder

NOTE: Sporadic and hereditary neurodegenerative diseases characterized by filamentous AS brain lesions. Disease in which AS lesions are the predominant or sole form of brain amyloid are shown in italics. Notably, AD is a triple brain amyloidosis because it is associated with lesions formed by deposits of fibrillar tau, $A\beta$, and AS.

abnormally aggregated AS filaments in these processes.[2–12] The following key observations support this new perspective on PD and related disorders:

(1) Mutations in the AS gene cause familial PD;

(2) Lewy bodies (LBs) and dystrophic Lewy neuritis are detected by anti-AS antibodies, but these hallmark PD amyloid lesions also occur in other disorders including Alzheimer's disease (AD), the LB variant of AD (LBVAD), and dementia with LBs (DLB);

(3) AS filaments are recovered from PD and DLB brains as well as from LBs purified from DLB brains;

(4) recombinant AS forms LB-like filaments with properties that are typical for amyloid fibrils and amino acids 71–82 in AS are essential for filament assembly;

(5) AS single transgenic (TG) mice and flies develop a neurodegenerative disease phenotype with filamentous AS amyloid deposits;

(6) cortical LBs detected with antibodies to AS correlate with dementia in PD, DLB, and LBVAD;

(7) anti-AS antibodies detect more LBs in familial AD, sporadic AD, and Down's syndrome brains with AD pathology than previously described using other antibodies, suggesting that LBs are present in most cases of sporadic and hereditary AD;

(8) AS forms filaments that aggregate into amyloid-like glial cytoplasmic inclusions (GCIs), which are hallmarks of neurodegeneration with brain iron accumulation type 1 (NBIA-1) and multiple system atrophy (MSA);

(9) epitope mapping studies with anti-AS antibodies demonstrate that regions spanning the entire length of AS are present in LBs and GCIs;

(10) filamentous AS aggregates in LBs, GCIs, and related lesions contain abnormally nitrated, phosphorylated, and ubiquitinated residues;

(11) cells transfected with AS followed by treatment with nitric oxide generators develop LB-like AS inclusions;

(12) double TG mice overexpressing mutant human amyloid-beta (Ab) precursor proteins and AS show an augmentation in AS inclusions;

(13) coexpression of heat shock proteins (HSPs) with AS in flies and of β-synuclein with AS in mice leads to an amelioration of the disease phenotype seen in single AS TG animals, while a drug (geldanamycin) that induces HSPs in AS TG flies prevents degeneration of LB-containing neurons following treatment of the TG flies with this drug.

Thus, prominent AS pathologies with the physical-chemical properties of amyloid deposits are the hallmark brain lesions of several neurodegenerative disorders that may represent different manifestations of nervous system degeneration due to common underlying disease mechanisms. Accordingly, these disorders are classified together as neurodegenerative synucleinopathies, and each of these disorders can be regarded as different forms of brain amyloidosis (TABLE 1).

The deleterious effects of AS aggregates on central nervous system (CNS) neurons (e.g., LBs) in PD or glial cells (e.g., GCIs) in MSA remain to be elucidated. However, LBs are likely to impair the function/viability of affected neurons based on studies of TG animal models of neurodegenerative diseases that have been engineered to overexpress AS in the CNS.[2,7–9] For example, AS filaments form a dense meshwork that could "trap" proteins destined for axonal transport, thereby depriving processes of trophic factors or other essential proteins. As a result of this cascade of events, axons arising from neurons harboring LBs may undergo a "dying back" process that disrupts synaptic transmission and eventually culminates in the degeneration of affected neurons. These speculations notwithstanding, the availability of TG animal models of LB-like inclusions generated by expressing mutant and wild-type human AS in the CNS will enable experimental tests of hypotheses about neurodegeneration in PD as well as the screening of new drugs that might reverse or prevent PD and related synucleiopathies.

In addition to synucleinopathies, emerging data implicate amyloid deposits formed by diverse proteins and peptides in the onset/progression of many other sporadic and hereditary neurodegenerative disorders (including AD, which is a triple brain amyloidosis, because it is associated with lesions formed by deposits of fibrillar tau, Aβ, and AS). Indeed, accumulating evidence suggests a mechanistic link between abnormal filamentous amyloid aggregates and the degeneration of affected brain regions in neurodegenerative disorders. Inexplicably, many of these neurodegenerative diseases share an enigmatic symmetry: that is, missense mutations in the gene encoding the disease protein cause an early-onset, highly aggressive familial disorder, as well as the hallmark brain amyloid lesions of the disease; but the same brain amyloid lesions also can be formed from the corresponding wild-type protein in sporadic variants of these conditions. Thus, clarification of this enigmatic symmetry in one disease could have a significant impact on understanding mechanisms underlying all of these disorders and on efforts to develop more effective therapies to treat them. Moreover, by addressing these important issues, it is likely that insights into the underlying mechanisms of PD and related synucleinopathies will emerge, and it may be possible to clarify the perplexing, but well-documented, cooccurrence of PD and AD in the same patient, which is more common than chance alone would predict.[7,13] More significantly, this research is likely to stimulate the discovery of innovative therapies designed to disrupt neurodegenerative mechanisms, including brain amyloidosis caused by the accumulation of filamentous AS aggregates; and thereby to block or retard the progression of PD and related synucleinopathies.

ACKNOWLEDGMENTS

The authors thank members of the Center for Neurodegenerative Disease Research (CNDR)—especially Drs. J. E. Duda, B. I. Giasson, and K. Uryu—as well as collaborators within and outside the University of Pennsylvania for their important contributions to the studies reviewed here; and the families of the many patients studied in CNDR who have made our research possible. The studies summarized here from CNDR were supported by grants from the National Institute on Aging of the National Institutes of Health and the Alzheimer's Association. For more information on these diseases, see the CNDR website (http://www.med.upenn.edu/cndr).

REFERENCES

1. LANG, A.E. & A.M. LOZANO. 1998. Parkinson's disease. New Engl. J. Med. **339:** 1044–1053 and 1130–1143.
2. BONINI, N.M. 2002. Chaperoning brain degeneration. Proc. Natl. Acad. Sci. USA **99:** 16407–16411.
3. CLAYTON, D.F. & J.M. GEORGE. 1999. Synucleins in synaptic plasticity and neurodegenerative disorders. J. Neurosci. Res. **58:** 120–129.
4. DICKSON, D.W. 2001. Alpha-synuclein and the Lewy body disorders. Curr. Opin. Neurol. **14:** 423–432.
5. FEANY, M.B. 2000. Studying neurodgenerative diseases in flies and worms. J. Neuropath. Exper. Neurol. **59:** 847–856.
6. GOEDERT, M. 2001. Alpha-synuclein and neurodegenerative diseases. Nat. Rev. Neurosci. **2:** 492–501.
7. TROJANOWSKI, J.Q. & V.M-Y. LEE. 2002. Parkinson's disease and related synucleinopathies are a new class of nervous system amyloidoses. Neurotoxicology **23:** 457–460.
8. AULUCK, P.K., H.Y.E. CHAN, J.Q. TROJANOWSKI, *et al.* 2002. Chaperone suppression of alpha-synuclein toxicity in a *Drosophila* model of Parkinson's disease. Science **295:** 865–868.
9. AULUCK, P.K. & N.M. BONINI. 2002. Pharmacological prevention of Parkinson's disease in Drosophila. Nat. Med. **8:** 1185–1186.
10. HASEGAWA, M., H. FUJIWARA, T. NONAKA, *et al.* 2002. Phosphorylated alpha-synuclein is ubiquitinated in alpha-synucleinopathy lesions. J. Biol. Chem. **277:** 49071–49076.
11. HASHIMOTO, M., E. ROCKENSTEIN, M. MANTEE, *et al.* 2001. Beta-synuclein inhibits alpha-synuclein aggregation: a possible role as an anti-parkinsonian factor. Neuron **32:** 213–223.
12. MASLIAH, E., E. ROCKENSTEIN, I. VEINBERGS, *et al.* 2001. Beta-amyloid peptides enhance alpha-synuclein accumulation and neuronal deficits in a transgenic mouse model linking Alzheimer's disease and Parkinson's disease. Proc. Natl. Acad. Sci. USA **98:** 12245–12250.
13. PERL, D.P., C.W. OLANOW & D. CALNE. 1998. Alzheimer's disease and Parkinson's disease: distinct entities or extremes of a spectrum of neurodegeneration. Ann. Neurol. **44:** S19–S31.

Mitochondrial Mechanisms of Neural Cell Death and Neuroprotective Interventions in Parkinson's Disease

GARY FISKUM,[a] ANATOLY STARKOV,[a,b] BRIAN M. POLSTER,[a,c] AND CHRISTOS CHINOPOULOS[a]

[a]Department of Anesthesiology, University of Maryland School of Medicine, Baltimore, Maryland 21201, USA

[c]Department of Molecular Microbiology and Immunology, The Johns Hopkins University School of Public Health, SHPH 5132, 615 N. Wolfe Street, Baltimore, Maryland 21205-2179, USA

ABSTRACT: Mitochondrial dysfunction, due to either environmental or genetic factors, can result in excessive production of reactive oxygen species, triggering the apoptotic death of dopaminergic cells in Parkinson's disease. Mitochondrial free radical production is promoted by the inhibition of electron transport at any point distal to the sites of superoxide production. Neurotoxins that induce parkinsonian neuropathology, such as MPP^+ and rotenone, stimulate superoxide production at complex I of the electron transport chain and also stimulate free radical production at proximal redox sites including mitochondrial matrix dehydrogenases. The oxidative stress caused by elevated mitochondrial production of reactive oxygen species promotes the expression and (or) intracellular distribution of the proapoptotic protein Bax to the mitochondrial outer membrane. Interactions between Bax and BH3 death domain proteins such as tBid result in Bax membrane integration, oligomerization, and permeabilization of the outer membrane to intermembrane proteins such as cytochrome c. Once released into the cytosol, cytochrome c together with other proteins activates the caspase cascade of protease activities that mediate the biochemical and morphological alterations characteristic of apoptosis. In addition, loss of mitochondrial cytochrome c stimulates mitochondrial free radical production, further promoting cell death pathways. Excessive mitochondrial Ca^{2+} accumulation can also release cytochrome c and promote superoxide production through a mechanism distinctly different from that of Bax. Ca^{2+} activates a mitochondrial inner membrane permeability transition causing osmotic swelling, rupture of the outer membrane, and complete loss of mitochondrial structural and functional integrity. While amphiphilic cations, such as dibucaine and propranolol, inhibit Bax-mediated cytochrome c release, transient receptor potential channel inhibitors inhibit mitochondrial swelling and cytochrome c release induced by the inner membrane permeability transi-

Address for correspondence: Dr. Gary Fiskum, Dept of Anesthesiology, Univ. of Maryland School of Medicine, 685 W. Baltimore St., MSTF 5.34, Baltimore, MD 21201. Voice: 410-706-3418; fax: 410-706-2550;
Gfisk001@umaryland.edu
[b]Current address: Department of Neurology, Weil Medical College, Cornell University, 510 E. 70th St., New York, NY 10021.

Ann. N.Y. Acad. Sci. 991: 111–119 (2003). © 2003 New York Academy of Sciences.

tion. These advances in the knowledge of mitochondrial cell death mechanisms and their inhibitors may lead to neuroprotective interventions applicable to Parkinsons's disease.

KEYWORDS: apoptosis; cytochrome c; calcium; excitotoxicity; Bax

INTRODUCTION

Parkinson's disease (PD) is a progressive neurodegenerative disease character-ized clinically by bradykinesia, rigidity, resting tremor, and ataxia. These symptoms are caused by decreased dopamine release in the striatum. Pathologically, PD is characterized primarily by the death of dopaminergic neurons in the substantia nigra pars compacta and the formation of ubiquitin- and α-synuclein–positive cytoplasmic inclusions (Lewy bodies). The molecular mechanisms responsible for these changes are not clearly understood. One theory is that mitochondrial dysfunction, due to ei-ther environmental or genetic factors, results in excessive oxidative stress that trig-gers apoptotic cell death.

EVIDENCE FOR A MITOCHONDRIAL ETIOLOGY OF PARKINSON'S DISEASE

Several lines of evidence support the hypothesis that mitochondrial dysfunction contributes to the etiology of Parkinson's disease. Electron transport chain complex I activity is reduced in PD substantia nigra autopsy specimens as well as in PD plate-lets.[1,2] A mitochondrial genomic etiology for defective complex I in PD is strongly suggested by the presence of altered complex I activity, abnormal mitochondrial morphology, and impaired mitochondrial energy-dependent activities in cybrid cell lines containing a normal nuclear genome but mitochondrial DNA from PD pa-tients.[3–5] Parkinson's disease cybrids are also more sensitive to death induced by MPP[+], a dopaminergic neuron-selective toxin that induces Parkinson-like lesions and symptoms in both humans and animals.[4] Additional evidence for a mitochondri-al etiology of PD is the finding that chronic systemic treatment of rats with rotenone, a highly specific complex I inhibitor, can induce Lewy body neuropathology in ad-dition to nigrostriatal dopaminergic degeneration and neurologic features of PD.[6]

MITOCHONDRIAL INITIATION OF NECROTIC AND APOPTOTIC CELL DEATH

Mitochondria have long been considered as mediators of cell death in neuro-degenerative disorders. The significance of mitochondrial injury was previously thought to be limited to the potential effects such injury has on maintaining sufficient cellular ATP to avoid necrotic cell death. However, we now understand that mito-chondria are the primary mediators of cell death caused by abnormal levels of intra-cellular Ca^{2+} elicited during excitotoxicity[7] and that mitochondrial mechanisms of neural cell death include oxidative stress and apoptosis in addition to metabolic fail-ure (FIG. 1). Relatively mild mitochondrial injury, where ATP levels are maintained

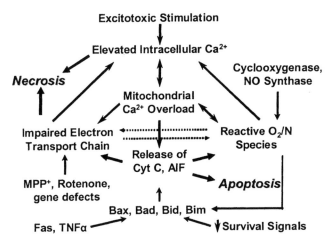

FIGURE 1. Mitochondrial mechanisms of neural cell death. Exitotoxic levels of intracellular Ca^{2+} accumulate within mitochondria, potentially causing metabolic failure, oxidative stress, and apoptosis via the release of cytochrome c and other proapoptotic mitochondrial proteins. Proteins, such as Bax, also mediate the release of mitochondrial cytochrome c, which, in addition to activating the caspase apoptotic cascade, can also stimulate mitochondrial free radical production. The levels and (or) subcellular distribution of these proteins is under the control of trophic factors and is also affected by oxidative stress. Mitochondrial free radical production is stimulated by the neurotoxins MPP^+ and rotenone and may be elevated by genomic or environmentally mediated alterations in electron transport chain activities.

near normal, results in mainly apoptotic cell death. More extensive injury that causes ATP depletion shifts the form of cell death toward necrosis. Excessive accumulation of Ca^{2+} that occurs during excitotoxic stimulation is likely not the only mediator of mitochondrial injury. Mitochondria are the targets of reactive oxygen species (ROS) generated by a number of different systems, including the mitochondrial electron transport chain (ETC), cyclooxygenases, Fe^{2+}-catalyzed hydroxyl radical ($OH^\bullet$) formation, and peroxynitrite formed from the reaction of nitric oxide ($NO^\bullet$) with superoxide (O_2^-). The levels and activities of mitochondrial antioxidant defense systems—for example, superoxide dismutase and glutathione peroxidase—and the redox state of mitochondrial NAD(P)H are therefore extremely important determinants of the extent of oxidative mitochondrial injury and neural cell survival.

THE INTRINSIC MITOCHONDRIAL PATHWAY OF APOPTOSIS

Discovery of the involvement of the release of mitochondrial cytochrome c in the activation of the cell death protease (caspase) cascade leading to apoptosis is one of the most important and certainly most unexpected events in the history of cell death research (FIG. 2). Release of several proapoptotic mitochondrial proteins, such as cytochrome c and apoptosis initiating factor (AIF), and their redistribution to the cytosol and nucleus during neural cell death *in vitro* and *in vivo* are well documented.[7] Sev-

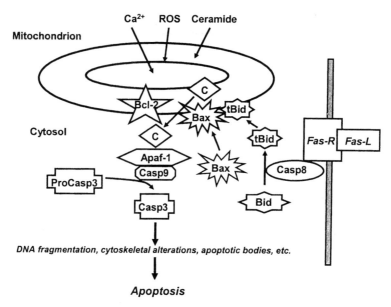

FIGURE 2. Mitochondrial participation in apoptosis. Agents, such as Ca^{2+}, ROS, and ceramide, as well as proapoptotic proteins, such as Bax, stimulate the release of other proapoptotic proteins—for example, cytochrome c (C in the figure)—from the mitochondrial intermembrane space into the cytosol. Cytochrome c and procaspase 9 together with apoptosis activating factor 1 (Apaf-1) form a multiprotein complex (apoptosome) that activates caspase 9, which then cleaves procaspase 3, forming active caspase 3. This caspase, together with other caspases it activates, proteolytically degrades a variety of proteins, causing the molecular and morphological alterations characteristic of apoptosis. Cell surface "death receptors," such as Fas, can activate caspase 3 directly through activation of caspase 8 (not shown) or participate in the mitochondrial pathway by processing Bid to form tBid, which greatly stimulates the release of cytochrome c by Bax. The antiapoptotic protein Bcl-2 is capable of inhibiting the release of cytochrome c mediated by either Ca^{2+} or Bax.

eral factors are capable of triggering the release of proapoptotic proteins from mitochondria, including elevated Ca^{2+}, ROS, ceramide, and other cell death proteins, such as Bax and tBid. Some apoptotic proteins, such as tBid, are activated by proteolytic cleavage and redistribute to the mitochondria in response to signals—for example, activation of the Fas and tumor necrosis factor (TNF)-α "cell death receptors." In addition to setting the mitochondrial pathway in motion, these receptors can trigger apoptosis via an "extrinsic pathway" by stimulating caspase 8–medated activation of caspase 3 through proteolytic cleavage. We obtained evidence for Fas receptor activation in the penumbra surrounding brain infarcts caused by closed head injury in humans.[8] The involvement of Fas and TNFα receptor activation in PD dopaminergic cell death is less clear. While the ligands for these receptors and other inflammatory cytokines are elevated in nigrostriatal dopaminergic regions and in the cerebrospinal fluid of PD patients,[9] these changes may reflect nonneuronal, proinflammatory cell activation.[10] Despite this controversy, abundant evidence obtained from patients and from animal models indicates that apoptosis plays a critical role in PD dopaminergic cell death and that the mitochondrial pathway of apoptosis is integrally involved.[11] Therefore, the molecular mechanisms responsible for the release of proapoptotic proteins from mitochondria are potential targets for therapeutic intervention in PD.

There are two fundamentally different mechanisms of mitochondrial protein release under consideration. The first involves physical disruption of the mitochondrial outer membrane and simple diffusion of cytochrome c from its normal exclusive location in the space located between the outer and inner mitochondrial membranes. The second mechanism involves transport of cytochrome c through a pore located in the outer membrane.

A likely cause for the physical disruption of the outer membrane is the osmotic swelling of the compartment surrounded by the inner membrane (matrix) due to an increased permeability of the inner membrane to small osmotically active solutes. There is a large body of literature describing this swelling phenomenon known as the mitochondrial membrane permeability transition (MPT).[12] This activity is triggered by abnormal mitochondrial Ca^{2+} accumulation and is promoted by oxidative stress and reactive metabolites, such as peroxynitrite. The MPT is generally defined as a relatively nonspecific increase in inner membrane permeability that results in a substantial increase in matrix volume and a decrease in mitochondrial membrane potential that can be inhibited by the presence of the drug cyclosporin A (CsA) and by overexpression of the antiapoptotic gene Bcl-2,[13] both of which protect against MPP+-induced dopaminergic cell death.[14,15] Although CsA is very effective at inhibiting the MPT for non neural cell mitochondria, Ca^{2+}-induced cytochrome c release from brain mitochondria is relatively resistant to inhibition by CsA in the presence of physiologically realistic concentrations of the cytosolic components Mg^{2+} and ATP.[16]

We recently found that 2-aminoethoxydiphenyl borate, an inhibitor of transient receptor potential (TRP) channels, is much more effective than CsA at protecting against Ca^{2+}-induced cytochrome c release from brain mitochondria.[17] This observation and others suggest that the MPT is associated with activation of Trp channels, a potential new class of targets for neuroprotection in PD and other brain disorders.

The MPT is an attractive mechanism of acute neural injury due to its activation by factors known to be associated with excitotoxicity and because of its sensitivity to inhibition by certain drugs and gene products known to be neuroprotective. However, increasing evidence indicates that the mechanism by which proapoptotic proteins such as Bax and tBid release cytochrome c and cause other forms of mitochondrial dysfunction is independent of the MPT and involves either pore formation or lipid alterations at the mitochondrial outer membrane.[18–20] The potential importance of Bax in PD is illustrated by the observation that Bax-knockout mice are resistant to nigrostriatal cell death induced by MPP+.[21]

The Bax-mediated mechanism of cytochrome c release is not inhibited by CsA but is inhibited by specific amphiphilic cations, such as dibucaine and propranolol, known to affect membrane lipid–protein interactions.[22] In addition to activation of proapoptotic proteins like Bid by cell death receptors, expression of the genes coding for these proteins and mitochondrial–protein interactions are promoted by high Ca^{2+} and ROS through their stimulation of complex signal transduction cascades.[23] Therefore, Ca^{2+} together with oxidative stress can promote cytochrome c release and apoptosis by both the MPT- and Bax-mediated molecular mechanisms that exhibit different pharmacologic sensitivities.

Mechanisms of mitochondrial proapoptotic protein release in addition to the MPT- and Bax-dependent pathways should also be considered. As AIF release appears downstream of cytochrome c release and caspase activation,[24] it is possible that proteolytic cleavage of AIF or an anchoring protein might be necessary. Also, as cytochrome c release stimulates mitochondrial generation of reactive oxygen species,[25] the oxidative modification of mitochondrial membrane lipids or proteins could be another event responsible for or promoting release of proapoptotic mitochondrial proteins.

A possible key to the development of mitochondrial neuroprotective interventions is the understanding of the mechanisms by which the antiapoptotic, mitochondrial protein Bcl-2 inhibits cytochrome c release mediated by both MPT-dependent and -independent pathways. Bcl-2 and its close relative Bcl-X_L exert some form of antioxidant activity that confers cytoprotection against ROS that may also inhibit activation of the MPT.[13,26] In contrast, Bcl-2 inhibition of Bax appears to involve direct protein–protein interaction, impairment of Bax oligomerization, and consequently inhibition of pore formation.[27] Stimulation of Bcl-2 expression has been demonstrated in several ischemic preconditioning paradigms and may represent a primary mechanism of neuroprotection by estrogen.[28] Investigators have also utilized protein transduction domains to deliver exogenous Bcl-X_L to cells throughout the brain and have demonstrated neuroprotection when these fusion proteins were administered by intraperitoneal injection up to 1 hour following the occlusion of the middle cerebral artery of mice.[29] Delivery of neuroprotective proteins, such as Bcl-2 and glial cell line–derived neurotrophic factor (GDNF), as a therapeutic approach for neurodegenerative disorders like Parkinson's disease is therefore possible and may prove to be effective.

MITOCHONDRIAL MECHANISMS OF REACTIVE OXYGEN SPECIES GENERATION

As several lines of evidence suggest that elevated mitochondrial ROS production contributes to the etiology of Parkinson's disease and as oxidative stress is a potent activator of apoptosis, understanding the mechanisms of mitochondrial free radical production is critically important in elucidating the pathophysiology of Parkinson's and other neurodegenerative diseases. The two most commonly cited sites of mitochondrial ROS production are ubisemiquinone (during complex III reduction) and complex I, although others, such as complex II, may also contribute.[30] The site of mitochondrial ROS production implicated most strongly in Parkinson's disease is complex I of the electron transport chain. Some neurotoxins that induce PD neuropathology *in vivo*, such as MPP^+ and rotenone, are inhibitors of complex I and stimulate ROS generation *in vitro*.[31] Acting along with hydroxyl radical ($OH^{\bullet}$) and peroxynitrite ($HNOO^-$), these ROS species can cause oxidative damage and inhibition of mitochondrial enzyme activities, including those of complex I and alpha-ketoglutarate dehydrogenase complex (αKGDC) (FIG. 3).[32,33] This inhibition can lead to metabolic failure through impairment of electron transport–dependent generation of the proton-motive force that drives the synthesis of ATP. Complete detoxification of superoxide depends on the enzymes superoxide dismutase (SOD), glutathione peroxidase (GPX), and glutathione reductase (GR) together with glutathione and a

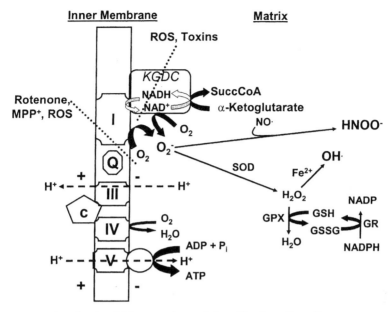

FIGURE 3. Mitochondrial generation and detoxification of reactive oxygen species. The site of mitochondrial reactive oxygen species (ROS) production most widely implicated in Parkinson's disease is complex I of the electron transport chain. Indirect evidence for involvement of complex I includes the observations that neurotoxins capable of inducing Parkinson's symptoms and neuropathology *in vivo*, such as MPP^+ and rotenone, are inhibitors of complex I and stimulate ROS generation *in vitro*. However, these same agents result in inhibition of the overall enzyme activity of α-ketoglutarate dehydrogenase complex (αKGDC), a multisubunit complex that can also catalyze superoxide (O_2^-) and consequently H_2O_2 production. The ROS metabolites most likely to mediate oxidative injury to mitochondria and other cellular constituents are hydroxyl radical ($OH^\bullet$) and peroxynitrite ($HNOO^-$). These agents can cause oxidative damage and inhibition of mitochondrial enzyme activities, including those of complex I and αKGDC. This inhibition can lead to metabolic failure through impairment of electron transport–dependent generation of the proton-motive force that drives the synthesis of ATP at complex V (F_1F_0 ATP synthetase). Complete detoxification of superoxide depends on the enzymes superoxide dismutase (SOD), glutathione peroxidase (GPX), and glutathione reductase (GR) together with glutathione and a sufficiently reduced redox state of NAD(P)H to drive the reduction of glutathione and consequently the reduction of H_2O_2 to H_2O.

sufficiently reduced redox state of NAD(P)H to drive the reduction of glutathione and consequently the reduction of H_2O_2 to H_2O.

Our recent observations indicate that in addition to complex I, several tricarboxylic acid cycle dehydrogenases are potential sources of ROS, with αKGDH appearing the most active.[34] In particular, the rate of ROS production by isolated brain mitochondria measured under a state of rapid metabolism, as normally exists in neurons, was highest with α-ketoglutarate as respiratory substrate, even though several other substrates support higher rates of respiration. Zinc also promotes ROS production by the lipoamide dehydrogenase component of aKGDH, but it inhibits overall enzyme activity.[35] Considering the findings that environmental exposure to zinc is a risk factor for Parkinson's disease and that αKGDH enzyme activity is reduced in PD and in Alzheimer's disease,[36] the relationships between this enzyme complex, ROS production, and dopaminergic cell death in cellular and animal models of PD require further investigation.

REFERENCES

1. PARKER, W.D.J., S.J. BOYSON & J.K. PARKS. 1989. Abnormalities of the electron transport chain in idiopathic Parkinson's disease. Ann. Neurol. **26:** 719–723.
2. SHULTS, C.W., R.H. HAAS, D. PASSOV & M.F. BEAL. 1997. Coenzyme Q10 levels correlate with the activities of complexes I and II/III in mitochondria from parkinsonian and nonparkinsonian subjects. Ann. Neurol. **42:** 261–264.
3. SWERDLOW, R.H., J.K. PARKS, S.W. MILLER, et al. 1996. Origin and functional consequences of the complex I defect in Parkinson's disease. Ann. Neurol. **40:** 663–671.
4. SHEEHAN, J.P., R.H. SWERDLOW, S.W. MILLER, et al. 1997. Calcium homeostasis and reactive oxygen species production in cells transformed by mitochondria from individuals with sporadic Alzheimer's disease. J. Neurosci. **17:** 4612–4622.
5. TRIMMER, P.A., R.H. SWERDLOW, J.K. PARKS, et al. 2000. Abnormal mitochondrial morphology in sporadic Parkinson's and Alzheimer's disease cybrid cell lines. Exp. Neurol. **162:** 37–50.
6. BETARBET, R., T.B. SHERER, G. MACKENZIE, et al. 2000. Chronic systemic pesticide exposure reproduces features of Parkinson's disease. Nat. Neurosci. **3:** 1301–1306.
7. FISKUM, G. 2000. Mitochondrial participation in ischemic and traumatic neural cell death. J. Neurotrauma **17:** 843–855.
8. QIU, J., M.J. WHALEN, P. LOWENSTEIN, et al. 2002. Upregulation of the Fas receptor death-inducing signaling complex after traumatic brain injury in mice and humans. J. Neurosci. **22:** 3504–3511.
9. NAGATSU, T., M. MOGI, H. ICHINOSE & A. TOGARI. 2000. Changes in cytokines and neurotrophins in Parkinson's disease. J. Neural Transm. Suppl. 277–290.
10. FERRER, I., R. BLANCO, B. CUTILLAS & S. AMBROSIO. 2000. Fas and Fas-L expression in Huntington's disease and Parkinson's disease. Neuropathol. Appl. Neurobiol. **26:** 424–433.
11. DAWSON, T.M. & V.L. DAWSON. 2002. Neuroprotective and neurorestorative strategies for Parkinson's disease. Nat. Neurosci. **5** Suppl.: 1058–1061.
12. FRIBERG, H. & T. WIELOCH. 2002. Mitochondrial permeability transition in acute neurodegeneration. Biochimie **84:** 241–250.
13. KOWALTOWSKI, A.J., A.E. VERCESI & G. FISKUM. 2000. Bcl-2 prevents mitochondrial permeability transition and cytochrome c release via maintenance of reduced pyridine nucleotides. Cell Death. Differ. **7:** 903–910.
14. SEATON, T.A., J.M. COOPER & A.H. SCHAPIRA. 1998. Cyclosporin inhibition of apoptosis induced by mitochondrial complex I toxins. Brain Res. **809:** 12–17.
15. YANG, L., R.T. MATTHEWS, J.B. SCHULZ, et al. 1998. 1-Methyl-4-phenyl-1,2,3,6-tetrahydropyride neurotoxicity is attenuated in mice overexpressing Bcl-2. J. Neurosci. **18:** 8145–8152.
16. ANDREYEV, A. & G. FISKUM. 1999. Calcium induced release of mitochondrial cytochrome c by different mechanisms selective for brain versus liver. Cell Death. Differ. **6:** 825–832.
17. CHINOPOULOS, C., A.A. STARKOV & G. FISKUM. 2003. Cyclosporin A-insensitive permeability transition in brain mitochondria: inhibition by 2-aminoethoxydiphenyl borate. J. Biol. Chem. In press.
18. KORSMEYER, S.J., M.C. WEI, M. SAITO, et al. 2000. Pro-apoptotic cascade activates BID, which oligomerizes BAK or BAX into pores that result in the release of cytochrome c. Cell Death Differ. **7:** 1166–1173.
19. KUWANA, T., M.R. MACKEY, G. PERKINS, et al. 2002. Bid, Bax, and lipids cooperate to form supramolecular openings in the outer mitochondrial membrane. Cell **111:** 331–342.

20. POLSTER, B.M., K.W. KINNALLY & G. FISKUM. 2001. Bh3 death domain peptide induces cell type-selective mitochondrial outer membrane permeability. J. Biol. Chem. **276:** 37887–37894.
21. VILA, M., V. JACKSON-LEWIS, S. VUKOSAVIC, *et al.* 2001. Bax ablation prevents dopaminergic neurodegeneration in the 1-methyl- 4-phenyl-1,2,3,6-tetrahydropyridine mouse model of Parkinson's disease. Proc. Natl. Acad. Sci. USA **98:** 2837–2842.
22. POLSTER, B.M. & G. FISKUM. 2003. Inhibition of Bax-induced cytochrome c release from neural cell and brain mitochondria by dibucaine and propranolol. J. Neurosci. **23:** 2735–2743.
23. MARTIN, L.J. 2001. Neuronal cell death in nervous system development, disease, and injury. Int. J. Mol. Med. **7:** 455–478.
24. ARNOULT, D., P. PARONE, J.C. MARTINOU, *et al.* 2002. Mitochondrial release of apoptosis-inducing factor occurs downstream of cytochrome c release in response to several proapoptotic stimuli. J. Cell Biol. **159:** 923–929.
25. STARKOV, A.A., B.M. POLSTER & G. FISKUM. 2002. Regulation of hydrogen peroxide production by brain mitochondria by calcium and Bax. J. Neurochem. **83:** 220–228.
26. OUYANG, Y., S. CARRIEDO & R. GIFFARD. 2002. Effect of Bcl-X(L) overexpression on reactive oxygen species, intracellular calcium, and mitochondrial membrane potential following injury in astrocytes. Free Radic. Biol. Med. **33:** 544.
27. CHENG, E.H., M.C. WEI, S. WEILER, *et al.* 2001. BCL-2, BCL-X(L) sequester BH3 domain-only molecules preventing BAX- and BAK-mediated mitochondrial apoptosis. Mol. Cell **8:** 705–711.
28. ALKAYED, N.J., S. GOTO, N. SUGO, *et al.* 2001. Estrogen and Bcl-2: gene induction and effect of transgene in experimental stroke. J. Neurosci. **21:** 7543–7550.
29. CAO, G., W. PEI, H. GE, *et al.* 2002. In vivo delivery of a Bcl-xL fusion protein containing the TAT protein transduction domain protects against ischemic brain injury and neuronal apoptosis. J. Neurosci. **22:** 5423–5431.
30. BOVERIS, A. 1977. Mitochondrial production of superoxide radical and hydrogen peroxide. Adv. Exp. Med. Biol. **78:** 67–82.
31. LENAZ, G., C. BOVINA, M. D'AURELIO, *et al.* 2002. Role of mitochondria in oxidative stress and aging. Ann. N.Y. Acad. Sci. **959:** 199–213.
32. HILLERED, L. & L. ERNSTER. 1983. Respiratory activity of isolated rat brain mitochondria following in vitro exposure to oxygen radicals. J. Cereb. Blood Flow Metab. **3:** 207–214.
33. NULTON-PERSSON, A.C. & L.I. SZWEDA. 2001. Modulation of mitochondrial function by hydrogen peroxide. J. Biol. Chem. **276:** 23357–23361.
34. STARKOV, A. & G. FISKUM. 2002. Generation of reactive oxygen species by brain mitochondria mediated by alpha-ketoglutarate dehydrogenase. Soc. Neurosci. 194.17.
35. GAZARYAN, I.G., B.F. KRASNIKOV, G.A. ASHBY, *et al.* 2002. Zinc is a potent inhibitor of thiol oxidoreductase activity and stimulates reactive oxygen species production by lipoamide dehydrogenase. J. Biol. Chem. **277:** 10064–10072.
36. GIBSON, G.E., L.C. PARK, K.F. SHEU, *et al.* 2000. The alpha-ketoglutarate dehydrogenase complex in neurodegeneration. Neurochem. Int. **36:** 97–112.

Mitochondria, Oxidative Damage, and Inflammation in Parkinson's Disease

M. FLINT BEAL

*Department of Neurology and Neuroscience, Weill Medical College of Cornell University,
New York Presbyterian Hospital, New York, New York 10021, USA*

ABSTRACT: The pathogenesis of Parkinson's disease (PD) remains obscure, but there is increasing evidence that impairment of mitochondrial function, oxidative damage, and inflammation are contributing factors. The present paper reviews the experimental and clinical evidence implicating these processes in PD. There is substantial evidence that there is a deficiency of complex I activity of the mitochondrial electron transport chain in PD. There is also evidence for increased numbers of activated microglia in both PD postmortem tissue as well as in animal models of PD. Impaired mitochondrial function and activated microglia may both contribute to oxidative damage in PD. A number of therapies targeting inflammation and mitochondrial dysfunction are efficacious in the MPTP model of PD. Of these, coenzyme Q_{10} appears to be particularly promising based on the results of a recent phase 2 clinical trial in which it significantly slowed the progression of PD.

KEYWORDS: inflammation; microglia; mitochondria; oxidative damage; creatine; coenzyme Q_{10}

THE ROLE OF FREE RADICALS AND IMPAIRED ENERGY METABOLISM IN PARKINSON'S DISEASE

All aerobic organisms are continually exposed to oxidative stress.[1] Oxidative phosphorylation involves the transfer of electrons, which can lead to the generation of free radicals, independently existing species that contain one or more unpaired electrons. Most free radicals are unstable reactive species that can extract an electron from neighboring molecules to complete their own orbital. This leads to oxidation of neighboring molecules. Critical biologic molecules including DNA, proteins, and membrane lipids are subject to oxidative damage.

Mitochondria are believed to be the most important cellular source of free radicals generating superoxide radicals at ubiquinone and NADH dehydrogenase (complex I).[2] Superoxide is normally converted by superoxide dismutase (SOD) to H_2O_2. H_2O_2 reacts with transition metals to generate hydroxyl radicals, the prime mediators of cell damage. Superoxide can also react with nitric oxide to the form of per-

Address for correspondence: M. Flint Beal, M.D., Chairman, Department of Neurology and Neuroscience, Weill Medical College of Cornell University, 525 East 68th Street, Room F610, New York, NY 10021. Voice: 212-746-6575; fax: 212-746-8532.

fbeal@med.cornell.edu

Ann. N.Y. Acad. Sci. 991: 120–131 (2003). © 2003 New York Academy of Sciences.

oxynitrite (ONOO$^-$).[3] This reaction occurs at the rate of 6.7×10^9 M^{-1} S^{-1}, threefold faster than the rate of superoxide dismutation by superoxide dismutase. Peroxynitrite generation thus depends on the concentration of superoxide and nitric oxide in the cell. Peroxynitrite can exist in an activated "hydroxyl radical–like" transitional state. At physiologic pH, peroxynitrite may diffuse over several cell diameters to produce cell damage by oxidizing lipids, proteins, and DNA. Peroxynitrite can react with Cu,Zn SOD to form nitronium ion, which may then nitrate tyrosine residues.[4] The 3-nitrotyrosine so generated is an excellent biochemical marker of peroxynitrite-mediated oxidative damage.

Much of the current interest in the association between neurodegeneration and mitochondrial dysfunction/oxidative damage stems from studies of 1-methyl-4-phenyl-1,2,3,6-tetrahydropyridine (MPTP)-induced parkinsonism. The MPTP model of PD results in a clinical syndrome that replicates the major features of PD in man and nonhuman primates.[5] MPTP is metabolized to MPTP$^+$ and MPP$^+$ (1-methyl-4-phenylpyridinium) by the enzyme monoamine oxidase B. MPP$^+$ is subsequently selectively taken up by dopaminergic terminals and concentrated in neuronal mitochondria in the substantia nigra. *In vitro* experiments demonstrated that nicotinamide dehydrogenase (NADH), complex I of the electron transport chain, is weakly and reversibly inhibited by MPP$^+$, leading to reductions in mitochondrial ATP production.[6] MPP$^+$ can also cause irreversible inactivation of complex I by generating free radicals and increasing lipid peroxidation.[7] Inhibition of NADH dehydrogenase by MPP$^+$ leads to superoxide production in isolated bovine heart submitochondrial particles and *in vivo*.[8,9] Finally, MPTP-induced damage is attenuated in transgenic mice overexpressing superoxide dismutase.[10] We previously showed that mice deficient in either MnSOD or glutathione peroxidase show increased vulnerability to MPTP toxicity.[11,12] Thus, the MPTP model of parkinsonism has already set a precedent for a causal relationship between mitochondrial dysfunction and oxidative cellular damage.

Evidence extending this hypothesis to the pathogenesis of idiopathic PD comes from a 30–40% decrease in complex I activity in the substantia nigra.[13–16] Reduced staining for complex I subunits in PD substantia nigra, but preserved staining for subunits of the other electron transport complexes, has been demonstrated immunohistochemically.[17] Strong support for a mitochondrial DNA–encoded defect comes from studies that showed that complex I defects from PD platelets are transferable into mitochondrial-deficient cell lines.[18,19] These defects are associated with increased free radical production, increased susceptibility to MPP$^+$, and impaired mitochondrial calcium buffering.[20] Direct sequencing of mitochondrial complex I and tRNA genes, however, failed to show homoplasmic mutations.[21]

OXIDATIVE DAMAGE IN PD

A great deal of interest has been focused on the possibility that oxidative damage may play a role in the pathogenesis of PD. There are studies showing increased levels of malondialdehyde and cholesterol lipid hydroperoxides, markers for lipid peroxidation, in PD substantia nigra.[22,23] There are widespread increases in protein carbonyls in PD postmortem brain tissue.[24] Concentrations of 8-hydroxy-2-deoxyguanosine, a marker of oxidative damage to DNA, are significantly increased in PD substantia nigra and striatum.[25,26] However, attempts to detect increased free radicals using electron spin resonance have been unsuccessful. Evidence for nitrosyl radicals in PD substantia nigra was recently obtained.[27] Another means of looking for oxidative stress is to measure concentrations of reduced glutathione. Reduced glutathione is decreased in PD substantia nigra by approximately 50%.[28–31] Individuals with incidental Lewy body disease may have presymptomatic PD, and they have a 35% reduction in reduced glutathione as compared with age-matched controls.[32]

INFLAMMATION AND PD

There is increasing evidence that inflammation may contribute to PD pathogenesis. There is an increase in reactive microglia in the striatum and substantia nigra of patients with idiopathic PD.[33,34] Although gliosis may in some circumstances be beneficial, at other times it exerts deleterious effects. Microglial cells, which are the resident macrophages in the brain, respond to many insults with rapid proliferation, hypertrophy, and expression of a number of cytokines.[35,36] The brain area that encompasses the substantia nigra has the highest density of microglia in the brain.[37] Activated microglia upregulate cell surface markers such as the macrophage antigen complex-I (MAC-1), and they produce a variety of proinflammatory cytokines. There appears to be a graded response with differential expression depending on the severity of the insult.[36] A consequence of activation of microglia is the production of reactive oxygen species. They can originate from NADPH oxidase, which produces superoxide ($O_2^\bullet$); COX-2, which produces free radicals as a byproduct of prostaglandin synthesis; and from inducible nitric oxide synthase (iNOS), which generates $NO^\bullet$. iNOS, because it does not require Ca^{2+} for activity, produces much higher levels of $NO^\bullet$ for longer periods (hours) than do the endothelial and neuronal isoforms of NOS, which require Ca^{2+} for activity. NADPH-oxidase is a major source of activity-dependent superoxide.[38] The reaction of $O_2^\bullet$ with $NO^\bullet$ generates peroxynitrite $ONOO^-$, which is strongly implicated in PD pathogenesis. Prior studies showed that Lewy body–positive substantia nigra neurons in PD stain with antibodies to 3-nitrotyrosine, which is thought to be a specific marker for peroxynitrite-mediated damage.[39] More recent studies showed that Lewy bodies react with antibodies to nitrated α-synuclein, the major protein component of Lewy bodies.[40]

It was reported in a small number of cases that the mRNA for the Clq and C9 components of complement are increased in PD substantia nigra.[41] A number of cytokines including interleukin (IL)-1, IL-6, and tumor necrosis factor (TNF)-α contribute to inflammatory processes. Studies of TNFα showed it to be increased 366% in the striatum and 432% in the cerebrospinal fluid (CSF) of PD patients.[42] Furthermore, an increase in TNFα imunoreactive glial cells was reported in the substantia nigra of PD patients, as compared to controls.[43,44]

The density of glial cells expressing IL-1β and interferon (IFN)-γ was also increased in PD substantia nigra.[44] Others found increased levels of Il-1β and IL-6 in the caudate, putamen, and cerebral cortex of postmortem PD brains.[45] Both IL-1β and IL-6 were also found to be increased in the CSF of PD patients.[46] Another group found an increase in IL-6 in the CSF of PD patients and reported that levels inversely correlate with the severity of PD.[47] Last, an IL-1β polymorphism was reported to increase the risk of PD.[48,49]

INFLAMMATION IN ANIMAL MODELS

Although there has been tremendous progress in genetic models of PD, they are not yet ideal in producing the cardinal features of PD.[5] The most experience has been with toxin models of PD including MPTP, rotenone, and 6-hydroxydopamine. An activation of microglia in both the striatum and in the substantia nigra has been well documented to occur in the MPTP model of PD.[50–52] The microglial activation was associated with elevated IL-6 levels.[50] MPTP toxicity is also associated with increases in IL-1β.[53] We demonstrated that mice deficient in IL-1β converting enzyme are markedly resistant to MPTP neurotoxicity.[54] A recent study showed that minocycline prevented MPTP-induced activation of microglia, as well as the formation of IL-1β, activation of NADPH-oxidase, and induction of iNOS.[52] This was associated with reduced 3-nitrotyrosine formation, and reduced loss of substantia nigra dopaminergic neurons.[52] Another group showed protection as well[55] but suggested that minocycline may also have direct neuroprotective effects. This was recently shown to be the case with direct effects on the mitochondrial permeability transition and cytochrome c release.[56] The importance of inflammation was underscored by a study of humans exposed to MPTP in which persistent activation of microglia was associated with oxidative degeneration of substantia nigra neurons.[57] Recently systemic administration of rotenone to rats was shown to produce an excellent animal model of PD.[58] Studies of rotenone toxicity in neuron/glia cultures from rat mesencephalon show enhanced neurodegeneration in the presence of glia.[59] A critical feature of the toxicity was the release of $O_2^\bullet$ from microglia, which was attenuated by inhibitors of NADPH oxidase.

There is also substantial evidence for neuroinflammation playing a role in progressive neurodegeneration following administration of 6-hydroxydopamine.[60] Studies using PET and PK1195 (a ligand for activated microglia) showed that an increase in activated microglia occurs coincident with loss of dopaminergic neurons.[61] Minocycline was reported to inhibit microglial activation and to protect nigral cells after 6-OHDA injection into mouse striatum.[62] Chronic infusion of lipopolysaccharide for 2 weeks into the substantia nigra results in rapid activation of microglia, followed by a delayed and gradual loss of nigral neurons beginning at 4–6 weeks and reaching 70% at 10 weeks.[63]

ANTIINFLAMMATORY AGENTS FOR NEUROPROTECTION

A number of antiinflammatory agents have shown promise for the amelioration of degeneration of dopaminergic neurons induced by MPTP. Approaches have utilized both transgenic mice as well as pharmacologic agents. MPTP-induced activation of microglia is associated with an upregulation of iNOS and 3-nitrotyrosine formation.[64] Studies in iNOS-deficient mice show that degeneration of dopaminergic neurons is significantly attenuated; but there is no protection of dopaminergic terminals.[64,65] However, there have been no reports of the effects of pharmacologic inhibition of iNOS on MPTP neurotoxicity. Another inflammatory pathway implicated in neurodegeneration is cyclooxygenase 2 (COX-2). COX-2 is expressed and regulated in glial cells by cytokines and lipopolysaccharide.[66] However, in excitotoxic lesions, synaptic excitation, apoptotic neuronal death, and cerebral ischemia

COX-2 is expressed primarily in neurons.[67–70] Cyclooxygenase catalyzes the formation of prostaglandins, which involves reduction of the hydroperoxide resulting in the generation of free radicals. Superoxide radicals, a COX-2 reaction product, can react with NO$^{\bullet}$ to form the strong oxidant peroxynitrite. A recent study showed that overexpression of COX-2 can activate cell cycle genes, which may contribute to apoptotic cell death.[71] Mice overexpressing COX-2 show increased vulnerability to kainic acid and have elevated lipid peroxidation. COX-2 inhibitors inhibit lipopolysaccharide-induced increases in TNF-α, which can stimulate astrocytic glutamate release.[72,73] Neuronal death mediated by N-methyl-D-aspartate (NMDA) is diminished in a dose-dependent manner by COX-2 inhibitors in primary neuronal cultures.[74] Transgenic mice that are deficient in COX-2 show reduced susceptibility to focal ischemia and to NMDA neurotoxicity.[75] The COX-2 inhibitor meloxicam significantly attenuated both the reduction of striatal dopamine levels and the depletion of substantia nigra dopaminergic neurons.[76] In COX-2–deficient mice, however, there was protection against loss of dopaminergic neurons in the substantia nigra, but no protective effect against lowering of striatal dopamine levels.[77]

Another promising approach is to use thalidomide. Thalidomide reduces COX-2 levels and also inhibits TNFα production.[78-80] Mice deficient in both TNFα receptors are resistant to MPTP toxicity.[81] Thalidomide has been reported to attenuate MPTP-induced decreases in striatal dopamine levels, but the numbers of dopaminergic neurons in the substantia nigra were not examined.[82] Another approach is to use phosphodiesterase IV inhibitors, which inhibit the breakdown of cAMP. Phosphodiesterase IV is selectively localized to immune cells and the central nervous system. Type IV phosphodiesterase inhibitors are effective against inflammatory lesions in the central nervous system, such as those produced in experimental autoimmune encephalomyelitis.[83,84] Rolipram inhibits lipopolysaccharide-induced increases in plasma levels of TNFα in rats.[85] Phosphodiesterase IV inhibitors are also neuroprotective against MPTP neurotoxicity.[86] In these studies, several phosphodiesterase IV inhibitors produced neuroprotection against both MPTP-induced depletion of striatal dopamine and as loss of substantia nigra neurons.

Last, peroxisome proliferator–activated receptor (PPAR)–γ agonists show good antiinflammatory effects. A broad range of proinflammatory genes are transcriptionally regulated by the nuclear hormone receptor PPAR-γ. PPARs are a subfamily of ligand-activated transcription factors structurally related to the steroid and retinoic acid receptor families.[87] The PPAR-γ isoform is expressed in adipocytes, where it regulates lipid metabolism and reduces insulin resistance. Newly developed drugs of the thiazolidinedione class target the PPAR-γ receptor and reduce plasma glucose in type 2 diabetics, although they do not alter glucose levels in nondiabetic animals and humans.[88] PPAR-γ agonists suppress the expression of the proinflammatory cytokines IL-1β, TNFα, and IL-6,[89, 90] as well as of MMP-9 and iNOS.[91–93] The PPAR-γ agonist troglitazone reduces cell death in cultured cerebellar neurons after glutamate exposure.[94] The PPAR-γ agonist pioglitazone reduced the severity and incidence of experimental allergic encephalomyelitis.[95] Pioglitazone was recently shown to exert neuroprotective effects against MPTP-induced degeneration of substantia nigra neurons; however, it did not protect against striatal dopamine depletion.[96] Lipopolysaccharide induces iNOS expression and release of nitric oxide in microglia, and COX-2 expression in neurons.[97] PPAR-γ agonists inhibit lipopolysaccharide-induced cell death as well as increases in nitric oxide and COX-2 activity.[97]

COENZYME Q_{10} AND CREATINE AS POTENTIAL THERAPIES FOR PD

Coenzyme Q_{10}, which is also known as ubiquinone, is an essential cofactor of the electron transport chain, where it accepts electrons from complexes 1 and 2.[98] Coenzyme Q_{10} also serves as an important antioxidant in both mitochondria and lipid membranes.[99,100] It is a lipid-soluble compound composed of redox-active quinone as well as a hydrophobic tail. It is soluble and mobile in the hydrophobic core of the phospholipid bilayer of the inner membrane of the mitochondria.

Considerable interest has been shown in the potential utility of coenzyme Q_{10} for treatment of mitochondrial disorders.[101] There have been several reports of beneficial effects in patients with mitochondrial defects; and we have demonstrated that coenzyme Q_{10} increased brain mitochondrial coenzyme Q_{10} concentrations in mature and older animals.[102] It also decreased α-tocopherol concentrations in mitochondria consistent with a sparing effect. We found that coenzyme Q_{10} exerts neuroprotective effects against the mitochondrial toxins malonate and 3-nitropropionic acid.[103,104] It also showed neuroprotective effects against MPTP toxicity in older mice.[105] We found that coenzyme Q_{10} levels were significantly reduced in mitochondria from PD patients.[106] We also demonstrated that coenzyme Q_{10} supplementation significantly increased plasma levels in PD patients. Recently a small phase II clinical trial was undertaken.[107] Patients were assigned to placebo or coenzyme Q_{10} at 300, 600, or 1200 mg daily. They were evaluated using the Unified Parkinson's Disease Rating Scale at screening, baseline, and up to 16 months. In this pilot trial the administration of coenzyme Q_{10} showed a significant slowing of disease progression.

We also investigated whether creatine can exert neuroprotective effects. The creatine kinase system can shuttle high-energy phosphates such as phosphocreatine (PCr) to sites of energy usage in the cell, such as ion pumps in organelles, the plasma membranes, and the endoplasmic reticulum.[108,109] Creatine may exert neuroprotective effects by increasing PCr levels and thereby providing extra energy for ion homeostasis and the functional and structural integrity of mitochondria. Creatine exerts neuroprotective effects *in vitro* as well as *in vivo*. Creatine protects against both glutamate and β-amyloid toxicity in rat hippocampal neurons.[110,111] Creatine also protects against 3-nitropropionic acid and glutamate neurotoxicity in rat hippocampal and striatal neurons.[112] We found that creatine protects against both malonate and 3-nitropropionic acid striatal neurotoxicity *in vivo*;[102] and against MPTP toxicity in a dose-dependent manner.[111] Creatine administration also exerts neuroprotective effects in transgenic mouse models of both amyotrophic lateral sclerosis and Huntington's disease.[113–115] We recently demonstrated that creatine can exert additive neuroprotective effects when administered in combination with COX-2 inhibitors against MPTP neurotoxicity (unpublished data).

CONCLUSIONS

The pathogenesis of PD is unknown, but a substantial body of evidence implicates both mitochondrial dysfunction, oxidative damage, and inflammation in disease pathogenesis. Agents targeting both mitochondrial dysfunction and inflammation are effective in attenuating damage to dopaminergic neurons in the

MPTP model of PD. One of these agents, coenzyme Q_{10}, has shown initial promise as an agent to slow the progression of PD. Clinical trials of other agents to slow the progress of PD are urgently needed. We suspect that combinations of agents targeting different disease mechanisms may produce additive or synergistic neuroprotective effects that will lead to effective therapies to slow or halt PD.

ACKNOWLEDGMENTS

I wish to thank Sharon Melanson for secretarial assistance. This work was supported by grants from The Department of Defense and the Parkinson's Disease Foundation.

REFERENCES

1. HALLIWELL, B. 1992. Reactive oxygen species and the central nervous system. J. Neurochem. **59:** 1609–1623.
2. TURRENS, J.F., A. ALEXANDRE & A.L. LEHNINGER. 1985. Ubisemiquinone is the electron donor for superoxide formation by complex III of heart mitochondria. Arch. Biochem. Biophys. **237:** 408–414.
3. BECKMAN, J.S. & J.P. CROW. 1993. Pathological implications of nitric oxide superoxide and peroxynitrite formation. Biochem. Soc. Trans. **21:** 330–334.
4. ISCHIROPOULOS, H., L. ZHU, J. CHEN, et al. 1992. Peroxynitrite-mediated tyrosine nitration catalyzed by superoxide dismutase. Arch. Biochem. Biophys. **298:** 431–437.
5. BEAL, M.F. 2001. Experimental models of Parkinson's disease. Nat. Rev. Neurosci. **2:** 325–334.
6. SINGER, T.P., N. CASTAGNOLI, R.R. RAMSAY & A.J. TREVOR. 1987. Biochemical events in the development of parkinsonism induced by MPTP. J. Neurochem. **49:** 1–8.
7. CLEETER, M.J.W., J.M. COOPER & A.H.V. SCHAPIRA. 1992. Irreversible inhibition of mitochondrial complex I by 1-methyl-4-phenylpyridium: evidence for free radical involvement. J. Neurochem. **58:** 786–789.
8. HASEGAWA, E., K. TAKESHIGE, T. OISHI, et al. 1990. MPP^+ induces NADH dependent superoxide formation and enhances NADH dependent lipid peroxidation in bovine heart submitochondrial particles. Biochem. Biophys. Res. Commun. **170:** 1049–1055.
9. SRIRAM, K., K.S. PAI, M.R. BOYD & V. RAVINDRANATH. 1997. Evidence for generation of oxidative stress in brain by MPTP: in vitro and in vivo studies in mice. Brain Res. **749:** 44–52.
10. PRZEDBORSKI, S., V. KOSTIC, V. JACKSON-LEWIS, et al. 1992. Transgenic mice with increased Cu/Zn-superoxide dismutase activity are resistant to N-methyl-4-phenyl-1,2,3,6-tetrahydropyridine-induced neurotoxicity. J. Neurosci. **12:** 1658–1667.
11. ANDREASSEN, O.A., R.J. FERRANTE, A. DEDEOGLU, et al. 2001. Mice with a partial deficiency of manganese superoxide dismutase show increased vulnerability to the mitochondrial toxins malonate, 3- nitropropionic acid, and MPTP. Exp. Neurol. **167:** 189–195.
12. KLIVENYI, P., O.A. ANDREASSEN, R.J. FERRANTE, et al. 2000. Inhibition of neuronal nitric oxide synthase protects against MPTP toxicity. Neuroreport **11:** 1265–1268.
13. BINDOFF, L.A., M. BIRCH-MARTIN, N.E.F. CARTLIDGE, et al. 1989. Mitochondrial function in Parkinsons disease. Lancet **1:** 49.
14. SCHAPIRA, A.H.V., J.M. COOPER, D. DEXTER, et al. 1990. Mitochondrial complex I deficiency in Parkinson's disease. J. Neurochem. **54:** 823–827.
15. JANETZKY, B., S. HAUCK, M.B.H. YOUDIM, et al. 1994. Unaltered aconitase activity, but decreased complex I activity, in substantia nigra pars compacta of patients with Parkinson's disease. Neurosci. Lett. **169:** 126–128.
16. MANN, V.M., J.M. COOPER, D. KRIGE, et al. 1992. Brain, skeletal muscle, and platelet homogenate mitochondrial function in Parkinson's disease. Brain **115:** 333–342.

17. HATTORI, N., M. TANAKA, T. OZAWA & Y. MIZUNO. 1991. Immunohistochemical studies on complexes I, II, III and IV of mitochondria in Parkinson's disease. Ann. Neurol. **30:** 563–571.
18. SWERDLOW, R.H., J.K. PARKS, S.W. MILLER, et al. 1996. Origin and functional consequences of the complex I defect in Parkinson's disease. Ann. Neurol. **40:** 663–671.
19. GU, M., J.M. COOPER, J.W. TAANMAN & A.H.V. SCHAPIRA. 1998. Mitochondrial DNA transmission of the mitochondrial defect in Parkinson's disease. Ann. Neurol. **44:** 177–186.
20. SHEEHAN, J.P., R.H. SWERDLOW, W.D. PARKER, et al. 1997. Altered calcium homeostasis in cells transformed by mitochondria from individuals with Parkinson's disease. J. Neurochem. **68:** 1221–1233.
21. SIMON, D.K., R. MAYEUX, K. MARDER, et al. 2000. Mitochondrial DNA mutations in complex I and tRNA genes in Parkinson's disease. Neurology **54:** 703–709.
22. DEXTER, D.T., C.J. CARTER, F.R. WELLS, et al. 1989. Basal lipid peroxidation in substantia nigra is increased in Parkinson's disease. J. Neurochem. **52:** 381–389.
23. DEXTER, D.T., A.E. HOLLY, W.D. FLITTER, et al. 1994. Increased levels of lipid hydroperoxides in the Parkinsonian substantia nigra: an HPLC and ESR study. Mov. Disord. **9:** 92–97.
24. ALAM, Z.I., S.E. DANIEL, A.J. LEES, et al. 1997. A generalised increase in protein carbonyls in the brain in Parkinson's but not incidental Lewy body disease. J. Neurochem. **69:** 1326–1329.
25. ALAM, Z.I., A. JENNER, S.E. DANIEL, et al. 1997. Oxidative DNA damage in the Parkinsonian brain: an apparent selective increase in 8-hydroxyguanine levels in substantia nigra. J. Neurochem. **69:** 1196–1203.
26. SANCHEZ-RAMOS, J.R., E. OVERVIK & B.N. AMES. 1994. A marker of oxyradical-mediated DNA damage (8-hydroxy-2′ deoxyguanosine) is increased in nigro-striatum of Parkinson's disease brain. Neurodegeneration. **3:** 197–204.
27. SHERGILL, J.K., R. CAMMACK, C.E. COOPER, et al. 1996. Detection of nitrosyl complexes in human substantia nigra, in relation to Parkinson's disease. Biochem. Biophys. Res. Commun. **228:** 298–305.
28. PERRY, T.L., D.V. GODIN & S. HANSEN. 1982. Parkinson's disease: a disorder due to nigral glutathione deficiency? Neurosci. Lett. **33:** 305–310.
29. PERRY, T.L. & V.W. YONG. 1986. Idiopathic Parkinson's disease, progressive supranuclear palsy and glutathione metabolism in the substantia nigra of patients. Neurosci. Lett. **67:** 269–274.
30. RIEDERER, P., J.-W. PARK & B. AMES. 1989. Transition metals, ferritin, glutathione, and ascorbic in parkinsonian brains. J. Neurochem. **52:** 515–520.
31. SOFIC, E., K.W. LANGE, K. JELLINGER & P. RIEDERER. 1992. Reduced and oxidized glutathione in the substantia nigra of patients with Parkinson's disease. Neurosci. Lett. **142:** 128–130.
32. DEXTER, D.T., J. SIAN, S. ROSE, et al. 1994. Indices of oxidative stress and mitochondrial function in individuals with incidental Lewy body disease. Ann. Neurol. **35:** 38–44.
33. MCGEER, P.L., S. ITAGAKI, B.E. BOYES & E.G. MCGEER. 1988. Reactive microglia are positive for HLA-DR in the substantia nigra of Parkinson's and Alzheimer's disease brains. Neurology **38:** 1285–1291.
34. MIRZA, Z.N., M. KATO, H. KIMURA, et al. 2002. Fenoterol inhibits superoxide anion generation by human polymorphonuclear leukocytes via beta-adrenoceptor-dependent and -independent mechanisms. Ann. Allergy Asthma Immunol. **88:** 494–500.
35. FLOYD, R.A. 1999. Antioxidants, oxidative stress, and degenerative neurological disorders. Proc. Soc. Exp. Biol. Med. **222:** 236–245.
36. RAIVICH, G., L.L. JONES, A. WERNER, et al. 1999. Molecular signals for glial activation: pro- and anti-inflammatory cytokines in the injured brain. Acta Neurochir. Suppl. **73:** 21–30.
37. KIM, W.G., R.P. MOHNEY, B. WILSON, et al. 2000. Regional difference in susceptibility to lipopolysaccharide-induced neurotoxicity in the rat brain: role of microglia. J. Neurosci. **20:** 6309–6316.
38. BABIOR, B.M. 1999. NADPH oxidase: an update. Blood **93:** 1464–1476.

39. GOOD, P.F., A. HSU, P. WERNER, et al. 1998. Protein nitration in Parkinson's disease. J. Neuropathol. Exp. Neurol. **57:** 338–339.
40. GIASSON, B.I., J.E. DUDA, I.V. MURRAY, et al. 2000. Oxidative damage linked to neurodegeneration by selective alpha-synuclein nitration in synucleinopathy lesions. Science **290:** 985–989.
41. MCGEER, P.L., K. YASOJIMA & E.G. MCGEER. 2001. Inflammation in Parkinson's disease. Adv. Neurol. **86:** 83–89.
42. MOGI, M., M. HARADA, P. RIEDERER, et al. 1994. Tumor necrosis factor-alpha (TNF-alpha) increases both in the brain and in the cerebrospinal fluid from parkinsonian patients. Neurosci. Lett. **165:** 208–210.
43. BOKA, G., P. ANGLADE, D. WALLACH, et al. 1994. Immunocytochemical analysis of tumor necrosis factor and its receptors in Parkinson's disease. Neurosci. Lett. **172:**151–154.
44. HUNOT, S., N. DUGAS, B. FAUCHEUX, et al. 1999. FcepsilonRII/CD23 is expressed in Parkinson's disease and induces, in vitro, production of nitric oxide and tumor necrosis factor-alpha in glial cells. J. Neurosci. **19:** 3440–3447.
45. MOGI, M., M. HARADA, T. KONDO, et al. 1994. Interleukin-1 beta, interleukin-6, epidermal growth factor and transforming growth factor-alpha are elevated in the brain from parkinsonian patients. Neurosci. Lett. **180:** 147–150.
46. BLUM-DEGEN, D., T. MULLER, W. KUHN, et al. 1995. Interleukin-1 beta and interleukin-6 are elevated in the cerebrospinal fluid of Alzheimer's and de novo Parkinson's disease patients. Neurosci. Lett. **202:** 17–20.
47. MULLER, T., D. BLUM-DEGEN, H. PRZUNTEK & W. KUHN. 1998. Interleukin-6 levels in cerebrospinal fluid inversely correlate to severity of Parkinson's disease. Acta Neurol Scand. **98:** 142–144.
48. MCGEER, P.L., K. YASOJIMA & E.G. MCGEER. 2002. Association of interleukin-1beta polymorphisms with idiopathic Parkinson's disease. Neurosci. Lett. **326:** 67–69.
49. SCHULTE, T., L. SCHOLS, T. MULLER, et al. 2002. Polymorphisms in the interleukin-1 alpha and beta genes and the risk for Parkinson's disease. Neurosci. Lett. **326:** 70–72.
50. KOHUTNICKA, M., E. LEWANDOWSKA, I. KURKOWSKA-JASTRZEBSKA, et al. 1998. Microglial and astrocytic involvement in a murine model of Parkinson's disease induced by 1-methyl-4-phenyl-1,2,3,6-tetrahydropyridine (MPTP). Immunopharmacology **39:** 167–180.
51. KURKOWSKA-JASTRZEBSKA, I., A. WRONSKA, M. KOHUTNICKA, et al. 1999. The inflammatory reaction following 1-methyl-4-phenyl-1,2,3, 6-tetrahydropyridine intoxication in mouse. Exp. Neurol. **156:** 50–61.
52. WU, H., S.B. KANATOUS, F.A. THURMOND, et al. 2002. Regulation of mitochondrial biogenesis in skeletal muscle by CaMK. Science. **296:** 349–352.
53. MOGI, M., A. TOGARI, M. OGAWA, et al. 1998. Effects of repeated systemic administration of 1-methyl-4-phenyl- 1,2,3,6-tetrahydropyridine (MPTP) to mice on interleukin-1beta and nerve growth factor in the striatum. Neurosci. Lett. **250:** 25–28.
54. KLIVENYI, P., R.J. FERRANTE, R.T. MATTHEWS, et al. 1999. Neuroprotective effects of creatine in a transgenic animal model of amyotrophic lateral sclerosis. Nature Med. **5:** 347–350.
55. DU, Y., Z. MA, S. LIN, et al. 2001. Minocycline prevents nigrostriatal dopaminergic neurodegeneration in the MPTP model of Parkinson's disease. Proc. Natl. Acad. Sci. USA **98:** 14669–14674.
56. ZHU, S., I.G. STAVROVSKAYA, M. DROZDA, et al. 2002. Minocycline inhibits cytochrome c release and delays progression of amyotrophic lateral sclerosis in mice. Nature **417:** 74–78.
57. LANGSTON, J.W., L.S. FORNO, J. TETRUD, et al. 1999. Evidence of active nerve cell degeneration in the substantia nigra of humans years after 1-methyl-4-phenyl-1,2,3,6-tetrahydropyridine exposure. Ann. Neurol. **46:** 598–605.
58. BETARBET, R., T.B. SHERER, G. MACKENZIE, et al. 2000. Chronic systemic pesticide exposure reproduces features of Parkinson's disease. Nat. Neurosci. **3:** 1301–1306.
59. GAO, H.M., J. JIANG, B. WILSON, et al. 2002. Microglial activation-mediated delayed and progressive degeneration of rat nigral dopaminergic neurons: relevance to Parkinson's disease. J. Neurochem. **81:** 1285–1297.

60. Akiyama, H. & P.L. McGeer. 1989. Microglial response to 6-hydroxydopamine-induced substantia nigra lesions. Brain Res. **489:** 247–253.
61. Cicchetti, F., A.L. Brownell, K. Williams, *et al.* 2002. Neuroinflammation of the nigrostriatal pathway during progressive 6- OHDA dopamine degeneration in rats monitored by immunohistochemistry and PET imaging. Eur. J. Neurosci. **15:** 991–998.
62. He, Q.-P., M.-L. Smith, P.-A. Li & B.K. Siesjo. 1997. Necrosis of the substantia nigra, pars reticulate, in flurothyl-induced status epilepticus is ameliorated by the spin trap α phenyl-N-*tert*-butyl nitrone. Free Radic. Biol. Med. **22:** 917–922.
63. Gao, H.M., J.S. Hong, W. Zhang & B. Liu. 2002. Distinct role for microglia in rotenone-induced degeneration of dopaminergic neurons. J. Neurosci. **22:** 782–790.
64. Liberatore, G.T., V. Jackson-Lewis, S. Vukosavic, *et al.* 1999. Inducible nitric oxide synthase stimulates dopaminergic neurodegeneration in the MPTP model of Parkinson disease. Nature Med. **5:** 1403–1409.
65. Dehmer, T., J. Lindenau, S. Haid, *et al.* 2000. Deficiency of inducible nitric oxide synthase protects against MPTP toxicity in vivo. J. Neurochem. **74:** 2213–2216.
66. Cao, X. & J. Phillis. 1994. α-Phenyl-tert-butyl nitrone reduced cortical infarct and edema in rats subjected to focal ischemia. Brain Res. **644:** 267–272.
67. Adams, J., Y. Collaco-Moraes & J. de Belleroche. 1996. Cyclooxygenase-2 induction in cerebral cortex: an intracellular response to synaptic excitation. J. Neurochem. **66:** 6–13.
68. Ho, L., H. Osaka, P.S. Aisen & G.M. Pasinetti. 1998. Induction of cyclooxygenase (COX)-2 but not COX-1 gene expression in apoptotic cell death. J. Neuroimmunol. **89:** 142–149.
69. Planas, A.M., M.A. Soriano, C. Justicin & E. Rodriguez-Farre. 1999. Induction of cyclooxygenase-2 in the rat brain after a mild episode of focal ischemia without tissue inflammation or neural cell damage. Neurosci. Lett. **275:** 141–144.
70. Tocco, G., J. Freire-Moar, S.S. Schreiber, *et al.* 1997. Maturational regulation and regional induction of cyclooxygenase-2 in rat brain: implications for Alzheimer's disease. Exp. Neurol. **144:** 339–349.
71. Mirjany, M., L. Ho & G.M. Pasinetti. 2002. Role of cyclooxygenase-2 in neuronal cell cycle activity and glutamate-mediated excitotoxicity. J. Pharmacol. Exp. Ther. **301:** 494–500.
72. Araki, E., C. Forster, J.M. Dubinsky, *et al.* 2001. Cyclooxygenase-2 inhibitor ns-398 protects neuronal cultures from lipopolysaccharide-induced neurotoxicity. Stroke **32:** 2370–2375.
73. Bezzi, P., M. Domercq, L. Brambilla, *et al.* 2001. CXCR4-activated astrocyte glutamate release via TNFalpha: amplification by microglia triggers neurotoxicity. Nat. Neurosci. **4:** 702–710.
74. Hewett, S.J., T.F. Uliasz, A.S. Vidwans & J.A. Hewett. 2000. Cyclooxygenase-2 contributes to N-methyl-D-aspartate-mediated neuronal cell death in primary cortical cell culture. J. Pharmacol. Exp. Ther. **293:** 417–425.
75. Iadecola, C., K. Niwa, S. Nogawa, *et al.* 2001. Reduced susceptibility to ischemic brain injury and N-methyl-D- aspartate-mediated neurotoxicity in cyclooxygenase-2-deficient mice. Proc. Natl. Acad. Sci. USA. **98:** 1294–1299.
76. Teismann, P. & B. Ferger. 2001. Inhibition of the cyclooxygenase isoenzymes COX-1 and COX-2 provide neuroprotection in the MPTP-mouse model of Parkinson's disease. Synapse **39:** 167–174.
77. Feng, Z., T. Wang, D. Li, *et al.* 2002. Cyclooxygenase-2-deficient mice are resistant to 1-methyl-4-phenyl1, 2, 3, 6-tetrahydropyridine-induced damage of dopaminergic neurons in the substantia nigra. Neurosci. Lett. **329:** 354.
78. Enomoto, M. & S. Nishiguchi. 2002. SEN viruses and treatment response in chronic hepatitis C virus. Lancet **359:** 1780–1781.
79. Fujita, K., Y. Kawarada, K. Terada, *et al.* 2000. Quantitative detection of apoptotic thymocytes in low-dose X-irradiated mice by an anti-single-stranded DNA antibody. J. Radiat. Res. (Tokyo) **41:** 139–149.
80. Moreira, A.L., L. Tsenova-Berkova, J. Wang, *et al.* 1997. Effect of cytokine modulation by thalidomide on the granulomatous response in murine tuberculosis. Tuber. Lung Dis. **78:** 47–55.

81. SRIRAM, K., J.M. MATHESON, S.A. BENKOVIC, et al. 2002. Mice deficient in TNF receptors are protected against dopaminergic neurotoxicity: implications for Parkinson's disease. FASEB J. **16:** 1474–1476.

82. BOIREAU, A., F. BORDIER, P. DUBEDAT, et al. 1997. Thalidomide reduces MPTP-induced decrease in striatal dopamine levels in mice. Neurosci. Lett. **234:** 123–126.

83. DINTER, H., J. TSE, M. HALKS-MILLER, et al. 2000. The type IV phosphodiesterase specific inhibitor mesopram inhibits experimental autoimmune encephalomyelitis in rodents. J. Neuroimmunol. **108:** 136–146.

84. MARTINEZ, I., C. PUERTA, C. REDONDO & A. GARCIA-MERINO. 1999. Type IV phosphodiesterase inhibition in experimental allergic encephalomyelitis of Lewis rats: sequential gene expression analysis of cytokines, adhesion molecules and the inducible nitric oxide synthase. J. Neurol. Sci. **164:** 13–23.

85. DUTTA, P., D.E. RYAN & R. TABRIZCHI. 2001. The influence of phosphodiesterase inhibitor, rolipram, on hemodynamics in lipopolysaccharide-treated rats. Jpn. J. Pharmacol. **85:** 241–249.

86. HULLEY, P., J. HARTIKKA, S. ABDEL'AL, et al. 1995. Inhibitors of type IV phosphodiesterases reduce the toxicity of MPTP in substantia nigra neurons in vivo. Eur. J. Neurosci. **7:** 2431–2440.

87. LEMBERGER, T., O. BRAISSANT, C. JUGE-AUBRY, et al. 1996. PPAR tissue distribution and interactions with other hormone-signaling pathways. Ann. N.Y. Acad. Sci. **804:** 231–251.

88. FUJISAWA, H., T. OGURA, A. HOKARI, et al. 1995. Inducible nitric oxide synthase in a human glioblastoma cell line. J. Neurochem. **64:** 85–91.

89. JIANG, C., A.T. TING & B. SEED. 1998. PPAR-gamma agonists inhibit production of monocyte inflammatory cytokines. Nature **391:** 82–86.

90. RICOTE, M., A.C. LI, T.M. WILLSON, et al. 1998. The peroxisome proliferator-activated receptor-gamma is a negative regulator of macrophage activation. Nature **391:** 79–82.

91. KITAMURA, Y., J. KAKIMURA, Y. MATSUOKA, et al. 1999. Activators of peroxisome proliferator-activated receptor-gamma (PPARgamma) inhibit inducible nitric oxide synthase expression but increase heme oxygenase-1 expression in rat glial cells. Neurosci. Lett. **262:** 129–132.

92. MARX, N., F. MACH, A. SAUTY, et al. 2000. Peroxisome proliferator-activated receptor-gamma activators inhibit IFN-gamma-induced expression of the T cell-active CXC chemokines IP-10, Mig, and I-TAC in human endothelial cells. J. Immunol. **164:** 6503–6508.

93. SHU, H., B. WONG, G. ZHOU, et al. 2000. Activation of PPARalpha or gamma reduces secretion of matrix metalloproteinase 9 but not interleukin 8 from human monocytic THP-1 cells. Biochem. Biophys. Res. Commun. **267:** 345–349.

94. URYU, S., S. TOKUHIRO, T. MURASUGI & T. ODA. 2002. A novel compound, RS-1178, specifically inhibits neuronal cell death mediated by beta-amyloid-induced macrophage activation in vitro. Brain Res. **946:** 298–306.

95. FEINSTEIN, D.L., E. GALEA, V. GAVRILYUK, et al. 2002. Peroxisome proliferator-activated receptor-gamma agonists prevent experimental autoimmune encephalomyelitis. Ann. Neurol. **51:** 694–702.

96. BREIDERT, T., J. CALLEBERT, M.T. HENEKA, et al. 2002. Protective action of the peroxisome proliferator-activated receptor-gamma agonist pioglitazone in a mouse model of Parkinson's disease. J. Neurochem. **82:** 615–624.

97. KIM, M.O., Q. SI, J.N. ZHOU, et al. 2002. Interferon-beta activates multiple signaling cascades in primary human microglia. J. Neurochem. **81:** 1361–1371.

98. DALLNER, G. & P.J. SINDELAR. 2000. Regulation of ubiquinone metabolism. Free Radic. Biol. Med. **29:** 285–294.

99. NOACK, H., U. KUBE & W. AUGUSTIN. 1994. Relations between tocopherol depletion and coenzyme Q during lipid peroxidation in rat liver mitochondria. Free Radic. Res. **20:** 375–386.

100. LASS, A. & R.S. SOHAL. 1998. Electron transport-linked ubiquinone-dependent recycling of α-tocopherol inhibits autooxidation of mitochondrial membranes. Arch. Biochem. Biophys. **352:** 229–236.

101. BEAL, M.F. 2002. Coenzyme Q10 as a possible treatment for neurodegenerative diseases. Free Radic. Res. **36:** 455–460.
102. MATTHEWS, R.T., L. YANG, B.G. JENKINS, *et al.* 1998. Neuroprotective effects of creatine and cyclocreatine in animal models of Huntington's disease. J. Neurosci. **18:** 156–163.
103. BEAL, M.F., R. HENSHAW, B.G. JENKINS, *et al.* 1994. Coenzyme Q_{10} and nicotinamide block striatal lesions produced by the mitochondrial toxin malonate. Ann. Neurol. **36:** 882–888.
104. MATTHEWS, R.T., L. YANG, S. BROWNE, *et al.* 1998. Coenzyme Q10 administration increases brain mitochondrial concentrations and exerts neuroprotective effects. Proc. Natl. Acad. Sci. USA **95:** 8892–8897.
105. BEAL, M.F., R.T. MATTHEWS, A. TIELEMAN & C.W. SHULTS. 1998. Coenzyme Q10 attenuates the 1-methyl-1,2,3-etrahydropyridine (MPTP) induced loss of striatal dopamine and dopaminergic axons in aged mice. Brain Res. **783:** 109–114.
106. SHULTS, C.W., R.H. HAAS, D. PASSOV & M.F. BEAL. 1997. Coenzyme Q_{10} is reduced in mitochondria from parkinsonian patients. Ann. Neurol. **42:** 261–264.
107. SHULTS, J. & A.L. MORROW. 2002. Use of quasi-least squares to adjust for two levels of correlation. Biometrics **58:** 521–530.
108. DUNANT, Y., F. LOCTIN, J. MARSAL, *et al.* 1988. Energy metabolism and quantal acetylcholine release: effects of botulinum toxin, 1-fluoro-2,4-dinitrobenzene, and diamide in the *Torpedo* electric organ. J. Neurochem. **50:** 431–439.
109. HEMMER, W. & T. WALLIMANN. 1993. Functional aspects of creatine kinase in brain. Dev. Neurosci. **15:** 249–260.
110. BREWER, G.J. & T.W WALLIMANN. 2000. Protective effect of the energy precursor creatine against toxicity of glutamate and β-amyloid in rat hippocampal neurons. J. Neurochem. **74:** 1968–1978.
111. MATTHEWS, R.T., R.J. FERRANTE, P. KLIVENYI, *et al.* 1999. Creatine and cyclocreatine attenuate MPTP neurotoxicity. Exp. Neurol. **157:** 142–149.
112. BRUSTOVETSKY, N., T. BRUSTOVETSKY & J.M. DUBINSKY. 2001. On the mechanisms of neuroprotection by creatine and phosphocreatine. J. Neurochem. **76:** 425–434.
113. FERRANTE, R.J., O.A. ANDREASSEN, B.G. JENKINS, *et al.* 2000. Neuroprotective effects of creatine in a transgenic mouse model of Huntington's disease. J. Neurosci. **20:** 4389–4397.
114. KLEVENYI, P., O. ANDREASSEN, R.J. FERRANTE, *et al.* 1999. Transgenic mice expressing a dominant negative mutant interleukin-1beta converting enzyme show resistance to MPTP neurotoxicity. Neuroreport **10:** 635–638.
115. ANDREASSEN, O.A., A. DEDEOGLU, R.J. FERRANTE, *et al.* 2001. Creatine increase survival and delays motor symptoms in a transgenic animal model of Huntington's disease. Neurobiol. Dis. **8:** 479–491.

Apoptosis Inducing Factor and PARP-Mediated Injury in the MPTP Mouse Model of Parkinson's Disease

HONGMIN WANG, MIKA SHIMOJI, SEONG-WOON YU, TED M. DAWSON, AND VALINA L. DAWSON

Department of Neurology, Neuroscience, and Physiology, Institute for Cell Engineering, Johns Hopkins University School of Medicine, Baltimore, Maryland 21287, USA

ABSTRACT: Experimental intoxication models are used to study the more common sporadic form of Parkinson's disease (PD). 1-Methyl-4-phenyl-1,2,3,6-tetrahydropyrimidine (MPTP) animal models of PD provide a valuable and predictive tool to probe the molecular mechanisms of dopamine neuronal cell death in PD. MPTP is a powerful neurotoxin that induces neuronal degeneration in the substantia nigra pars compacta and produces PD-like symptoms in several mammalian species tested, a feat not yet accomplished in genetically engineered mice expressing human genetic mutations. The mechanisms of MPTP-induced neurotoxicity are not yet fully understood but involve activation of N-methyl-D-aspartate (NMDA) receptors by glutamate, production of NO by nNOS and iNOS, oxidative injury to DNA, and activation of the DNA damage-sensing enzyme poly (ADP-ribose) polymerase (PARP). Recent experiments indicate that translocation of a mitochondrial protein apoptosis inducing factor (AIF) from mitochondria to the nucleus depends on PARP activation and plays an important role in excitotoxicity-induced cell death. This article briefly reviews the experimental findings regarding excitotoxicity, PARP activation, and AIF translocation in MPTP toxicity and dopaminergic neuronal cell death.

KEYWORDS: Parkinson's disease; apoptosis inducing factor; MPTP mouse model

INTRODUCTION

Parkinson's disease (PD) is a neurological disorder characterized by slowness of movement, resting tremors, rigidity, and difficulty with balance.[1–3] These clinical features are primarily due to the progressive loss of dopaminergic neurons in the substantia nigra pars compacta (SNpc).[4] The degeneration of dopaminergic neurons is associated with the characteristic Lewy body formation (α-synuclein aggregation with eosinophilic intraneuronal inclusions).[5–8] Although there are temporary therapeutic approaches available such as dopamine replacement and surgical treatment to alleviate PD symptoms, no current treatment strategy can stop the progression of this disease.

Address for correspondence: Valina L. Dawson, Ph.D., Department of Neurology, 600 North Wolfe Street, Carnegie 214, Baltimore, MD 21287. Voice: 410-614-3359; fax: 410-614-9568. vdawson@jhmi.edu

Ann. N.Y. Acad. Sci. 991: 132–139 (2003). © 2003 New York Academy of Sciences.

The identification of genetic mutants that lead to PD in familial cases is a wonderful advancement for PD research and allows the generation of genetically engineered mice to study the disease. However, it must not be forgotten that familial PD is a relatively rare event and the majority of patients suffer from sporadic PD. Experimental intoxication models have been to study the more common sporadic form of PD. 1-Methyl-4-phenyl-1,2,3,6-tetrahydropyrimidine (MPTP) animal models of PD provide a valuable and predictive tool to probe the molecular mechanisms of dopamine neuronal cell death in PD. MPTP is a powerful neurotoxin that induces neuronal degeneration in SNpc and produces PD-like symptoms in several mammalian species tested,[6–11] a feat not yet accomplished in genetically engineered mice expressing human genetic mutations. The mechanisms of MPTP induced neurotoxicity are not yet fully understood, but overexcitation of N-methyl-D-aspartate (NMDA) receptors by glutamate plays an important role in MPTP-induced parkinsonism.[12–15] Excessive NMDA-receptor stimulation leads to activation of neuronal nitric oxide synthase (nNOS) and production of NO and other free radicals that cause DNA damage and subsequent activation of the DNA damage sensing enzyme, poly (ADP-ribose) polymerase (PARP).[16–21] PARP overactivation in response to MPTP administration plays a critical role in striatal neuronal cell death. Our recent experiments indicate that translocation of a mitochondrial protein, apoptosis-inducing factor (AIF) from mitochondria to the nucleus depends on PARP activation and plays an important role in excitotoxicity-induced cell death.[22] This article briefly reviews the experimental findings regarding excitotoxicity, PARP activation, and AIF translocation in MPTP toxicity and dopaminergic neuronal cell death.

EXCITOTOXICITY, NO, AND ACTIVATION OF PARP IN MPTP-INDUCED NEURONAL CELL DEATH

MPTP is used to generate animal models for the investigation of sporadic PD as MPTP exposure in mammals replicates parkinsonian mortoric signs.[5] MPTP penetrates the blood-brain barrier and is converted, primarily in glial cells, into the active agent, 1-methyl-4-phenylpyridinium (MPP+) by monoamine oxidase. MPP+ is selectively taken up into dopaminergic neurons via the high-affinity and energy-dependent dopamine transporters.[23,24] Once in dopaminergic neurons, free cytosolic MPP+ enters mitochondria by an energy-dependent mechanism and is then concentrated in the organelle.[25,26] MPP+ is a selective and potent mitochondrial complex I inhibitor of the electron transport chain and impairs mitochondrial functions leading to decrements in cellular ATP levels. Energetic failure in dopaminergic neurons induces depolarization of neuronal membrane potential and release of the excitotoxic neurotransmitter, glutamate. In addition, decrements in cellular ATP pools impair the uptake of extracellular glutamate. These functional changes trigger excessive glutamate accumulation in the extracellular space and cause overstimulation of glutamate receptors. *In vivo* experiments show that administration of certain selective NMDA antagonists such as AP7, CPP, and MK801 provide significant protection against MPP+ induced toxicity. Repeated application of these NMDA antagonists can also result in long-term protection after intranigral administration of MPP+.[12] These results strongly support the notion that excitotoxicity plays an important role in MPTP-induced toxicity.

MPTP-induced excitotoxicity is mediated mainly via formation of NO and other free radicals. Overactivation of NMDA receptors causes a large amount of calcium influx into neuronal cells and activating nNOS to produce NO. NO can combine with superoxide anion to form the very toxic compound, peroxynitrite.[5,27–29] There exists compelling evidence that the generation of NO radical plays a prominent role in MPTP-induced neurotoxicity. Inhibition of the activity of NOS can protect neurons from MPTP-induced reduction of striatal dopamine and its metabolites, homovanillic acid (HVA) and dihydroxyphenylacetic acid (DOPAC).[28] Studies using the NOS inhibitor, 7-nitroindasazole show that the protective effect is dose-dependent. NOS inhibition can protect mice against MPTP-induced loss of dopaminergic neurons in the MPTP mouse model.[28] Finally, mice lacking the gene for nNOS show significant resistance to MPTP-induced dopaminergic neurotoxicity.[28] Taken together these data indicate that NO is key player in MPTP-induced neurotoxicity.

NO and peroxynitrite-mediated neurotoxicity in the MPTP mouse model is believed to damage DNA, which subsequently activates the nuclear enzyme, PARP.[29–31] PARP is a DNA binding protein and it can sense the nick of DNA molecule induced by free radicals or other damaging reagents. The activity of PARP is completely dependent on the number of DNA breaks and it is totally inactive in the absence of DNA nicks.[17–21] Among more than ten different PARPs, PARP-1 is the most abundant being expressed at approximately one molecule per 1,000 DNA base pairs.[32] The damaged DNA in dopaminergic neurons is detectable in both wild type and PARP-1 knockout (KO) neurons after MPTP administration.[33] Stimulation of NMDA receptors preferentially causes the activation of PARP in wild type of mice, whereas in our experiments we failed to observe the activation of PARP-1 in the mice lacking the gene for nNOS, suggesting that formation of NO is critical in activating PARP.[22,31] Activation of PARP plays an important role in MPTP-induced neurotoxicity in mice. Following MPTP administration, mitochondrial complex I of the electron transport chain is inhibited, leading to decrements in intracellular ATP levels. When PARP is activated, NAD is depleted via poly(ADP-ribosyl)ation of nuclear proteins, and ATP is further depleted in an effort to resynthesize NAD. Some reports indicate that PARP inhibitors, such as benzamide and DHIQ, can significantly protect the brain from MPTP-induced decreases in ATP and NAD levels, as well as decrements in striatal dopamine and its metabolites, DOPAC and HVA.[34–37] In the PARP-/- mice MPTP exposure fails to produce the reductions of dopamine, HVA, and DOPAC in striatum by 80–90% as observed in wild type mice.[31] MPTP also causes a 60% reduction of both tyrosine hydroxylase (TH) and Nissl-stained neurons in SNpc in the wild type of mice, whereas these neurons are spared in PARP-/- mice. In addition, the time course of PARP activation and the presence of PAR polymer in cells correlates with dopaminergic neuronal cell death.[31] These results taken together implicate PARP activation as a principal determinant of MPTP-induced dopaminergic cell death.

PARP ACTIVATION INDUCED NEURONAL CELL DEATH IS MEDIATED VIA APOPTOSIS INDUCING FACTOR TRANSLOCATION

Overactivation of PARP triggers a cell death cascade resulting in tissue damage. In wild-type mice, intrastriatal microinjection of NMDA produces well-delineated lesions. In contrast, microinjection of NMDA does not produce a visible lesion in the PARP-/- mice. In addition, cultured PARP-/- cortical neurons are remarkably resistant to excitotoxicity induced by NMDA-receptor stimulation.[38] These results link production of NO and other free radical species to PARP activation and to the cell death and tissue damage after an excitotoxic insult. However, it is still uncertain how activation of PARP triggers the cell death cascade. Recent investigations indicate that excitotoxicity followed by PARP activation is likely mediated via apoptosis inducing factor (AIF) and its translocation from mitochondria to the nucleus.[22]

AIF is a mitochondrial flavoprotein that mediates caspase-independent cell death.[39] In response to toxic stimuli, AIF initiates cell death by translocation from mitochondria to the nucleus to induce nuclear condensation and DNA fragmentation.[39–41] Results from our group support a link between AIF in PARP-mediated cell death.[22] We observe that NMDA mediated excitotoxicity is caspase independent and PARP dependent. In cultured cortical neurons, five-minutes of NMDA (500 µM) exposure elicits neurotoxicity in a delayed manner. Neuronal cell death induced by NMDA is significantly reduced by PARP inhibitors including, DPQ and completely blocked in cortical cultures from mice lacking PARP-1 gene. In contrast, neuronal cell death caused by NMDA receptor overstimulation cannot be prevented by the broad-spectrum caspase inhibitors, boc-aspartyl-fmk (BAF) and Z-VAD.fmk.[22,42] Following PARP activation AIF translocates from mitochondria to the nucleus, preceding cytochrome c release and activation of the major execution caspase, caspase 3. 15 min after NMDA receptor stimulation, AIF translocation can be detected in the nucleus. In contrast, release of cytochrome c and activation of caspase-3 is detected 1-2 hours after NMDA treatment. The time course of AIF translocation is coincident with changes in nuclear morphology (nuclear condensation) and DNA damage. Accompanying AIF translocation is mitochondrial membrane depolarization and phosphatidylserine exposure on the cell surface. In response to NMDA receptor stimulation, AIF translocation is also coincident with PARP activation in NMDA treated neurons. PARP activation can be easily detected 15 minutes after NMDA receptor stimulation. In contrast, in PARP-1 knockout cortical neurons AIF translocation does not occur, the nucleus remains undisturbed and the cells do not die following NMDA-receptor stimulation.[42,43] These results taken together suggest that AIF and its translocation triggered via PARP activation may play a prominent role in NMDA excitotoxicity. To investigate the functional the role of AIF in excitotoxcity, AIF translocation was blocked by overexpression of Bcl-2, an anti-apoptotic protein that prevents AIF translocation.[39] Overexpression of Bcl-2 protein protects cells against PARP dependent death.[22,43] In a more direct experiment, addition of neutralizing antibodies to AIF provides substantial cytoprotection against PARP dependent cell death.[22] In total, these observations make a compelling argument for PARP-dependent death being mediated by via mitochondrial release of AIF and its translocation to the nucleus.

AIF IN THE MPTP MODEL OF PD

Consistent with the *in vitro* studies, our *in vivo* observations indicate that translocation of AIF into the nucleus may play an important role in MPTP induced toxicity. Exposure of mice to MPTP results in significant and persistent decreases in dopam-

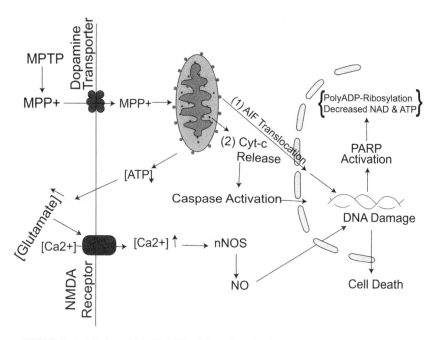

FIGURE 1. Model of PARP AND AIF actions in the MPTP model of dopaminergic neurotoxicity. MPTP can penetrate the blood-brain barrier and is converted to MPP+. MPP+ is transported into dopaminergic neurons by the dopamine transporter and accumulates in mitochondria, where it inhibits mitochondrial complex I of the electron transport chain. The blockade of oxidative phosphorylation results in loss of cellular ATP levels, neuronal excitability, glutamate release, and activation of NMDA receptors. Calcium flows through NMDA receptors, activating nNOS to produce NO. NO reacts with superoxide anion to form peroxynitrite, which in turn damages DNA and activates PARP. PARP activation results in synthesis of PAR polymers, ribosylation of proteins, and consumption of NAD and ATP. These PARP-dependent events signal to the mitochondria to induce AIF release and translocation to the nucleus. In the nucleus AIF triggers large-scale DNA fragmentation and nuclear condensation. These nuclear changes in neurons are likely the final commitment point in the neurotoxic cascade.

ine and its metabolites in the striatum, and tyrosine hydroxylase (TH) immunoreactivity. MPTP exposure results in irreversible dopaminergic neurodegeneration in the SNcp.[6–11] In the MPTP-treated mice, we find AIF in the nucleus in the TH positive neurons as soon as 2 hours after the last MPTP injection. However, AIF translocation is not seen in PARP-1 KO mice injected with MPTP.[44] With the mounting evidence that AIF plays a critical role in PARP-dependent death and the observations for a major role for PARP activation in mediating MPTP-induced dopaminergic neurotoxicity, these observations of AIF translocation in wild type but not PARP-1 KO mice following MPTP exposure implicates AIF as a candidate molecule in the MPTP triggered death cascade. The MPTP neurotoxic cascade may proceed in the following manner (FIG. 1). When administered to mice, MPTP can penetrate the blood-brain barrier. In brain, MPTP is converted to MPP+ by monoamine oxidase B.[23,26] MPP+ is selectively taken up by dopaminergic neurons via the dopamine transporter and accumulates in mitochondria of dopaminergic neurons. In mitochondria, MPP+ selectively inhibits the mitochondrial complex I of the electron transport chain and blocks the oxidative phosphorylation, leading to drop in cellular ATP levels, which indirectly causes neuronal depolarization, release of glutamate and overexcitation of NMDA receptors. Overstimulation of NMDA receptors by excessive extracellular glutamate results in opening the calcium channels and elevations in intracellular calcium. Elevated intracellular calcium activates nNOS to synthesize NO. NO reacts with superoxide anion to form peroxynitrite, which is a potent DNA damaging agent. DNA damage, in turn, activates PARP. PARP activation produces PAR polymers and at the same time consumes NAD and ATP. The generation of PAR polymers, the ribosylation of proteins and the loss of NAD and ATP and/or other factors caused by PARP activation signal to the mitochondria to induce AIF release and translocation. These events precede cytochrome c release and caspase activation. The translocation of AIF is associated with DNA fragmentation and nuclear condensation. The dismantling of the nuclear structure is likely the final commitment point to cell death.

SUMMARY

Research in Parkinson's disease is entering a new era. Advances in understanding the molecular mechanisms of cell death and the pathogenesis of sporadic and familial Parkinson's disease is creating new therapeutic opportunities for the treatment of this disease. It is likely that both neuroprotective and neurorestorative therapies will be necessary to elicit complete recovery from the devastating effects of PD. A better understanding of the basic processes involved in neurotoxicity is a prerequisite to derive new therapeutic interventions. AIF appears to be a central executioner of neuronal cell death and may be an engaging target for new therapeutic interventions to rescue neuronal cells.

ACKNOWLEDGMENTS

The secretarial assistance of Weza Cotman is gratefully acknowledged. This work was supported by the National Institutes of Health, the American Heart Association, the Robert Packard Center for ALS Research and the Mary Lou McIlhaney scholarship. We apologize to our colleagues whose work was not discussed in detail or referenced due to space limitations.

REFERENCES

1. DAWSON, T.M. 2000. New animal models for Parkinson's disease. Cell **101:** 115–118.
2. LANG, A.E. & A.M. LOZANO. 1998. Parkinson's disease. First of two parts. N. Engl. J. Med. **339:** 1044–1053.
3. LANG, A.E. & A.M. LOZANO. 1998. Parkinson's disease. Second of two parts. N. Engl. J. Med. **339:** 1130–1143.
4. LEE, C.S., M. SCHULZER, E.K. MAK, *et al.* 1994. Clinical observations on the rate of progression of idiopathic parkinsonism. Brain **117:** 501–507.
5. DAWSON, V.L. & T.M. DAWSON. 1996. Nitric oxide neurotoxicity. J. Chem. Neuroanat. **10:** 179–190.

6. FORNO, L.S., J.W. LANGSTON, L.E. DELANNEY, et al. 1986. Locus ceruleus lesions and eosinophilic inclusions in MPTP-treated monkeys. Ann. Neurol. **20:** 449–455.
7. MIZUNO, Y., N. SONE & T. SAITOH. 1987. Effects of 1-methyl-4-phenyl-1,2,3,6-tetrahydropyridine and 1-methyl-4- phenylpyridinium ion on activities of the enzymes in the electron transport system in mouse brain. J. Neurochem. **48:** 1787–1793.
8. DEXTER, D.T., I. NANAYAKKARA, M.A. GOSS-SAMPSON, et al. 1994. Nigral dopaminergic cell loss in vitamin E deficient rats. Neuroreport **5:** 1773–1776.
9. SCHAPIRA, A.H. 1996. Neurotoxicity and the mechanisms of cell death in Parkinson's disease. Adv. Neurol. **69:** 161–165.
10. LANGSTON, J.W. 1996. The etiology of Parkinson's disease with emphasis on the MPTP story. Neurology **47:** S153–160.
11. HEIKKILA, R.E., B.A. SIEBER, L. MANZINO & P.K. SONSALLA. 1989. Some features of the nigrostriatal dopaminergic neurotoxin 1-methyl-4-phenyl-1,2,3,6-tetrahydropyridine (MPTP) in the mouse. Mol. Chem. Neuropathol. **10:** 171–183.
12. TURSKI, L., K. BRESSLER, K.J. RETTIG, et al. 1991. Protection of substantia nigra from MPP+ neurotoxicity by N-methyl-D- aspartate antagonists. Nature **349:** 414–418.
13. SONSALLA, P.K., D.S. ALBERS & G.D. ZEEVALK. 1998. Role of glutamate in neurodegeneration of dopamine neurons in several animal models of parkinsonism. Amino Acids **14:** 69–74.
14. BEAL, M.F. 1998. Excitotoxicity and nitric oxide in Parkinson's disease pathogenesis. Ann. Neurol. **44:** S110–114.
15. SHERER, T.B., R. BETARBET & J.T. GREENAMYRE. 2001. Pathogenesis of Parkinson's disease. Curr. Opin. Investig. Drugs **2:** 657–662.
16. JUAREZ-SALINAS, H., J.L. SIMS & M.K. JACOBSON. 1979. Poly(ADP-ribose) levels in carcinogen-treated cells. Nature **282:** 740–741.
17. BENJAMIN, R.C. & D.M. GILL. 1980. Poly(ADP-ribose) synthesis in vitro programmed by damaged DNA. A comparison of DNA molecules containing different types of strand breaks. J. Biol. Chem. **255:** 10502–10508.
18. MILAM, K.M. & J.E. CLEAVER. 1984. Inhibitors of poly(adenosine diphosphate-ribose) synthesis: effect on other metabolic processes. Science **223:** 589–591.
19. BERGER, N.A. 1985. Poly(ADP-ribose) in the cellular response to DNA damage. Radiat. Res. **101:** 4–15.
20. THRAVES P.J., U. KASID & M.E. SMULSON. 1985. Selective isolation of domains of chromatin proximal to both carcinogen-induced DNA damage and poly-adenosine diphosphate-ribosylation. Cancer Res. **45:** 386–391.
21. SZABO, C. & V.L. DAWSON. 1998. Role of poly(ADP-ribose) synthetase in inflammation and ischaemia-reperfusion. Trends Pharmacol. Sci. **19:** 287–298.
22. YU, S.W., H. WANG, M.F. POITRAS, et al. 2002. Mediation of poly(ADP-ribose) polymerase-1-dependent cell death by apoptosis-inducing factor. Science **297:** 259–263.
23. PIFL, C., B. GIROS & M.G. CARON. 1993. Dopamine transporter expression confers cytotoxicity to low doses of the parkinsonism-inducing neurotoxin 1-methyl-4-phenylpyridinium. J. Neurosci. **13:** 4246–4253.
24. DUNNETT, S.B. & A. BJORKLUND. 1999. Prospects for new restorative and neuroprotective treatments in Parkinson's disease. Nature **399:** A32–39.
25. RAMSAY, R.R., S.O. SABLIN, S.O. BACHURIN & T.P. SINGER. 1993. Oxidation of tetrahydrostilbazole by monoamine oxidase A demonstrates the effect of alternate pathways in the kinetic mechanism. Biochemistry **32:** 9025–9030.
26. BLUM, D., S. TORCH, M.F. NISSOU & J.M. VERNA. 2001. 6-Hydroxydopamine-induced nuclear factor-kappa B activation in PC12 cells. Biochem. Pharmacol. **62:** 473–481.
27. BECKMAN, J.S. & J.P. CROW. 1993. Pathological implications of nitric oxide, superoxide and peroxynitrite formation. Biochem. Soc. Trans. **21:** 330–334.
28. PRZEDBORSKI, S., V. JACKSON-LEWIS, R. YOKOYAMA, et al. 1996. Role of neuronal nitric oxide in 1-methyl-4-phenyl-1,2,3,6- tetrahydropyridine (MPTP)-induced dopaminergic neurotoxicity. Proc. Natl. Acad. Sci. USA **93:** 4565–4571.
29. RADONS, J., B. HELLER, A. BURKLE, et al. 1994. Nitric oxide toxicity in islet cells involves poly(ADP-ribose) polymerase activation and concomitant NAD+ depletion. Biochem. Biophys. Res. Commun. **199:** 1270–1277.

30. ZHANG, J., V.L. DAWSON, T.M. DAWSON & S.H. SNYDER. 1994. Nitric oxide activation of poly(ADP-ribose) synthetase in neurotoxicity. Science **263:** 687–689.
31. MANDIR, A.S., S. PRZEDBORSKI, V. JACKSON-LEWIS, *et al.* 1997. Poly(ADP-ribose) polymerase activation mediates 1-methyl-4-phenyl-1, 2,3,6-tetrahydropyridine (MPTP)-induced parkinsonism. Proc. Natl. Acad. Sci. USA **96:** 5774–5779.
32. CHIARUGI, A. & M.A. MOSKOWITZ. 2002. Cell biology. PARP-1—a perpetrator of apoptotic cell death? Science **297:** 200–201.
33. TATTON, N.A. & S.J. KISH. 1997. In situ detection of apoptotic nuclei in the substantia nigra compacta of 1-methyl-4-phenyl-1,2,3,6-tetrahydropyridine-treated mice using terminal deoxynucleotidyl transferase labelling and acridine orange staining. Neuroscience **77:** 1037–1048.
34. COSI, C., F. COLPAERT, W. KOEK, *et al.* 1996. Poly(ADP-ribose) polymerase inhibitors protect against MPTP-induced depletions of striatal dopamine and cortical noradrenaline in C57Bl/6 mice. Brain Res. **729:** 264–269.
35. COSI, C., H. SUZUKI, S.D. SKAPER, *et al.* 1997. Poly(ADP-ribose) polymerase (PARP) revisited. A new role for an old enzyme: PARP involvement in neurodegeneration and PARP inhibitors as possible neuroprotective agents. Ann. N.Y. Acad. Sci. **825:** 366–379.
36. COSI, C. & M. MARIEN. 1999. Decreases in mouse brain NAD+ and ATP induced by 1-methyl-4-phenyl-1, 2,3,6-tetrahydropyridine (MPTP): prevention by the poly(ADP-ribose) polymerase inhibitor, benzamide. Brain Res. **809:** 58–67.
37. COSI, C. & M. MARIEN. 1999. Implication of poly (ADP-ribose) polymerase (PARP) in neurodegeneration and brain energy metabolism. Decreases in mouse brain NAD+ and ATP caused by MPTP are prevented by the PARP inhibitor benzamide. Ann. N.Y. Acad. Sci. **890:** 227–239.
38. MANDIR, A.S., M.F. POITRAS, A.R. BERLINER, *et al.* 2000. NMDA but not non-NMDA excitotoxicity is mediated by Poly(ADP-ribose) polymerase. J. Neurosci. **20:** 8005–8011.
39. SUSIN, S.A., H.K. LORENZO, N. ZAMZAMI, *et al.* 1999. Molecular characterization of mitochondrial apoptosis-inducing factor. Nature **397:** 441–446.
40. DAUGAS, E., S.A. SUSIN, N. ZAMZAMI, *et al.* 2000. Mitochondrio-nuclear translocation of AIF in apoptosis and necrosis. FASEB J. **14:** 729–739.
41. JOZA, N., S.A. SUSIN, E. DAUGAS, *et al.* 2001. Essential role of the mitochondrial apoptosis-inducing factor in programmed cell death. Nature **410:** 549–554.
42. WANG, H., S.W. YU, M.F. POITRAS, *et al.* 2001. Translocation of apoptosis-inducing factor is involved in NMDA excitotoxicity and is poly(ADP-ribose) polymerase dependent. Abstr. Soc. Neurosci. 96.16.
43. WANG, H., S.W. YU, M.F. POITRAS, *et al.* 2002. Apoptosis-inducing factor mediates poly(ADP-ribose) polymerase-1 dependent NMDA excitotoxicity. Abstr. Soc. Neurosci. 199.4.
44. SHIMOJI, M., L. ZHANG, A.S. MANDIR, *et al.* 2002. Investigation of inclusion body formation in the MPTP mouse model of Parkinson's disease. Abstr. Soc. Neurosci. 485.8.

Cellular Models to Study Dopaminergic Injury Responses

TIMOTHY J. COLLIER, KATHY STEECE-COLLIER, SUSAN McGUIRE, AND CARYL E. SORTWELL

Department of Neurological Sciences and the Research Center for Brain Repair, Rush Presbyterian-St. Luke's Medical Center, Chicago, Illinois 60612, USA

ABSTRACT: The study of immature midbrain dopamine (DA) neurons and dopaminergic cell lines in culture provides an opportunity to analyze mechanisms of cell death and avenues of potential intervention relevant to Parkinson's disease (PD) in a controlled environment. Use of cell culture models has provided evidence for different sets of intracellular changes associated with DA neuron death following exposure to the neurotoxins 6-hydroxydopamine and MPP+, supporting roles for oxidative stress and impaired energy metabolism as significant factors endangering these cells. Interference with death of cultured DA neurons has provided an initial test system that has yielded all the identified neurotrophic factors for DA neurons. More recent work suggests that combinations of molecules secreted by myelinating glial cells and their precursors provide even greater neuroprotection for DA neurons. Most recently, culture systems have been used to implicate microglial activation in DA neuron injury, providing impetus to the investigation of antiinflammatory agents as potential therapeutics for PD. Thus, cell culture models provide an important bidirectional link between mechanistic studies and clinically relevant observations.

KEYWORDS: culture; neurotoxin; apoptosis; oxidant stress; neurotrophic factors; microglia; inflammation; pramipexole

Symptoms of Parkinson's disease (PD) have been linked primarily to degeneration of dopamine (DA) neurons in the substantia nigra and the ensuing effects of striatal DA depletion on the activity of neurons within basal ganglia circuitry. While this relatively focal neurodegeneration is the culprit in PD, the cause of degeneration remains unknown. As inquiry into the etiology of PD goes on, one approach to prevention and therapy is identification of factors that specifically render DA neurons vulnerable to decay. While such studies are nearly impossible to conduct in populations of PD patients, models of the DA system, both in whole animals and isolated cells grown in culture, can be powerful tools. This brief review focuses upon

Address for correspondence: Timothy J. Collier, Ph.D., Dept. of Neurological Sciences, Rush Presbyterian-St. Luke's Medical Center, Tech 2000, Suite 200, 2242 W. Harrison St., Chicago, IL 60612. Voice: 312-563-3579; fax: 312-563-3571.

tcollier@rush.edu

Ann. N.Y. Acad. Sci. 991: 140–151 (2003). © 2003 New York Academy of Sciences.

the use of DA neurons held in the controlled environment of cell culture as a system for analyzing mechanisms of cell death and avenues for potential intervention relevant to PD.

CHARACTERISICS OF THE CELL CULTURE MODEL

At the outset, it is important to acknowledge the characteristics of cell culture systems that can impact the types of studies conducted and the interpretation of data obtained. Among these factors are types of cells, cell density, and culture environment.

Types of Cells

Cultures of both primary immature DA neurons and immortalized lines of cells exhibiting features of the DA neuron phenotype have been employed to study degeneration and neuroprotection relevant to PD. Each type of culture presents attributes and limitations. Dopaminergic cell lines by their nature are altered from the normal state of the DA neuron to provide cells with the capacity for continuous proliferation. The impact of this proliferative state on the expression of differentiated features of the DA phenotype remains a question in studies using these cells. However, cell lines provide a homogeneous population of cells for study, allowing for reproducibility across experiments, and sufficient numbers of DA-like neurons to enable certain molecular analyses that would be difficult on primary cultures. The ability to bank these cells promotes the ease and lowers the costs of experimentation. Primary cultures are derived from tissue harvested from embryonic or early postnatal donors. As such, the main advantage of these cultures is that they contain authentic DA neurons cultured in the context of their naturally occurring neighboring cell types. The region of the developing ventral mesencephalon containing the substantia nigra can be surgically isolated from donors, yielding cultures that include the specific type of DA neuron of relevance to PD. However, the use of primary cells is considerably more challenging than working with cell lines. The numbers and types of cells comprising the cultures rely upon the precision and reproducibility of the surgical isolation. Even in the hands of skilled practitioners DA neurons comprise less than 5% of cells in primary culture. This lack of enrichment in DA neurons and heterogeneity of cells in culture complicate certain types of analysis. Measurements used must be able to detect the DA neuron "signal" against the background "noise" of many other cells. Primary DA neurons harvested are usually postmitotic, limiting the life span of the cultures and requiring new harvests with each new study. Cultured DA neurons are immature and may not accurately reflect responses of adult DA neurons.

Cell Density

One pervasive variable in cell culture work is the density at which cells are plated. Plating density is of particular importance in primary cultures containing DA neurons due to demonstrated trophic effects of the resident glial cells for DA neurons,[1–3] and DA neurons for each other.[4] For example, we have found that the density of cells in primary cultures significantly affects their response to insult. Microisland cultures,[5] containing 30,000 cells, were significantly more resistant to withdrawal of serum from the culture medium than were cultures with 1/4 of this density. Similarly, when one evaluates results of cell culture experiments one must understand that the ability to manipulate cell density can significantly impact the experimental outcome. For example, the experimenter has the option to use low-density cultures when investigating agents that may increase DA neuron survival in order to provide a greater opportunity to detect survival effects against the background of suboptimal conditions. While this approach is common, it biases the experiment toward detection of modest effects and may exaggerate their biological significance. Work in our laboratory has shown that treatment of primary cultures plated at 7500 cells/well enables the detection of a significant enhancement of DA neuron survival in the presence of the caspase inhibitor acetyl-tyrosinyl-valyl-alanyl-aspartyl-chloro-methylketone (Ac-YVAD-cmk) that is not present in denser cultures plated at 30,000 cells/well. The two culture conditions yield entirely different conclusions concerning the potential efficacy of this agent in the prevention of DA neuron degeneration.

Culture Environment

The environment of cells in culture is accessible to manipulation in several ways, each of which can influence the experimental outcome. The physical interaction of cells with the culture well can yield notable differences in cell density within a single culture. In our experience, cells plated in fluid that fills the well produce preferential survival of DA neurons around the outer edge, with sparse survival in the center of the well. As noted above, cell density can impact experimental outcomes, and variable density within a single well can be problematic. An alternative method is the microisland culture technique,[5] in which cells are plated in a drop of fluid in the center of the culture well, not contacting an edge. Cells settle and attach to the dish in small circular cultures that present greater uniformity of cell density and no "edge effect." Multiple types of culture medium are available that, depending upon the recipe, can promote or inhibit the survival of glial cells and the general viability of cultured neurons. Filter floor inserts can be used to introduce an additional cell type and to study interactions by secreted diffusible factors as compared to physical cell–cell interactions. Cultured cells are bathed in a fluid environment through which experimental agents can be delivered. This provides direct access to the cells, but may not simulate delivery of agents to cells in the intact nervous system. It has become increasingly clear that all aspects of the culture environment may significantly impact experimental observations. Standard procedure has been to provide cultures with 20% oxygen within the incubators in which cells are maintained. It has become clear that this oxygen level is far in excess of the approximately 1–3% oxygen these cells experience in the environment of the developing brain, yielding a persistent environment of oxidative stress while in culture. Any experimental manipulations are superimposed upon this undefined background of cellular stress. Perhaps one of the most interesting examples of the effects of the culture environment on cells involves the concept of *in vitro* replicative senescence, or the Hayflick limit.[6] This is the finding that proliferative cell types held in culture divide a finite number of times and then enter growth arrest, or cellular senescence. This phenomenon has long been believed to be a reflection of an intrinsic cellular mechanism of aging. Recent reports indicate that replicative senescence is a consequence of "culture shock," or suboptimal conditions, and that alterations in the culture environment can yield unlimited proliferation of normal cells.[7,8]

With these caveats in mind, it remains true that cell culture models provide an important research tool. Cultures provide direct access to the DA neuron, allowing study of intracellular mechanisms of toxicity and neurotrophism, dose–response studies of experimental agents, and rapid screening of potential novel therapeutics. Cell culture provides an important bidirectional link between mechanistic studies and clinically relevant observations. The remainder of this review will discuss examples of the use of primary DA neuron cultures for identifying factors that endanger DA neurons and may provide avenues for development of novel therapeutics.

NEUROTOXINS FOR DOPAMINE NEURONS

A variety of evidence suggests that two important factors that may mediate degeneration of DA neurons in PD are oxidative stress and impaired energy metabolism.[9,10] The neurotoxins 6-hydroxydopamine (6-OHDA) and 1-methyl-4-phenyl-1,2,3,6-tetrahydropyridine (MPTP) are widely used to generate animal models of PD and when administered *in vivo* can produce relatively selective degeneration of the mesostriatal DA system. Accordingly, better understanding of mechanisms of DA neuron degeneration in response to these toxins may provide clues to mechanisms of cell death in PD. Culture systems are well suited to this type of analysis, and detailed studies of the response of cultured primary DA neurons to these agents have been pursued.[11–13] The findings of these experiments suggest that 6-OHDA and MPTP endanger DA neurons via distinct mechanisms. Cultures of embryonic day 14 (E14) mouse ventral mesencephalon, containing the relevant developing DA neurons, were exposed to concentrations of each toxin determined to yield 50–70% death of DA neurons over 24–48 hours. To determine whether the toxins were producing apoptotic cell death, cultures were stained for the presence of annexin-V, an early marker of apoptosis and indicator of translocation of phosphatidylserine residues from the inner to the outer leaflet of the plasma membrane. At 6 hours after exposure to the toxins, 83% of DA neurons exposed to 6-OHDA stained positive for annexin-V, while none were positive after exposure to the toxic metabolite of MPTP, MPP+. Similarly, treatment of toxin-exposed cultures with the caspase inhibitor BAF significantly protected DA neurons exposed to 6-OHDA (78.7% recovery), with no effect on DA neurons exposed to MPP+. By these measures, 6-OHDA, but not MPP+, kills DA neurons via apoptotic mechanisms. Additional experiments used fluorophores to assess mitochondrial membrane potential and generation of reactive oxygen species. These measures indicated that both neurotoxins generate bursts of reactive oxygen species within minutes of exposure. Disparate effects were detected for mitochondrial membrane potential. 6-OHDA induced a transient collapse of the mitochondrial membrane potential followed by hyperpolarization, consistent with rapid oxidative inactivation of components of metabolic pathways and a pattern typical of apoptosis. In contrast, MPP+ produced depolarization of the membrane potential that was delayed by 12–24 hours. This pattern is consistent with inhibition of complex I and a delayed metabolic death. Several other possible participants in MPP+-mediated DA neuron death did not appear to be significant. Blockade of excitotoxicity with a variety of glutamate receptor blockers and calcium channel blockers had no effect on MPP+ toxicity. Treatment of cultures with alternate metabolic sources to address impaired energy metabolism and with nitric oxide synthase inhibitors provided only modest protection from MPP+ toxicity. So while the findings are consistent with 6-OHDA endangering DA neurons via increased oxidative stress and induction of apoptosis, mechanisms associated with MPP+ appear to be different and less clear.

Interestingly, these culture findings did suggest a role of reactive oxygen species in the action of both neurotoxins. Accordingly, the investigators tested the protective effects of a potent antioxidant in the culture model, the carboxyfullerene compound C_3. Effects were compared to the DA neurotrophic factor glial cell line–derived neurotrophic factor (GDNF). This molecule arguably has received the most attention as a potential therapeutic for PD. C_3 treatment produced potent rescue of DA neurons in 6-OHDA–exposed cultures (92% recovery) and partial protection of MPP+ treated cultures (37.5% recovery). This is consistent with the primary role of oxidant stress in 6-OHDA toxicity and its participation in MPP+ toxicity. In both instances GDNF was less effective, rescuing 38% and 29% of DA neurons treated with 6-OHDA and MPP+, respectively. Thus, studies of DA neurotoxin actions using cell culture models support the role of oxidant stress in the demise of DA neurons and suggest the potential efficacy of carboxyfullerene derivatives as potential therapeutic protectants in PD.

INFLAMMATION AND DOPAMINE NEURONS

Recently, interest has turned to the role of inflammation in a host of neurodegenerative diseases. Large numbers of activated microglia are present in the substantia nigra in PD[14,15] and MPTP-induced parkinsonism.[16] Whether activated microglia participate in the pathogenesis of PD has been a matter of conjecture. Proinflammatory cytokines, including interleukin (IL)-1β, interferon (INF)-γ, and tumor necrosis factor (TNF)-α, are elevated in PD substantia nigra and cerebrospinal fluid.[15,17–19] Still, it remains to be determined whether microglia can provoke or enhance DA neuron degeneration in PD, or whether they are present as phagocytes. Another use of cell culture models is in the study of such interactions between two defined cell populations.

In a clever series of experiments, investigators exploited the propensity of microglia to tightly adhere to plastic to generate a purified population of microglia from 3–4-day-old rat brain.[20] To determine conditions for activating microglia, cultures were exposed to either bacterial lipopolysaccharide (LPS) or immunoglobulins (IgGs) from serum of PD patients, and release of IL-1β and TNF-α into culture medium were measured as markers of microglial activation. After exposure to either activating agent, inflammatory cytokine levels increased approximately 20-fold, with an accompanying 15-fold increase in release of reactive oxygen species detected in culture medium. The investigators then cocultured either resting microglia or activated microglia with cells of a dopaminergic cell line, MES 23.5 cells, or primary cultures of E14 rat ventral mesencephalon. Coculture with resting microglia had no effect on either type of dopaminergic neuron. However, coculture of MES 23.5 cells with activated microglia reduced tyrosine hydroxylase (TH) activity, a marker of the DA phenotype, by approximately 65%. Cocultures then were incubated with neutralizing antibodies to the inflammatory cytokines and selective inhibitors of reactive oxygen species to determine the factors contributing to microglial-mediated cytotoxicity. The results indicated that the reactive oxygen species nitric oxide (NO) and hydrogen peroxide (H_2O_2), but not the cytokines, were responsible for dopaminergic cell injury. For primary cultures of ventral mesencephalon, at 2 days after coculture with activated microglia, approximately 85% of TH-positive DA neurons were lost. Thus, evidence derived from use of cell culture models supports the view that activated microglia may initiate or amplify oxidative stress contributing to DA neuron degeneration in PD. In addition, therapeutic strategies that incorporate prevention of inflammation, and specifically microglial activation, may be beneficial in treatment of PD.

NEUROPROTECTIVE STRATEGIES

Cell culture systems historically have provided the initial test system for novel therapeutic molecules. For PD, virtually every neurotrophic molecule for DA neurons has been characterized using cell cultures.[21] Experimental agents are tested for their capacity to improve baseline survival and differentiated features of cultured DA neurons, as well as their capacity to protect DA neurons against insults such as serum deprivation and addition of toxins. Two examples of potential therapeutic approaches developed in cell culture models are reviewed briefly here.

The first example is pramipexole (PPX), a D3-type DA receptor agonist. PPX has sevenfold higher affinity for the D3 receptor than for D2 or D4 receptors.[22] At low concentrations PPX decreases DA synthesis, release, and the firing of DA neurons, thereby decreasing extracellular DA concentrations.[23] PPX also has antioxidant activity.[24] Both actions would reduce oxidative stress and could benefit survival of DA neurons. In fact, when added to primary cultures of ventral mesencephalon exposed to neurotoxic concentrations of levodopa (l-dopa),[25,26] PPX reduced DA neuron death in a dose-dependent manner.[27] In order to assess the individual contributions of actions via the D3 receptor versus antioxidant properties, a number of pharmacological experiments were performed.[28,29] Experiments utilized 7-OH-DPAT, a D3 agonist without intrinsic antioxidant properties, and antioxidants including tocopherol. Addition of 7-OH-DPAT to cultures treated with l-dopa and PPX potentiated the protection of DA neurons. Addition of the D3 antagonist U99194 decreased the protective effect of PPX. Addition of agents affecting D2 receptor function were without effect. In contrast, 7-OH-DPAT did not by itself protect DA neurons in l-dopa–treated cultures but did provide protection when combined with low levels of tocopherol. Interestingly, treatment of cultures containing DA neurons with either PPX or 7-OH-DPAT produced conditioned medium that, when placed on sister cultures, increased the number and growth of DA neurons. Taken together, the effects of PPX appear to be attributable to a combination of antioxidant actions and actions at the D3 DA receptor that stimulates secretion of neurotrophic activity for DA neurons. Further studies suggest that the D3-stimulated neurotrophic activity is oxidant labile. Thus, PPX may present the unique capacity to stimulate DA neurotrophic activity and protect that activity from inactivation in the presence of prooxidants such as l-dopa via its additional antioxidant properties.

The second example is the identification of DA neurotrophic activity produced by the glial progenitor cell type O2A (oligodendrocyte–type 2 astrocyte precursor). Several reports in the literature document that striatal target tissue exerts trophic effects on DA neurons in coculture systems.[4,30–35] Our own experience in transplantation paradigms confirmed that implanting grafts of embryonic striatal tissue near grafts of DA neurons improved their survival and influenced the directionality of DA neurite extension.[36] A preliminary report in the literature suggested that striatal cultures enriched in O2A progenitor cells released activity into the culture medium that protected cultured DA neurons from death produced by serum deprivation.[37] We pursued this finding in a series of culture experiments of our own.[38]

We exploited a prior finding that exposure of cultures to a combination of the mitogens platelet-derived growth factor (PDGF)-AA and basic fibroblast growth factor (bFGF) induced proliferation of O2A progenitor cells and enriched cultures in this cell type.[39] Accordingly, we collected tissue from E14 rat striatum (lateral ganglionic eminence, LGE), dispersed the cells, plated them in culture, and exposed the cultures to fresh mitogens at 48-hour intervals for 1 month. As cultures became confluent during this interval cells were divided and replated. After 1 month of enrichment in O2A progenitors, mitogens were discontinued; and we collected culture medium containing factors secreted by the cells at 24-hour intervals for several days. Cultures stained with the O2A progenitor cell marker A2B5+ confirmed that mitogen-treated cultures contained numerous dense clusters of O2A cells. Staining for markers of neurons, astrocytes, and mature oligodendrocytes confirmed their presence as well, but with much reduced prevalence in comparison to O2A cells.

Striatal O2A (SO2A) conditioned medium (CM) was aliquoted and diluted to achieve concentrations of 0, 25, 50, 75, and 100% SO2A CM. When primary micro-island cultures of E14 rat ventral mesencephalon were exposed to increasing concentrations of SO2A CM during the first 4 days in culture, TH+ DA neurons increased in number in a dose-dependent manner, achieving a 400% increase at concentrations $\geq$75% SO2A CM. CM from striatal cultures not enriched in O2A cells produced only modest increases in DA neuron survival that did not reach statistical significance. In addition to increasing the number of TH+ neurons in cultures, SO2A CM increased the expression of TH in individual neurons by 43%.

As discussed earlier, culture conditions can be manipulated to yield different populations of cells. In the present experiments, mesencephalic cultures were maintained in hormone-supplemented serum-free (HSSF) medium. These conditions do not support mesencephalic astrocytes, and staining for the marker glial fibrillary acidic protein (GFAP) confirmed that cultures were essentially free of astrocytes. Treatment with SO2A CM did not increase the number of glia. Thus, the effects of CM on the number of TH+ neurons was not attributable to an indirect effect mediated by astrocytes. Counts of all neurons, visualized by staining for microtuble-associated protein (MAP)-2, revealed no significant increase in numbers in cultures exposed to SO2A CM. This finding supports a relatively specific effect of CM on TH+ DA neurons and is consistent with their known prevalence at approximately 5% of the neurons in culture.

The increased number of TH+ cells in cultures exposed to SO2A CM could represent an effect on cell survival or be a function of increased TH expression. Increased TH expression was documented and would allow visualization of cells with levels of TH below the limit of detection by the immuncytochemical technique. Accordingly we examined the effects of SO2A CM on cell death by visualizing the number of apoptotic profiles in culture using the TdT-mediated dUTP-biotin nick end labeling (TUNEL) technique and measuring levels of lactate dehydrogenase in the culture medium. For both measures, increasing concentrations of SO2A CM yielded corresponding dose-related decreases in markers of cell death. Thus, while SO2A CM clearly increases expression of TH, its effects on numbers of DA neurons in culture also can be related to inhibition of cell death.

In a final experiment we compared the effects of SO2A CM and another glial conditioned medium, Schwann cell conditioned medium (SCCM),[40] to known neurotrophic factors for DA neurons. Microisland cultures were plated and held in HSSF medium supplemented with published optimal concentrations of neurotrophic factors (GDNF, 50ng/mL; brain-derived neurotrophic factor [BDNF], 50 ng/mL; neurotrophin [NT]-4, 10 ng/mL; NT3, 10 ng/mL; neurturin [NTN], 10 ng/mL; bFGF, 10 ng/mL; epidermal growth factor [EGF], 10 ng/mL) or 75% CM from confluent cultures of SO2A cells or rat Schwann cells collected at 24-hour intervals. Cultures were fixed and stained for TH on day 4 *in vitro*. In these culture conditions, only GDNF, SO2A CM, and SCCM significantly increased DA neuron survival, with

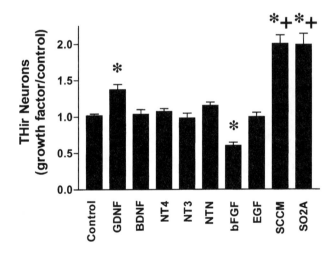

FIGURE 1. Neurotrophic effects of known factors and conditioned medium from Schwann cells and striatal O2A progenitor cells for embryonic DA neurons in microisland cultures. In these culture conditions, survival-promoting effects of several known growth factors were modest and not statistically significant. Only GDNF and cell conditioned media significantly enhanced the number of TH+ DA neurons in culture at 4 days *in vitro*. In addition, the combinations of molecules secreted by striatal O2A cells and Schwann cells significantly outperformed GDNF. These natural mixtures of molecules appear to provide an improved source of dopamine neurotrophic activity over any single identified molecule. *$P < 0.05$ as compared to control. [+]$P < 0.0001$ as compared to GDNF. Data presented is mean + SEM of cell counts in treatment conditions/control conditions. ABBREVIATIONS: THir = TH immunoreactive; GDNF = glial cell line–derived neurotrophic factor; BDNF = brain-derived neurotrophic factor; NT4 = neurotrophin 4; NT3 = neurotrophin 3; NTN = neurturin; bFGF = basic fibroblast growth factor; EGF = epidermal growth factor; SCCM = Schwann cell conditioned medium (75%); SO2A = striatal O2A progenitor cell conditioned medium (75%).

SO2A CM and SCCM exhibiting significantly better effects than GDNF (FIG. 1). bFGF had a significant detrimental effect on the number of TH+ neurons. To our knowledge this is the only example of such a comparison of the effects of DA neurotrophic factors in microisland cultures, and it is an example of the impact of culture conditions on experimental outcome measures. As discussed earlier, potential survival-promoting factors often are screened purposely in suboptimal culture conditions that favor detection of a positive effect. However, such conditions may exaggerate the biological significance of a given outcome. It is of interest that with microisland cultures, a condition in which the cultured cells are maintained in closer physical proximity to one another, effects of many of the identified neurotrophic molecules for DA neurons were modest and did not reach statistical significance. Of these, only GDNF exerted a significant effect on the number of DA neurons and was significantly outperformed by the natural combinations of molecules secreted by cultured SO2A and Schwann cells. This comparison suggests that these cell-derived mixtures are more potent than any individual molecule and may be of significant therapeutic interest.

CONCLUSIONS

In this brief review we have summarized the main issues related to the use of cell culture systems to study DA neurons and have provided examples of the use of culture models to examine mechanisms of DA neuron degeneration and to identify potential therapeutics. It is reasonable to ask whether cell culture findings effectively translate into valuable approaches *in vivo*. For the examples provided here, cell culture findings have been predictive of results in animal models of PD and in some cases have been studied for relevance in the disease itself. The response of cultured DA neurons to neurotoxins supports the important roles of oxidative stress and impaired mitochondrial energy metabolism. These continue to be important themes in the development of therapeutic approaches, although simple use of the antioxidant tocopherol has proved ineffective in PD.[41,42] The identification of activated microglia as active participants in DA neuron degeneration, as suggested by culture findings, has been confirmed in animal models of PD[43,44] and generated interest in clinical application of antiinflammatory drugs for PD. For the neuroprotective strategies, pramipexole has been shown to diminish DA neuron death in an animal model of PD[45] and has demonstrated efficacy as a monotherapy in mild-to-moderate PD.[46] Finally, neurotrophic activity derived from SO2A cells or Schwann cells has been shown to augment survival and function of transplanted embryonic DA neurons in a rat model of PD[47–49] and to stimulate TH expression in adult DA neurons of rats and monkeys.[50,51] Thus, the unique access to the DA neuron provided by cell culture systems serves as an important setting for analyzing cellular mechanisms, as well as a valuable prelude to preclinical animal studies and clinical trials.

ACKNOWLEDGMENTS

The authors are grateful for the technical contributions of Brian Daley, Matthew Fleming, Michelle Gartland, and Mark Gallagher. This work was supported by National Institutes of Health Grants AG08133, NS24032, AG10851, AG00844, and Department of Defense Grant DAMD 17-99-1-9543.

REFERENCES

1. ENGELE, J. & M.C. BOHN. 1991. The neurotrophic effects of fibroblast growth factors on dopaminergic neurons in vitro are mediated by mesencephalic glia. J. Neurosci. **11:** 3070–3078.
2. O'MALLEY, E.K., I.B. BLACK & C.F. DREYFUS. 1991. Local support cells promote survival of substantia nigra dopaminergic neurons in culture. Exp. Neurol. **112:** 40–48.
3. TAKESHIMA, T., J.M JOHNSTON & J.W. COMMISSIONG. 1994. Mesencephalic type 1 astrocytes rescue dopaminergic neurons from death induced by serum deprivation. J. Neurosci. **14:** 4769–4779.
4. DAL TOSO, R., O. GIORGI, C. SORANZO, *et al.* 1988. Development and survival of neurons in dissociated fetal mesencphalic serum-free cell cultures: I. Effects of cell density and of an adult mammalian striatal-derived neurontrophic factor (SDNF). J. Neurosci. **8:** 733–745.
5. TAKESHIMA, T., K. SHIMODA, J.M. JOHNSTON, *et al.* 1996. Standardized methods to bioassay neurotrophic factors for dopaminergic neurons. J. Neurosci Methods **67:** 27–41.
6. HAYFLICK, L. 1965. The limited in vitro lifetime of human diploid cell strains. Exp. Cell Res. **37:** 614–636.
7. MATHON, N.F., D.S. MALCOLM, M.C. HARRISINGH, *et al.* 2001. Lack of replicative senescence in normal rodent glia. Science **291:** 872–875.
8. TANG, D.G., Y.M. TOKUMOTO, J.A. APPERLY, *et al.* 2001. Lack of replicative senescence in cultured rat oligodendrocyte precursor cells. Science **291:** 868–871.
9. JENNER, P. 1998. Oxidative mechanisms in nigral cell death in Parkinson's disease. Mov. Disord. **13:** 24–34.
10. OLANOW, C.W. 1992. An introduction to the free radical hypothesis in Parkinson's disease. Ann. Neurol. **32:** S2–S9.
11. LOTHARIUS, J., L.L. DUGAN & K. L. O'MALLEY. 1999. Distinct mechanisms underlie neurotoxin-mediated cell death in cultured dopaminergic neurons. J. Neurosci. **19:** 1284–1293.
12. CHOI, W.S., S.Y. YOON, T.H. OH, *et al.* 1999. Two distinct mechanisms are involved in 6-hydroxydopamine- and MPP+-induced dopaminergic neuronal cell death: role of caspases, ROS, and JNK. J. Neurosci. Res. **57:** 86–94.
13. OH, J.H., W.S. CHOI, J.E. KIM, *et al.* 1998. Overexpression of HA-Bax but not Bcl-2 or Bcl-XL attenutates 6-hydroxydopamine-induced neuronal apoptosis. Exp. Neurol. **154:** 193–198.
14. MCGEER, P.L., S. ITAGAKI, B.E. BOYES, *et al.* 1988. Reactive microglia positive for HLA-DA in the substantia nigra of Parkinson's and Alzheimer's disease brain. Neurology **38:** 1285–1291.
15. HIRSCH, E.C., S. HUNOT, P. DAMIER, *et al.* 1998. Glia cells and inflammation in Parkinson's disease: a role in neurodegeneration. Ann. Neurol. **44:** S115–S120.
16. LANGSTON, J.W., L.S. FORNO, J. TETRUD, *et al.* 1999. Evidence of active nerve cell degeneration in the substantia nigra of humans years after 1-methyl-4-phenyl-1,2,3,6-tetrahydropyridine exposure. Ann. Neurol. **46:** 598–605.
17. MOGI, M., M. HARADA, H. NARABAYASHI, *et al.* 1996. Interleukin (IL)-1 beta, IL-2, IL-4, IL-6 and transforming growth factor-alpha levels are elevated in ventriucular cerebrospinal fluid in juvenile parkinsonism and Parkinson's disease. Neurosci. Lett. **211:** 13–16.
18. MOGI, M., M. HARADA, P. RIEDERER, *et al.* 1994. Tumor necrosis factor-alpha (TNF-alpha) increases both in the brain and in the cerebrospinal fluid from parkinsonian patients. Neurosci. Lett. **165:** 208–210.
19. LE, W.D., D.B. ROWE, J. JANKOVIC, *et al.* 1999. Effects of cerebrospinal fluid from patiens with Parkinson disease on dopaminergic cells. Arch. Neurol. **56:** 194–200.
20. LE, W.D., D. ROWE, W. XIE, *et al.* 2001. Microglial activation and dopaminergic cell injury: an in vitro model relevant to Parkinson's disease. J. Neurosci. **21:** 8447–8455.

21. COLLIER, T.J. & C.E. SORTWELL. 1999. Therapeutic potential of nerve growth factors in Parkinson's disease. Drugs Aging 14: 261–287.
22. PIERCEY, M.F., W.E. HOFFMAN, M.W. SMITH, et al. 1996. Inhibition of dopamine neuron firing by pramipexole, a dopamine D3 receptor-preferring agonist: comparison to other dopamine receptor agonists. Eur. J. Pharmacol. 312: 35–44.
23. CARTER, A.J. & R.E. MULLER. 1991. Pramipexole, a dopamine D2 autoreceptor agonist, decreases the extracellular concentration of dopamine in vivo. Eur. J. Pharmacol. 200: 65–72.
24. PIERCEY, M.F. 1998. Pharmacology of pramipexole, a dopamine D3-preferring agonist useful in treating Parkinson's disease. Clin. Neuropharmacol. 21: 141–151.
25. ALEXANDER, T., C.E. SORTWELL, C.D. SLADEK, et al. 1997. Comparison of neurotoxicity following repeated administration of L-DOPA, D-DOPA, and dopamine to embryonic mesencephalic dopamine neurons in cultures derived from Fisher 344 and Sprague-dawley donors. Cell Transplant. 6: 309–315.
26. ZIV, I., R. ZILKHA-FALB, D. OFFEN, et al. 1997. Levodopa induces apoptosis in cultured neuronal cells—a possible accelerator of nigrostriatal degeneration in Parkinson's disease? Mov. Disord. 12: 17–23.
27. CARVEY, P.M., S. PIERI & Z.D. LING. 1997. Attenuation of levodopa-induced toxicity in mesencephalic cultures by pramipexole. J. Neural Transm. 104: 209–228.
28. LING, Z.D., H.C. ROBIE, C.W. TONG, et al. 1999. Both the antioxidant and D3 agonist actions of pramipexole mediate its neuroprotective actions in mesencephalic cultures. J. Pharmacol. Exp. Ther. 289: 202–210.
29. CARVEY, P.M., S.O. MCGUIRE & Z.D. LING. 2001. Neuroprotective effects of D3 dopamine receptor agonists. Parkinsonism Relat. Disord. 7: 213–223.
30. PROCHIANTZ, A., U. DI PORZIO, A. KATO, et al. 1979. In vitro maturation of mesencephalic dopaminergic neurons from mouse embryos is enhanced in the presence of their striatal target cells. Proc. Natl. Acad. Sci. USA 76: 5387–5391.
31. DAGUET, M.-C., U. DIPORZIO, A. PROCHIANTZ, et al. 1980. Release of dopamine from dissociated mesencephalic dopaminergic neurons in primary cultures in absence or presence of striatal target cells. Brain Res. 191: 564–568.
32. HEMMENDINGER, L.M., B.B. GARBER, P.C. HOFFMAN, et al. 1981. Target neuron-specific process formation by embryonic mesencepahlic dopamine neurons in vitro. Proc. Natl., Acad. Sci. USA 78: 1264–1268.
33. HOFFMAN, P.C., L.M. HEMMENDINGER, C. KOTAKE, et al. 1983. Enhanced dopamine cell survival in reaggregates containing telencephalic targets. Brain Res. 274: 275–281.
34. TOMOZAWA, Y. & S.H. APPEL. 1986. Soluble striatal extracts enhance development of mesencephalic dopaminergic neurons in vitro. Brain Res. 399: 111–124.
35. DONG, J.F., A. DETTA, M.H.M. BAKKER, et al. 1993. Direct interaction with target-derived glia enhances survival but not differentiation of human fetal mesencephalic dopaminergic neurons. Neuroscience 56: 53–60.
36. SORTWELL, C.E., T.J. COLLIER & J.R. SLADEK, JR. 1997. Co-grafted embryonic striatum increases the survival of grafted embryonic dopamine neurons. J. Comp. Neurol. 399: 530–540.
37. TAKESHIMA, T., J.M. JOHNSTON & J.W. COMMISSIONG. 1994. Oligodendrocyte-type-2 astrocyte (O2A) progenitors increase the survival of rat mesencephalic, dopaminergic neurons from death induced by serum deprivation. Neurosci. Lett. 166: 178–182.
38. SORTWELL, C.E., B.F. DALEY, M.R. PITZER, et al. 2000. Oligodendrocyte-type 2 astrocyte-derived trophic factors increase survival of developing dopamine neurons through the inhibition of apoptotic cell death. J. Comp. Neurol. 426: 143–153.
39. BOGLER, O.,D. WREN, S.C. BARNETT, et al. 1990. Cooperation between two growth factors promotes extended self-renewal and inhibits differentiation of oligodendrocyte-type-2-astrocyte (O2A) progenitor cells. Proc. Natl. Acad. Sci. USA 87: 6368–6372.
40. COLLIER, T.J., C.D. SLADEK, M.J. GALLAGER, et al. 1990. Diffusible factor(s) from adult rat sciatic nerve increases cell number and neurite outgrowth of cultured embryonic ventral mesencephalic tyrosine hydroxylase-positive neurons. J. Neurosci. Res. 27: 394–399.
41. THE PARKINSON STUDY GROUP. 1993. Effects of tocopherol and deprenyl on the progression of disability in early Parkinson's disease. N. Engl. J. Med. 328: 176–183.

42. SHOULSON, I. 1998. DATATOP: a decade of neuroprotective inquiry. Ann. Neurol. **44:** S160–166.
43. WU, D.C., V. JACKSON-LEWIS, M. VILA, *et al.* 2002. Blockade of microglial activation is neuroprotective in the 1-methyl-4-phenyl-1,2,3,6-tetrahydropyridine mouse model of Parkinson's disease. J. Neurosci. **22:** 1763–1771.
44. HE, Y., W.-D. LE & S.H. APPEL. 2002. Role of Fc-gamma receptors in nigral cell injury induced by Parkinson disease immunoglobulin injection into mouse substantia nigra. Exp. Neurol. **176:** 322–327.
45. VU, T.Q., Z.D. LING, S.Y. MA, *et al.* 2000. Pramipexole attenuates the dopaminergic cell loss induced by intraventricular 6-hydroxydopamine. J. Neural Trans. **107:** 159–176.
46. SHANNON, K.M., J.P.J. BENNETT & J.H. FRIEDMAN. 1997. Efficacy of pramipexole, a novel dopamine agonist, as monotherapy in mild to moderate Parkinson's disease. Neurol. **49:** 724–728.
47. VAN HORNE, C.G., I. STROMBERG, D. YOUNG, *et al.* 1991. Functional enhancement of intrastriatal dopamine-containing grafts by the co-transplantation of sciatic nerve tissue in 6-hydroxydopamine-lesioned rats. Exp. Neurol. **113:** 143–154.
48. COLLIER, T.J. & J.E. SPRINGER. 1991. Co-grafts of embryonic dopamine neurons and adult sciatic nerve into the denervated striatum enhance behavioral and morphological recovery in rats. Exper. Neurol. **114:** 343–350.
49. SORTWELL, C.E., B.F. DALEY & T.J. COLLIER. 1998. Time course of apoptotic cell death in Mesencephalic suspension grafts: early trophic influence of O-2A progenitor-enriched Striatal co-grafts. Soc. Neurosci. Abstr. 421.7, **24:** 1056.
50. COLLIER, T.J. & P.N. MARTIN. 1993. Schwann cells as a source of neurotrophic activity for dopamine neurons. Exp. Neruol. **124:** 129–133.
51. COLLIER, T.J., J.D. ELSWORTH, J.R. TAYLOR, *et al.* 1994. Peripheral nerve-dopamine neuron co-grafts in MPTP-treated monkeys: augmentation of tyrosine hydroxylase-positive fiber staining and dopamine content in host systems. Neurosci. **61:** 875–889.

Convergent Pathobiologic Model of Parkinson's Disease

KATHLEEN A. MAGUIRE-ZEISS AND HOWARD J. FEDEROFF

Department of Neurology and the Center for Aging and Developmental Biology,
University of Rochester School of Medicine and Dentistry,
Rochester, New York 14642, USA

ABSTRACT: The etiology of Parkinson's disease (PD) has yet to be delineated. Human genetic studies as well as neurotoxicant and transgenic animal models of PD suggest that multiple events trigger the initiation of this progressive age-related neurodegenerative disorder. In addition, we propose that despite disparate disease triggers a convergent pathobiologic pathway exists leading to cell death. The common pathway model posits that both familial and sporadic forms of Parkinson's disease obligately share a common pathophysiological substrate. Herein we discuss the evidence for a common pathway model of Parkinson's disease through a review of synuclein transgenic models and outline an approach for the idenfication of shared therapeutic targets. We end with a discussion of a potential alternative therapy for Parkinson's disease.

KEYWORDS: Parkinson's disease; synuclein; single-chain antibodies; transgenic animals

The etiologic basis of Parkinson's disease (PD), the second most prevalent neurodegenerative disorder, is unknown. Several lines of evidence point to both genetic and environmental components in the development of this disease.[1–18] Originally described by James Parkinson as "shaking palsy," PD is typified by motoric dysfunction resulting in both tremor and rigidity.[19] Neuropathologically, PD cases manifest intracytoplasmic inclusions known as Lewy bodies, gliosis, and neuronal loss specific to the nigrostriatal system. Lewy bodies are composed of aggregated proteins, most notably α-synuclein and ubiquitin. α-Synuclein has received considerable attention in etiopathogensis following the description of several kindreds in which dominantly inherited mutations in the human gene result in early-onset PD.[20–25] However, these familial forms account for a very small percentage of the total PD cases. Environmental factors including pesticides, herbicides, and industrial chemicals have also been flagged as potential risk factors for PD.[11,14–16,26,27] Together, genetic and environmental factors may act synergistically to initiate a series of cellular events leading to the parkinsonian syndrome.

Address for correspondence: Howard J. Federoff, M.D., Ph.D., Professor of Neurology, Center for Aging and Developmental Biology, Box 645, University of Rochester School of Medicine and Dentistry, 601 Elmwood Ave., Rochester, NY 14642. Voice: 716-273-2190; fax: 716-442-6646.

howard_federoff@urmc.rochester.edu

Ann. N.Y. Acad. Sci. 991: 152–166 (2003). © 2003 New York Academy of Sciences.

Although the initiating triggers for sporadic PD may be disparate, the pathological result is uniformly described as a pronounced loss of dopaminergic neurons (DAN) in the nigrostriatal pathway. The consequence of this loss is a decrease in the neurotransmitter dopamine (DA) and motor dysfunction. Patients in the early stages of PD are aided by treatment with the drug levodopa, which is converted centrally to DA. However, as the disease progresses most patients become refractory to levodopa therapy. Thus, there is a great need to better understand the molecular mechanisms of PD and to design new therapies that would rescue, protect, and/or possibly generate new DAN. To elucidate the molecular events important in PD requires disease models that faithfully recapitulate the disorder. Many laboratories have produced a number of toxicant and genetic models that reproduce many of the pathological features of PD.[1,3,7,28] Herein we review the evidence for a common pathway model for PD through examination of models and outline an approach for the identification of potential shared therapeutic targets.

COMMON PATHWAY MODEL OF PD

Mutations in both α-synuclein and parkin appear sufficient to produce, respectively, rare dominant and recessive familial forms of PD. In addition, neurotoxicants including classes of pesticides, herbicides, and industrial chemicals are potential risk factors. The "common pathway" model posits that all PD must share a common pathobiologic course. Whether triggered by rare genetic mutations, pure toxicant

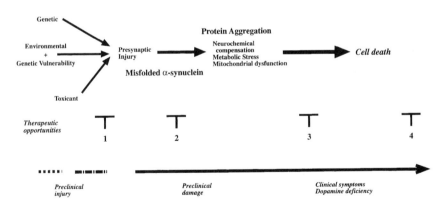

FIGURE 1. Schematic diagram depicting the common pathway model for PD. Environmental factors such as pesticides, herbicides, and industrial chemicals have been identified as potential risk factors for PD; whereas specific genetic mutations appear sufficient to produce rare familial PD, suggesting that the majority of idiopathic cases will result from an interplay between environmental exposure and inherited vulnerability. Thus multiple triggers produce the common clinical PD syndrome. Possible therapeutic targets are highlighted: (1) specific triggering mechanisms; (2) shared early pathway step prior to presynaptic dopamine dysfunction; targeting misfolded α-synuclein; (3) shared later pathway step when dopaminergic neuron dysfunction occurs; (4) restoring dopamine biosynthesis in denervated striatum. (Adapted from W.J. Bowers, et al.[5])

forms, or interactions between environmental toxicant and genetic vulnerability, all PD is postulated to be mechanistically convergent (FIG. 1 and Ref. 5). These multiple initiating mechanisms trigger cellular events, the first step of which results in presynaptic injury and dysfunction of the nigrostriatal tract. We surmise that presynaptic injury is clinically silent. Presynaptic injury is envisioned to stimulate cellular compensation, during which we predict that intracellular proteins such as α-synuclein initiate pathologic folding and consequent cell injury, perhaps by compromising proteosomal function. Progressive injury wrought by impaired disposal of possibly toxic abnormally folded and oxidized proteins are believed to evolve over years. As compensatory responses fail, neurochemical dysfunction (e.g., diminished DA release, uptake, and vesicular loading) are attended by bioenergetic failure, marked reactive oxygen species (ROS) generation, and finally cell death.

Clinical and pathological evidence support this common pathway model independently of the triggering mechanism. First, all PD patients have a selective and profound loss of ventral midbrain dopamine neurons. Second, the invariant loss of DA-releasing nigrostriatal presynaptic terminals precedes cell body loss in the substantia nigra.[29–32] Third, loss of these dopaminergic projection neurons results in the cardinal PD clinical features: bradykinesia, akinesia, tremor, rigidity, and postural reflex impairment (reviewed in Ref. 33). Fourth, neuropathology reveals the presence of α-synuclein and ubiquitin containing Lewy bodies.[34–39] Finally, systemic absorption of exogenous neurotoxicants best exemplified by MPTP induce in mouse, monkey, and man a clinical, biochemical, and pathological parkinsonian syndrome.[12,40,41] Taken together, these data indicate that disparate triggers elicit a cellular, biochemical, and presumably molecular response that results in the familiar parkinsonian syndrome.

Additional support for a convergent model of PD and the role of α-synuclein derives from recently developed animal models of familial α-synuclein mutations. Although rare, mutations in the α-synuclein gene cause intracytoplasmic α-synuclein inclusions and early-onset disease.[20–25] These autosomal-dominant cases directly implicate specific coding region mutations (A30P, A53T) in α-synuclein aggregation and/or degradation. Moreover, diminished protein processing is further supported by mutations in *parkin* and *ubiquitin carboxy-terminal-hydrolase-L1 (UCHL1)* two proteins involved in ubiquitin-dependent proteosomal function.[10,20,42–52] Linkage of toxicant injury to protein aggregation has been provided by recent evidence that MPTP stimulates production and oxidative modification of α-synuclein.[53–55]

TRANSGENIC MODELS OF PD

In our common pathway model α-synuclein plays an important role in DAN-specific dysfunction and death. To better appreciate its role in PD several laboratories are using transgenic technology to overexpress wild-type and mutant α-synuclein (see TABLE 1 and Refs.1,3,4,7).

Transgenic mouse models that use promoters capable of widespread expression such as PDGF, prion, and Thy1 generally result in increased protein accumulation, motor signs, abnormal axons, and neurites in multiple brain regions.[56–58] Transgenic mice employing the Thy1.2 promoter to drive α-synuclein overexpression display swollen neurites in the cerebellar Purkinje layer, nucleus dentatus, hippocampus, neocortex, and brain stem.[56] A second Thy1:α-synuclein transgenic mouse demon-

TABLE 1. Comparison of α-synuclein transgenic animals

Transgenic model human α-synuclein	Promoter	NT function	Protein accum.	Neuronal abnorm.	Motor dysf.	Ref.
WT	human PDGF-β	ND	(+)	(+)	(+)	58
WT A53T A30P	rat TH	(−)	(+)	(−)	(−)	60
WT A30P	mouse Thy1.2	ND	(+)	ND	(+)	56
WT A53T	mouse Thy1	ND	(+)	(+)	(+)	59
WT	rat TH	(+)	(−)	(−)	(+)	61
A53T/A30P	rat TH	(+)	(−)	(+)	(+)	61
WT A53T A30P	prion	ND	(+)	(+)	(+)	57

ABBREVIATIONS: NT = neurotransmitter; accum. = accumulation; Neuronal abnorm. = neuronal abnormalities, such as swollen neurites; Motor dysf. = motor dysfunction, such as alterations in behavioral tests of motor function.

strated neuropathologic α-synuclein aggregates and inclusions in an equally wide range of brain regions but most notably not in the substantia nigra pars compacta.[59] In fact, this transgene fails to express in ventral midbrain dopaminergic neurons, suggesting that these mice may be a more appropriate model for diffuse Lewy body disease rather than for PD (personal communication and Ref. 59). Cytoplasmic inclusions and α-synuclein aggregates, but no fibrillar material, were also observed in the neocortex, hippocampus, and substantia nigra of transgenic mice using the human PDGF-β promoter.[58] When driven by the mouse prion promoter, transgene product accumulation in the midbrain, cerebellum, brain stem, and spinal cord was correlated with an earlier onset of disease and death.[57]

To more faithfully recapitulate pathogenesis including neuroanatomical, neurochemical, and neuropathological changes in DAN *only*, two laboratories have developed transgenic animal models in which the catecholaminergic promoter tyrosine hydroxylase drives α-synuclein expression. One group reported modest α-synuclein accumulation without inclusions or neurochemical change when wild-type, A53T, or A30P α-synuclein was overexpressed.[60] On the other hand, our laboratory engineered two TH-driven transgenic lines that overexpress wild-type (hα-syn) or doubly mutated (hm²α-syn) human α-synuclein. The doubly-mutated α-synuclein transgene contains both the A53T and A30P mutations within the same open reading frame[61] (see FIG. 2, panel A). Transgenic animals were evaluated neuroanatomically, neurochemically, behaviorally, and neuropathologically.[61] Overexpression of either α-synuclein resulted in an age-dependent phenotype that included a range of motoric dysfunction, abnormal neurites, and neurotransmitter alterations, but no Lewy body inclusions. We have shown that α-synuclein mRNA is highly expressed in the substantia nigra (SN) in these animals by *in situ* hybridization analysis (FIG. 2, panel B).

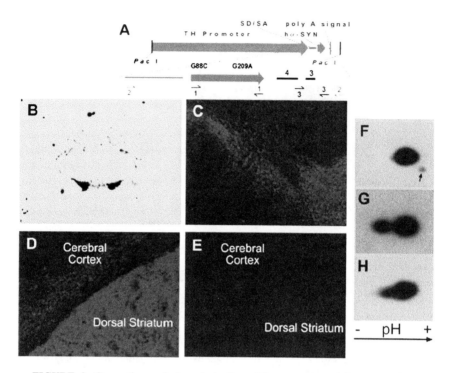

FIGURE 2. Generation and characterization of human α-synuclein transgenic mice. **(A)** Map of the human double mutant α-synuclein construct used for engineering the transgenic mice. **(B)** α-Synuclein mRNA Expression. Image of *in situ* hybridization from hm²α-SYN at the level of the SN. **(C–E)** Immunohistochemistry using a human specific polyclonal antibody to α-synuclein **(C,D)** in hm²α-SYN line and **(E)** in nontransgenic littermates. This antibody detected only human α-synuclein protein but not mouse α-synuclein. Human α-synuclein was most highly expressed in the cell bodies and dendrites of the SN and VTA, their axons, and in the striatum. **(F–H)** Striatal protein was subjected to 2-D PAGE followed by Western blotting using a polyclonal Ab to α-syn that recognizes both mouse and human α-syn. **(F)** Nontransgenic littermate controls demonstrated a larger single spot migrating at approximately 15 kDa and a much smaller spot *(arrow)* migrating at a slightly smaller MW and at a slightly more basic pI suggestive of a dephosphorylated form of mouse α-syn. Lines hm²α-syn-39 **(G)** and hwα-syn-5 **(H)** demonstrated unique spots migrating at a similar MW to mouse α-syn, but at different and slightly more acidic pIs. (Reproduced from E.K. Rich-field, *et al.*[61] with permission.)

Both hα-syn and hm²α-syn express high levels of α-synuclein protein in midbrain DAN cell bodies and their striatal projections[61] (FIG. 2, panels C,D). α-Synuclein colocalized with TH in cell bodies and dendrites of the SN, ventral tegmental area, locus ceruleus; and projection fields in the dorsal striatum, nucleus accumbens, olfactory tubercle, and cerebral cortex. The subcellular distribution of α-synuclein is both nuclear and cytoplasmic compared to TH which is strictly cytoplasmic[61] (FIG. 3, panels D–F). Whether α-synuclein nuclear localization identifies a previously undisclosed action remains to be determined. Of interest, hm²α-syn axons in the median forebrain bundle were pathologically dilated and beaded, resembling Lewy

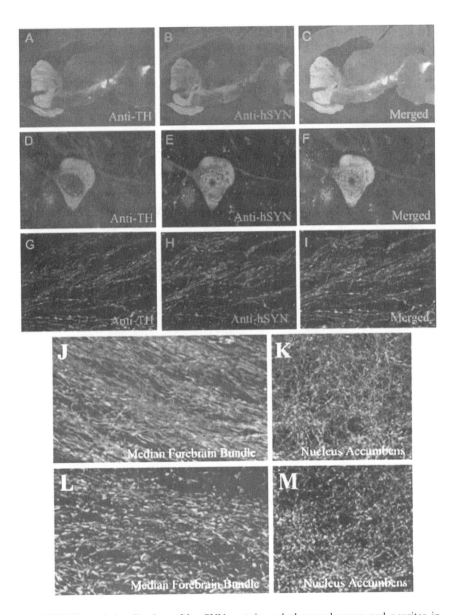

FIGURE 3. Colocalization of hα-SYN protein and abnormal axons and neurites in young hα-SYN transgenic mice. Double-label fluorescent IHC for TH (**A,D,G**), hα-SYN (**B,E,H**), both hα-SYN and TH (**C,F,I**) in a sagittal section from hm²α-SYN (**A–C**), a hwα-SYN SN neuron (**D–F**), or from hm²α-SYN median forebrain bundle (MFB, **G–I**). Confocal microscopy was used to image sections at 0.4-μm thickness using either the red or green filter (**D–I**) or routine fluorescent microscopy at 1.25× (**A–C**). The hα-SYN protein was present in dopaminergic cell bodies and dendrites (**B** and **E**) and nigrostriatal axons and terminals (**B** and **H**) in a distribution that matched that of TH (**A,D,G**). The hα-SYN protein was present in both the cytoplasm and the nucleus of neurons (**E**). Abnormal neurites were

neurites. However, no Lewy body-like inclusions were appreciated[61] (FIG. 3, panels J–M). Behavioral studies of these animals demonstrated an age-dependent decline in spontaneous activity and motor function, thus paralleling some of the clinical hallmarks of PD[61] (data not shown).

Why do different transgenic lines exhibit varying degrees of neuropathology? Our hm$^2\alpha$-syn model may represent a slower progress and possibly a more reflective model of the human disease, possibly because of TH promoter use. Most interestingly, our mice support the notion that the toxicity of α-synuclein does not require Lewy body formation but rather another, misfolded, protein structural state. This observation reinforces the concept of pathogenic stages as articulated in a common pathway model.

α-Synuclein transgenic animals are aiding in the identification of molecular mechanisms of PD pathogenesis, particularly the identification of cellular factors that regulate the aggregation and toxicity of α-synuclein. Although no model fully recapitulates all aspects of PD, the models appear to have great utility in addressing interactions between candidate neurotoxicants and α-synuclein itself. Indeed, our laboratory has shown that hα-syn and hm$^2\alpha$-syn mice manifest enhanced sensitivity to MPTP treatment. When treated, the transgenic mice exhibited markedly decreased locomotor activity and DAT density compared with nontransgenic littermates.[61]

To unravel the molecular basis of our staged convergent pathobiologic model we have embarked on an integrated and comparative bionomics analysis of striatum and substantia nigra in mouse models (α-synuclein transgenics and MPTP treatment) and human PD. This bipartite bionomics approach uses conventional high-density oligonucleotide microarray technology (Affymetrix) and a three-dimensional proteomics methodology to identify gene/gene product changes. Proteomics is accomplished by 2D-gel electrophoresis, differential spot detection, recovery, and digestion, followed by SELDI-TOF mass spectroscopy.

To discriminate pathophysiologically important changes we assert that the identified molecule must be expressed in the nigrostriatal pathway. Second, the molecule must be misregulated by neurotoxicant treatment and/or transgene expression in a temporally predictable manner. This combination of transcriptomic and proteomic methods will undoubtedly identify genes and gene products whose abundance is altered in PD and its models. Preliminary studies from the 2D-gel analysis followed by limited computer analysis demonstrates that five proteins are increased in hm$^2\alpha$-syn striatum, while four proteins are reduced compared to nontransgenic littermates (TABLE 2). Likewise five proteins were decreased in hm$^2\alpha$-syn substantia nigra

---

present in dendrites of SN and VTA neurons and axons to the striatum (G–I) and elsewhere. Fluorescent IHC for TH was performed in a nontransgenic littermate control mouse (J and K) or a hm$^2\alpha$-SYN mouse (L and M) in the MFB (J and L) or the nucleus accumbens (K and M). Confocal microscopy using a 100× objective at 0.5-μm steps was performed and a total of 10 sections stacked to make the final image. TH is normally present in MFB axons of control mice in a discontinuous manner, with the majority of axons having a uniform diameter with occasional modest dilations (J). In hm$^2\alpha$-SYN mice TH axons were more beaded and dilated in appearance, with more discontinuities (L). In the Acb, TH was present in smaller caliber processes and terminals of control mice (K). In hm$^2\alpha$-SYN mice the smaller caliber processes and terminals were more dilated and punctate (M). (Reproduced from E.K. Richfield, et al.[61] with permission.)

TABLE 2. Results of 2-D gel SELDI-TOF analysis

Brain region	Spot No.	MW	PI	-fold change
Striatum	111	52,265	5.86	+3.70
	156	42,069	5.98	+153.55
	165	39,657	5.88	+4.83
	177	39,167	7.38	+10.15
	264	28,882	5.52	−6.11
	277	25,937	5.18	+3.52
	356	15,096	5.43	−5.03
	358	14,687	6.42	−3.64
Substantia nigra	35	76,893	6.18	−7.85
	59	67,595	5.64	−3.13
	178	38,982	7.17	−3.09
	291	26,073	5.79	−3.35
	345	18,291	6.84	−4.79

NOTE: Striatum and substantia nigra were dissected from hm^{2}SYN and C57Bl/6 mice; protein lysates were prepared and run on a 2-D gel. 2-D electrophoresis was performed according to the method of O'Farrell[83] by Kendrick Labs, Inc. (Madison, WI) followed by limited computer comparison to determine differences between hm^{2}SYN and C57Bl/6 lysates. Protein spots of interest were excised from the Coomassie blue–stained gels, rehydrated, in-gel trypsinized, spotted onto Ciphergen H4 chips, and subjected to SELDI-TOF. Peptide molecular weights will be utilized for protein identification using peptide mass fingerprinting (ExPASy/PeptIdent).

(TABLE 2). These preliminary studies are indicative of the power of bionomic approaches combined with transgenic animal technology.

This bionomic approach must demonstrate that the identified dysregulated genes and their products are complicit in the pathophysiologic process. This will require using additional transgenesis and/or gene transfer to achieve gain and loss of function of the identified candidate molecules within the nigrostriatal pathway.

RATIONALE FOR MISFOLDED α-SYNUCLEIN AS A TARGET FOR MOLECULAR THERAPY

The precise mechanism(s) by which α-synuclein promotes injury and neurodegeneration is unknown. Insights gleaned from its apparent role in synaptic function and plasticity may delimit its potential pathologic contributions.[62–64] Synelfin, the avian homologue of α-synuclein, is developmentally regulated during the critical period of canary song learning development.[65] α-Synuclein is also developmentally regulated in mouse brain with a profile that is similar to those of other presynaptic proteins, such as synaptophysin, synaptotagmin I, and synapsin.[63,66] Interestingly, neuronal cells transfected to overexpress human α-synuclein exhibit reduced neurite outgrowth and alterations in cell adhesion capacity.[64] Whether such neuritic abnormalities are reflective of normal or pathologic α-synuclein function is unknown.

Other data disclose additional functions for α-synuclein including a role in oxidative stress. Binding and functional interaction of wild-type α-synuclein to the dopamine transporter (DAT) elicits membrane clustering of DAT, acceleration of DA uptake, and apoptosis.[67] This α-synuclein and DAT interaction could exacerbate toxicant-induced apoptosis. Inducible expression of wild-type and mutant α-synuclein (G209A) levels in HEK293 cells did not induce cell death, but toxic synergism between G209A mutant α-synuclein and dopamine was found.[68] Reports of DA-induced toxicity and cell death presumably results from the inherent reactivity of the neurotransmitter.[69,70] DA is readily oxidized to DA quinone resulting in the release of superoxide and hydrogen peroxide.[70,71] Furthermore, DA can covalently modify cysteine, forming S-cysteinyl dopamine on affected proteins, irreversibly modifying protein function.[72] DA terminals actively degenerate following DA-induced toxicity, and DA-derived orthoquinone (DAQ) forms covalent adducts with α-synuclein resulting in long-lived protofibril intermediates.[73,74] Taken together, these studies suggest that DA conspires with α-synuclein resulting in the generation of ROS and DA adduct formation on proteins leading to synaptic terminal dysfunction.

α-Synuclein misfolding is favored by mutation or oxidative damage and thus appears to be a central feature of the variously triggered forms of PD. Consistent with the idea that accumulation of aberrantly folded protein is integral to pathogenesis are the other familial forms that are characterized by loss of function mutations in the parkin and UCH-L1 genes. Since both gene products participate in the ubiquitin proteasome, it is evident that clearance of aberrantly folded proteins is slowed in parkinsonian dopaminergic neurons (reviewed in Ref. 46). Moreover, a nexus between toxicants such as MPTP and α-synuclein misfolding has also been established by experiments demonstrating that oxidative stress promotes the formation of α-synuclein aggregates and inclusions (reviewed in Refs. 17,75). This is also observed with other toxicants such as paraquat and rotenone.[6,9] A key question remains unanswered: which form(s) of α-synuclein compromise(s) neuronal function?

STEADY STATE α-SYNUCLEIN MODEL AND ALTERNATIVE THERAPIES FOR PD

We postulate that within DAN a steady state exists between the native α-synuclein (random coil), the preprotofibrillar conformer (β-sheet), and the aggregated form (FIG. 4). In this scenario either oxidative stress or the presence of A53T α-synuclein drives native conformers towards toxic oligomers. As a molecular instigator of PD, α-synuclein is analogous to amyloid beta (Aβ), which forms extracellular deposits and is a pathological hallmark of Alzheimer's disease.[76–78] Intracellular protein deposits are relevant to other neurological diseases as well, including amyotrophic lateral sclerosis and expanded polyglutamine disorders (reviewed in Ref. 79).

Under physiological conditions α-synuclein exists in a native random coil conformation and is normally targeted for degradation. Under conditions of oxidative stress, α-synuclein adopts an altered conformation (β-sheet; preprotofibrillar) that can serve as the nidus for pathophysiological seeding of toxic protein aggregates (preprotofibrils). The alteration in steady state towards a pathogenic β-sheet (preprotofibrillar)–containing population may represent a locus for therapeutic intervention. Furthermore, mutant α-synuclein relatively favors the β-sheet conformation without oxidative stress. Based on this evidence we suggest that therapies specifically designed to interact and reduce toxic α-synuclein conformers will attenuate dis-

(A)

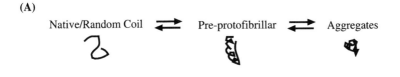

(B)

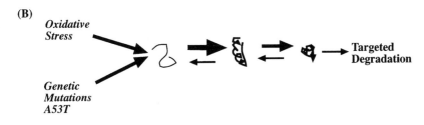

(C)

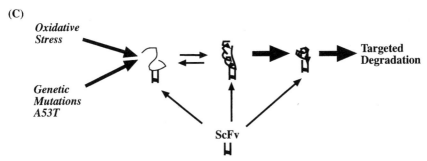

FIGURE 4. Schematic diagram of the dynamics between α-synuclein conformers. **(A)** Under normal physiological conditions a steady state exists between random coil, pre-protofibrillar, and aggregated α-synuclein conformers. **(B)** Under conditions of oxidative stress (neurotoxicant treatment) the steady state shifts toward the preprotofibrillar and aggregated α-synuclein conformers. Likewise, mutant α-synuclein (A53T) demonstrates a similar steady state shift. **(C)** ScFv's directed against conformer-specific forms of α-synuclein will either deplete the available pool of native or preprotofibrillar α-synuclein or target misfolded α-synuclein for degradation decreasing toxicity.

ease progression. Thus, preventing the formation of toxic preprotofibrillar forms of α-synuclein should be a goal of future therapeutics.

Our laboratory is pursuing a gene therapy approach whereby conformation-specific single-chain Fvs (scFvs) are expressed and intended to interfere with α-synuclein preprotofibrillar formation. ScFvs are composed of the minimal antibody binding site formed by noncovalent association of the V_H and V_L variable domains joined by a flexible polypeptide linker. Human scFv-phage libraries are available and allow for high-affinity human scFv antibodies to be selected from combinatorial libraries.[80] Antibody engineering makes it possible to manipulate the genes encoding the scFvs, allowing for antibody binding site expression *within* mammalian cells. Genetically fusing the scFv to intracellular targeting signals allows for specific subcellular expression.[81] These intracellular antibodies, termed intrabodies, are capable of modulating target protein function. Intrabodies have been used for both phenotypic and functional knockdown of target molecules. Perhaps most relevant to PD therapy through α-synuclein targeting is the recent work using human scFv intrabodies to disrupt huntingtin aggregation.[82] Huntingtin-specific scFvs bound to the N terminal polyglutamine residues and promoted solublilty of what otherwise would have been aggregated protein complexes.

In PD we suggest that protein aggregates forming within DAN are seeded, require the preprotofibrillar conformers of α-synuclein (β-sheet), and are cytotoxic. Identification of scFvs that will selectively recognize the preprotofibrillar conformers of α-synuclein is anticipated to attenuate protein toxicity (FIG. 4). In one case, scFvs could interact with α-synuclein prior to aggregation, thereby depleting the pool of available protein. In a second scenario scFvs bind to and deplete preprotofibrillar α-synuclein, thus attenuating aggregation. A third possibility is that scFvs interact with aggregated α-synuclein and efficiently target the complex for degradation. Each of these proposed strategies would decrease protein toxicity and potentially mitigate pathophysiologic damage.

SUMMARY

Transgenic models of α-synuclein overexpression will help to elucidate α-synuclein's role in PD pathogenesis. We postulate that combined genetic vulnerability and neurotoxicant exposure will provide mechanisms to examine sporadic PD. Our convergent pathobiologic model stipulates that disparate insults initiate a disease process that obligately share a common pathway leading to cell death. We further posit that α-synuclein misfolding is a proximal shared earlier step in the pathway. This critical step is suggested to induce cellular compensation that ultimately fails. The delineation of the transition from adaptive compensatory signaling to prodeath signaling affords the opportunity for therapeutic intervention. Our bionomic approach is formulated to identify both upstream (triggering stage) and downstream (compensatory or prodeath) targets involved in the convergent pathobiologic model. Genomic and proteomic methodologies in concert with innovative biologic approaches such as scFv gene transfer in transgenic/neurotoxicant models provide a basis to validate underlying pathogenic mechanisms and hold promise in the longer term for therapy.

ACKNOWLEDGMENT

This work was supported by NIH Grant R01-NS36420A to H.J.F.

REFERENCES

1. BEAL, M.F. 2001. Experimental models of Parkinson's disease. Nat. Rev. Neurosci. **2:** 325–334.
2. BETARBET, R., et al. 2000. Chronic systemic pesticide exposure reproduces features of Parkinson's disease. Nat. Neurosci. **3:** 1301–1306.

3. BETARBET, R., *et al.* 2002. Animal models of Parkinson's disease. Bioessays **24:** 308–318.
4. BOWERS, W.J., *et al.* 1997. Gene therapeutic strategies for neuroprotection: implications for Parkinson's disease. Exp Neurol. **144:** 58–68.
5. BOWERS, W.J., *et al.* 2001. Gene therapeutic approaches to the treatment of Parkinson's disease. Clin. Neurosci. Res. **1:** 483–495.
6. BROOKS, A.I., *et al.* 1999. Paraquat elicited neurobehavioral syndrome caused by dopaminergic neuron loss. Brain Res. **823:** 1–10.
7. DAWSON, T., *et al.* 2002. Animal models of PD: pieces of the same puzzle? Neuron **35:** 219–222.
8. KOWALL, N.W., *et al.* 2000. MPTP induces alpha-synuclein aggregation in the substantia nigra of baboons. Neuroreport **11:** 211–213.
9. MANNING-BOG, A.B., *et al.* 2002. The herbicide paraquat causes up-regulation and aggregation of alpha-synuclein in mice: paraquat and alpha-synuclein. J. Biol. Chem. **277:** 1641–1644.
10. MIZUNO, Y., *et al.* 1999. Genetic and environmental factors in the pathogenesis of Parkinson's disease. Adv. Neurol. **80:** 171–179.
11. OLANOW, C.W. & W.G. TATTON. 1999. Etiology and pathogenesis of Parkinson's disease. Annu. Rev. Neurosci. **22:** 123–144.
12. SCHMIDT, N. & B. FERGER. 2001. Neurochemical findings in the MPTP model of Parkinson's disease. J. Neural Transm. **108:** 1263–1282.
13. SCHWARTING, R.K. & J.P. HUSTON. 1996. The unilateral 6-hydroxydopamine lesion model in behavioral brain research. Analysis of functional deficits, recovery and treatments. Prog. Neurobiol. **50:** 275–331.
14. THIRUCHELVAM, M., *et al.* 2000. Potentiated and preferential effects of combined paraquat and maneb on nigrostriatal dopamine systems: environmental risk factors for Parkinson's disease? Brain Res. **873:** 225–234.
15. THIRUCHELVAM, M., *et al.* 2000. The nigrostriatal dopaminergic system as a preferential target of repeated exposures to combined paraquat and maneb: implications for Parkinson's disease. J. Neurosci. **20:** 9207–9214.
16. THIRUCHELVAM, M., *et al.* 2002. Developmental exposure to the pesticides paraquat and maneb and the Parkinson's disease phenotype. Neurotoxicology **23:** 621–633.
17. VILA, M., *et al.* 2000. Alpha-synuclein up-regulation in substantia nigra dopaminergic neurons following administration of the parkinsonian toxin MPTP. J. Neurochem. **74:** 721–729.
18. STEECE-COLLIER, K., *et al.* 2002. Etiology of Parkinson's disease: genetics and environment revisited. Proc. Natl. Acad. Sci. USA **99:** 13972–13974.
19. PARKINSON, J. 1817. An Essay on the Shaking Palsy. Sherwood, Neely, and Jones. London.
20. KITADA, T., *et al.* 1998. Mutations in the parkin gene cause autosomal recessive juvenile parkinsonism. Nature **392:** 605–608.
21. KRUGER, R., *et al.* 1998. Ala30Pro mutation in the gene encoding alpha-synuclein in Parkinson's disease. Nat. Genet. **18:** 106–108.
22. POLYMEROPOULOS, M.H., *et al.* 1996. Mapping of a gene for Parkinson's disease to chromosome 4q21-q23. Science **274:** 1197–1199.
23. POLYMEROPOULOS, M.H., *et al.* 1997. Mutation in the alpha-synuclein gene identified in families with Parkinson's disease. Science **276:** 2045–2047.
24. POLYMEROPOULOS, M.H. 2000. Genetics of Parkinson's disease. Ann. N.Y. Acad. Sci. **920:** 28–32.
25. SVEINBJORNSDOTTIR, S., *et al.* 2000. Familial aggregation of Parkinson's disease in Iceland. N. Engl. J. Med. **343:** 1765–1770.
26. GORELL, J.M., *et al.* 1998. The risk of Parkinson's disease with exposure to pesticides, farming, well water, and rural living. Neurology **50:** 1346–1350.
27. SEIDLER, A., *et al.* 1996. Possible environmental, occupational, and other etiologic factors for Parkinson's disease: a case-control study in Germany. Neurology **46:** 1275–1284.
28. CADET, J.L. 2001. Molecular neurotoxicological models of Parkinsonism: focus on genetic manipulation of mice. Parkinsonism Relat. Disord. **8:** 85–90.
29. MORRISH, P.K., *et al.* 1995. Clinical and [18F] dopa PET findings in early Parkinson's disease. J. Neurol. Neurosurg. Psychiatry **59:** 597–600.

30. PATE, B.D., *et al.* 1993. Correlation of striatal fluorodopa uptake in the MPTP monkey with dopaminergic indices. Ann. Neurol. **34:** 331–338.
31. SANCHEZ-PERNAUTE, R., *et al.* 2002. Functional imaging of the dopamine system: in vivo evaluation of dopamine deficiency and restoration. Neurotoxicology **23:** 469–478.
32. MAREK, K., *et al.* 2001. [123I]beta-CIT SPECT imaging assessment of the rate of Parkinson's disease progression. Neurology **57:** 2089–2094.
33. CENTONZE, D., *et al.* 1999. Neurophysiology of Parkinson's disease: from basic research to clinical correlates. Clin. Neurophysiol. **110:** 2006–2013.
34. MEZEY, E., *et al.* 1998. Alpha synuclein is present in Lewy bodies in sporadic Parkinson's disease. Mol. Psych. **3:** 493–499.
35. SPILLANTINI, M.G., *et al.* 1997. Alpha-synuclein in Lewy bodies. Nature **388:** 839–840.
36. SPILLANTINI, M.G., *et al.* 1998. alpha-Synuclein in filamentous inclusions of Lewy bodies from Parkinson's disease and dementia with lewy bodies. Proc. Natl. Acad. Sci. USA **95:** 6469–6473.
37. TROJANOWSKI, J.Q. & V.M. LEE. 1998. Aggregation of neurofilament and alpha-synuclein proteins in Lewy bodies: implications for the pathogenesis of Parkinson disease and Lewy body dementia. Arch. Neurol. **55:** 151–152.
38. WAKABAYASHI, K., *et al.* 1998. Accumulation of alpha-synuclein/NACP is a cytopathological feature common to Lewy body disease and multiple system atrophy. Acta Neuropathol. (Berl.) **96:** 445–452.
39. WAKABAYASHI, K., *et al.* 1998. Alpha-synuclein immunoreactivity in glial cytoplasmic inclusions in multiple system atrophy. Neurosci. Lett. **249:** 180–182.
40. LANGSTON, J.W., *et al.* 1983. Chronic Parkinsonism in humans due to a product of meperidine-analog synthesis. Science **219:** 979–980.
41. LANGSTON, J.W., *et al.* 1999. Evidence of active nerve cell degeneration in the substantia nigra of humans years after 1-methyl-4-phenyl-1,2,3,6-tetrahydropyridine exposure. Ann. Neurol. **46:** 598–605.
42. ABBAS, N., *et al.* 1999. A wide variety of mutations in the parkin gene are responsible for autosomal recessive parkinsonism in Europe. French Parkinson's Disease Genetics Study Group and the European Consortium on Genetic Susceptibility in Parkinson's Disease. Hum. Mol. Genet. **8:** 567–574.
43. HARHANGI, B.S., *et al.* 1999. The Ile93Met mutation in the ubiquitin carboxy-terminal-hydrolase-L1 gene is not observed in European cases with familial Parkinson's disease. Neurosci. Lett. **270:** 1–4.
44. HILKER, R., *et al.* 2001. Positron emission tomographic analysis of the nigrostriatal dopaminergic system in familial parkinsonism associated with mutations in the parkin gene. Ann. Neurol. **49:** 367–376.
45. ISHIKAWA, A. & S. TSUJI. 1996. Clinical analysis of 17 patients in 12 Japanese families with autosomal-recessive type juvenile parkinsonism. Neurology **47:** 160–166.
46. LEROY, E., *et al.* 1998. Deletions in the Parkin gene and genetic heterogeneity in a Greek family with early onset Parkinson's disease. Hum. Genet. **103:** 424–427.
47. LUCKING, C.B., *et al.* 2000. Association between early-onset Parkinson's disease and mutations in the parkin gene. French Parkinson's Disease Genetics Study Group. N. Engl. J. Med. 2000. **342:** 1560–1567.
48. RIESS, O. & R. KRUGER. 1999. Parkinson's disease—a multifactorial neurodegenerative disorder. J. Neural. Transm. Suppl. **56:** 113–125.
49. TANAKA, Y., *et al.* 2001. Inducible expression of mutant alpha-synuclein decreases proteasome activity and increases sensitivity to mitochondria-dependent apoptosis. Hum. Mol. Genet. **10:** 919–926.
50. VALENTE, E.M., *et al.* 2001. Localization of a novel locus for autosomal recessive early-onset parkinsonism, PARK6, on human chromosome 1p35-p36. Am. J. Hum. Genet. **68:** 895–900.
51. VAN DE WARRENBURG, B.P., *et al.* 2001. Clinical and pathologic abnormalities in a family with parkinsonism and parkin gene mutations. Neurology **56:** 555–557.
52. ZHANG, Y., *et al.* 2000. Oxidative stress and genetics in the pathogenesis of Parkinson's disease. Neurobiol. Dis. **7:** 240–250.

53. DONG, Z., *et al.* 2002. Overexpression of Parkinson's disease-associated alpha-synucleinA53T by recombinant adeno-associated virus in mice does not increase the vulnerability of dopaminergic neurons to MPTP. J. Neurobiol. **53:** 1–10.

54. GOMEZ-SANTOS, C., *et al.* 2002. MPP+ increases alpha-synuclein expression and ERK/MAP-kinase phosphorylation in human neuroblastoma SH-SY5Y cells. Brain Res. **935:** 32–39.

55. RATHKE-HARTLIEB, S., *et al.* 2001. Sensitivity to MPTP is not increased in Parkinson's disease-associated mutant alpha-synuclein transgenic mice. J. Neurochem. **77:** 1181–1184.

56. KAHLE, P.J., *et al.* 2000. Subcellular localization of wild-type and Parkinson's disease-associated mutant alpha-synuclein in human and transgenic mouse brain. J. Neurosci. **20:** 6365–6373.

57. LEE, M.K., *et al.* 2002. Human alpha-synuclein-harboring familial Parkinson's disease-linked Ala- 53→Thr mutation causes neurodegenerative disease with alpha-synuclein aggregation in transgenic mice. Proc. Natl. Acad. Sci. USA **99:** 8968–8973.

58. MASLIAH, E., *et al.* 2000. Dopaminergic loss and inclusion body formation in alpha-synuclein mice: implications for neurodegenerative disorders. Science **287:** 1265–1269.

59. VAN DER PUTTEN, H., *et al.* 2000. Neuropathology in mice expressing human alpha-synuclein. J. Neurosci. **20:** 6021–6029.

60. MATSUOKA, Y., *et al.* 2001. Lack of nigral pathology in transgenic mice expressing human alpha-synuclein driven by the tyrosine hydroxylase promoter. Neurobiol. Dis. **8:** 535–539.

61. RICHFIELD, E.K., *et al.* 2002. Behavioral and neurochemical effects of wild-type and mutated human alpha-synuclein in transgenic mice. Exp. Neurol. **175:** 35–48.

62. CLAYTON, D.F. & J.M. GEORGE. 1998. The synucleins: a family of proteins involved in synaptic function, plasticity, neurodegeneration, and disease. Trends Neurosci. **21:** 249–254.

63. HSU, L.J., *et al.* 1998. Expression pattern of synucleins (non-Abeta component of Alzheimer's disease amyloid precursor protein/alpha-synuclein) during murine brain development. J. Neurochem. **71:** 338–344.

64. TAKENOUCHI, T., *et al.* 2001. Reduced neuritic outgrowth and cell adhesion in neuronal cells transfected with human alpha-synuclein. Mol. Cell. Neurosci. **17:** 141–150.

65. GEORGE, J.M., *et al.* 1995. Characterization of a novel protein regulated during the critical period for song learning in the zebra finch. Neuron **15:** 361–372.

66. PRZEDBORSKI, S., *et al.* 1996. Role of neuronal nitric oxide in 1-methyl-4-phenyl-1,2,3,6- tetrahydropyridine (MPTP)-induced dopaminergic neurotoxicity. Proc. Natl. Acad. Sci. USA **93:** 4565–4571.

67. LEE, F.J., *et al.* 2001. Direct binding and functional coupling of alpha-synuclein to the dopamine transporters accelerate dopamine-induced apoptosis. FASEB J. **15:** 916–926.

68. TABRIZI, S.J., *et al.* 2000. Expression of mutant alpha-synuclein causes increased susceptibility to dopamine toxicity. Hum. Mol. Genet. **9:** 2683–2689.

69. LAI, C.T. & P.H. YU. 1997. Dopamine- and L-beta-3,4-dihydroxyphenylalanine hydrochloride (L-Dopa)-induced cytotoxicity towards catecholaminergic neuroblastoma SH-SY5Y cells. Effects of oxidative stress and antioxidative factors. Biochem. Pharmacol. **53:** 363–372.

70. SULZER, D. 2001. Alpha-synuclein and cytosolic dopamine: stabilizing a bad situation. Nat. Med. **7:** 1280–1282.

71. LAVOIE, M.J. & T.G. HASTINGS. 1999. Dopamine quinone formation and protein modification associated with the striatal neurotoxicity of methamphetamine: evidence against a role for extracellular dopamine. J. Neurosci. **19:** 1484–1491.

72. HASTINGS, T.G., *et al.* 1996. Role of oxidation in the neurotoxic effects of intrastriatal dopamine injections. Proc. Natl. Acad. Sci. USA **93:** 1956–1961.

73. CONWAY, K.A., *et al.* 2001. Kinetic stabilization of the alpha-synuclein protofibril by a dopamine-alpha-synuclein adduct. Science **294:** 1346–1349.

74. RABINOVIC, A.D., *et al.* 2000. Role of oxidative changes in the degeneration of dopamine terminals after injection of neurotoxic levels of dopamine. Neuroscience **101:** 67–76.
75. HASHIMOTO, M., *et al.* 1999. Oxidative stress induces amyloid-like aggregate formation of NACP/alpha-synuclein in vitro. Neuroreport **10:** 717–721.
76. MANN, D.M., *et al.* 1990. The prevalence of amyloid (A4) protein deposits within the cerebral and cerebellar cortex in Down's syndrome and Alzheimer's disease. Acta Neuropathol. (Berl.) **80:** 318–327.
77. OGOMORI, K., *et al.* 1989. Beta-protein amyloid is widely distributed in the central nervous system of patients with Alzheimer's disease. Am. J. Pathol. **134:** 243–251.
78. SUENAGA, T., *et al.* 1990. Modified Bielschowsky and immunocytochemical studies on cerebellar plaques in Alzheimer's disease. J. Neuropathol. Exp. Neurol. 1990. **49:** 31–40.
79. FORLONI, G., *et al.* 1995. Protein misfolding in Alzheimer's and Parkinson's disease: genetics and molecular mechanisms. Neurobiol. Aging **23:** 957.
80. MALONE, J. & M.A. SULLIVAN. 1996. Analysis of antibody selection by phage display utilizing anti-phenobarbital antibodies. J. Mol. Recognit. **9:** 738–745.
81. ZHU, Q., *et al.* 1999. Extended half-life and elevated steady-state level of a single-chain Fv intrabody are critical for specific intracellular retargeting of its antigen, caspase-7. J. Immunol. Methods **231:** 207–222.
82. LECERF, J.M., *et al.* 2001. Human single-chain Fv intrabodies counteract in situ huntingtin aggregation in cellular models of Huntington's disease. Proc. Natl. Acad. Sci. USA **98:** 4764–4769.
83. O'FARRELL, P.H. 1975. High resolution two-dimensional electrophoresis of proteins. J. Biol. Chem. **250:** 4007–4021.

The Relationship between Lewy Body Disease, Parkinson's Disease, and Alzheimer's Disease

JOHN HARDY

Laboratory of Neurogenetics, National Institute on Aging, National Institutes of Health, Bethesda, Maryland 20892, USA

ABSTRACT: The nosological relationship between Parkinson's disease, dementing syndromes with Lewy bodies, and Alzheimer's disease has been the subject of continuing debate. Here I argue, on the basis of recent data from families with hereditary versions of these diseases and from transgenic modeling, that these nosological debates are inevitable, impossible to resolve, and a product of the fact that we define diseases as entities rather than processes.

KEYWORDS: Lewy body disease; Parkinson's disease; Alzheimer's disease

Lewy bodies are eosinophilic lesions that are found in (presumably) damaged neurons. They have been considered to be the pathognomic lesion for Parkinson's disease[1] and clearly show a predilection for nigral neurons. This predilection, however, even in pure cases of clinically diagnosed Parkinson's disease, is not absolute. Lewy bodies in the nigra stain darkly, possibly because of the presence within them of oxidized catechols, and have been recognized there for many years. However, with the advent of, first, ubiquitin[2] and, more recently, α-synuclein[3] stains, it has become clear that their distribution is much wider and their frequency in brains much higher than was previously realized.

In 1984 Kosaka and colleagues[4] described an entity characterized by dementia and by Lewy bodies in cortical regions with a varying amount of "senile changes" (plaques and tangles). Since this first description, the nosological confusion between these diseases and Alzheimer's disease has continued, with many different names being proposed for entities with overlapping pathological and clinical phenotypes, including diffuse Lewy body disease,[4] Lewy body dementia,[5] senile dementia of Lewy body type,[6] and the Lewy body variant of Alzheimer's disease.[7] A consensus conference went some way toward simplifying the nomenclative confusion to dementia with Lewy bodies[8] but the boundaries of the disease with respect to Parkinson's disease and Alzheimer's disease remain unclear.[9] A key observation was that Lewy bodies were a common copathology with Aβ pathology in those cases of dementia where there were few tangles.[10]

Address for correspondence: John Hardy, Laboratory of Neurogenetics, National Institute on Aging, National Institutes of Health, Building 10, Room 6C103, MSC1589, Bethesda, MD 20892. Voice: 301-451-3829; fax: 301-480-0335.

hardyj@mail.nih.gov

Ann. N.Y. Acad. Sci. 991: 167–170 (2003). © 2003 New York Academy of Sciences.

Genetic analysis of kindred's autosomal-dominant diseases has shown the way that this conundrum can be understood. First, the realization that Lewy bodies can occur in families with amyloid precursor protein mutations[11] and in families with presenilin mutations[12] clearly shows that Lewy body formation can be initiated, relatively directly, by Aβ pathology. Second, genetic analysis of kindreds with Parkinson's disease[13] identified mutations in the α-synuclein gene[14] and led directly to the realization that α-synuclein was the primary constituent of Lewy bodies.[3] However, clinical investigation of these kindreds showed that, while parkinsonism was *usually* the presenting feature, in some cases dementia was the presenting feature,[14] and the pathology of these cases showed extensive cortical pathology.[15] In other words, from a genetic perspective, Parkinson's disease in these kindreds and "pure" dementia with Lewy bodies (with no amyloid pathology) are genetically closely related (one would say identical except that it must be likely that modifier genes alter the precise location of the pathology). Furthermore, genetic variability in α-synuclein expression contributes to the risk of sporadic disease,[16] suggesting that while the autosomal-dominant disease is rare, the lessons learned from its analysis can be more generally applied.

The production of transgenic mice with α-synuclein transgenes has been informative. While these mice do not develop Lewy bodies, they do develop subtle α-synuclein pathology.[17] In agreement with the human data showing that individuals with APP mutations also have Lewy bodies, crossing these mice with mice with APP mutations also potentiated this α-synuclein pathology.[18]

These data allow a simple synthesis (FIG. 1). In some individuals, for genetic reasons, Lewy bodies occur with a distribution that is often, but not always, nigracen-

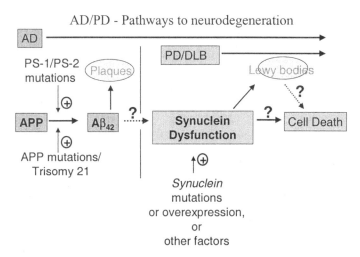

FIGURE 1. The relationship between pathologies: in Alzheimer's disease the Aβ pathology is upstream of, and can potentiate, the Lewy body pathology. This latter can be activated directly by α-synuclein mutations (or other genetic lesions). If an individual close to the threshold for developing Lewy bodies starts to develop Aβ pathology, this can initiate the cortical Lewy body formation (see Ref. 20). ABBREVIATIONS: AD = Alzheimer's disease; PD = Parkinson's disease; DLB = dementia with Lewy bodies.

tric.[19] However, Lewy body formation can be potentiated by Aβ pathology. This pathology is largely cortical. If this pathology occurs, it can potentiate Lewy body formation, especially in the cortical regions in which it occurs.

Conceptually, these ideas resemble those we have previously promulgated for the tauopathies; in particular, FIGURE 1 is derived from Reference 20. However, the parallels with tau pathologies are truly remarkable. Tangle pathology can be caused by APP[21] and presenilin mutations[22] and thus occur in the presence of Aβ pathology. Tangle pathology can be caused directly by tau mutations.[23] Tangle pathology can be predisposed to by tau haplotypes.[24,25] It is even the case that sporadic tangle disease has two variants—a common parkinsonian variant, progressive supranuclear palsy, and a less common, more dementing illness, corticobasal degeneration. The production of mice with tau mutations that develop tangles in the midbrain[26] but, when crossed with mice with APP mutations, develop cortical tangles[27] is particularly revealing and imitates the likely situation in the many cases of dementia with Lewy bodies, where amyloid pathology "pushes" cortical Lewy body pathology in someone who is genetically predisposed.

Under these circumstances, it can be seen that the nosological conundrum is insurmountable in that there is a continuum between these disease processes.[28] However, medicine is, of course, a pragmatic art; and making the best practical diagnosis is driven by the wish to ensure the best treatment. Arguments about nosology should be driven only by these pragmatic considerations.

Finally, this review does not take into account the likely cross-talk between tau and synuclein pathologies.[29] It is clear that such cross-talk occurs, but what underlies it is not yet understood.

REFERENCES

1. HUGHES, A.J., S.E. DANIEL & A.J. LEES. 1993. The clinical features of Parkinson's disease in 100 histologically proven cases. Adv. Neurol. **60:** 595–599.
2. LENNOX, G., et al. 1989. Anti-ubiquitin immunocytochemistry is more sensitive than conventional techniques in the detection of diffuse Lewy body disease. J. Neurol. Neurosurg. Psychiatry **52:** 67–71.
3. SPILLANTINI, M.G., et al. 1997. Alpha-synuclein in Lewy bodies. Nature **388:** 839–840.
4. KOSAKA, K., M. YOSHIMURA, K. IKEDA & H. BUDKA. 1984. Diffuse type of Lewy body disease: progressive dementia with abundant cortical Lewy bodies and senile changes of varying degree—a new disease? Clin. Neuropathol. **3:** 185–192.
5. GIBB, W.R., M.M. ESIRI & A.J. LEES. 1987. Clinical and pathological features of diffuse cortical Lewy body disease (Lewy body dementia). Brain **110:** 1131–1153.
6. PERRY, R.H., et al. 1990. Senile dementia of Lewy body type. A clinically and neuropathologically distinct form of Lewy body dementia in the elderly. J. Neurol. Sci. **95:** 119–139.
7. HANSEN, L., et al. 1990. The Lewy body variant of Alzheimer's disease: a clinical and pathologic entity. Neurology **40:** 1–8.
8. McKEITH, I.G., et al. 1996. Consensus guidelines for the clinical and pathologic diagnosis of dementia with Lewy bodies (DLB): report of the consortium on DLB international workshop. Neurology **47:** 1113–1124.
9. McKEITH, I.G., et al. 2003. Dementia with Lewy bodies. Semin. Clin. Neuropsychiatry **8:** 46–57.
10. LANTOS, P.L., et al. 1994. Lewy bodies in the brain of two members of a family with the 717 (Val to Ile) mutation of the amyloid precursor protein gene. Neurosci. Lett. **172:** 77–79.

11. HANSEN, L.A., E. MASLIAH, D. GALASKO & R.D. TERRY. 1993. Plaque-only Alzheimer disease is usually the lewy body variant, and vice versa. J. Neuropathol. Exp. Neurol. **52:** 648–654.
12. HARDY, J. 1994. Lewy bodies in Alzheimer's disease in which the primary lesion is a mutation in the amyloid precursor protein. Neurosci. Lett. **180:** 290–292.
13. LIPPA, C.F., et al. 1998. Lewy bodies contain altered alpha-synuclein in brains of many familial Alzheimer's disease patients with mutations in presenilin and amyloid precursor protein genes. Am. J. Pathol. **153:** 1365–1370.
14. MUENTER, M.D., et al. 1998. Hereditary form of parkinsonism-dementia. Ann. Neurol. **43:** 768–781.
15. GWINN-HARDY, K., et al. 2000. Distinctive neuropathology revealed by alpha-synuclein antibodies in hereditary parkinsonism and dementia linked to chromosome 4p. Acta Neuropathol. (Berl.) **99:** 663–672.
16. FARRER, M., et al. 2001. α-Synuclein gene haplotypes are associated with Parkinson's disease. Human Mol. Genet. **10:** 1847–1851.
17. MASLIAH, E., et al. 2000. Dopaminergic loss and inclusion body formation in alpha-synuclein mice: implications for neurodegenerative disorders. Science **287:** 1265–1269.
18. MASLIAH, E., et al. 2001. β-Amyloid peptides enhance alpha-synuclein accumulation and neuronal deficits in a transgenic mouse model linking Alzheimer's disease and Parkinson's disease. Proc. Natl. Acad. Sci. USA **98:** 12245–12250.
19. BRAAK, H., et al. 2003. Staging of brain pathology related to sporadic Parkinson's disease. Neurobiol. Aging **24:** 197–211.
20. HARDY, J., et al. 1998. Genetic dissection of Alzheimer's disease and related dementias: amyloid and its relationship to tau. Nat. Neurosci. **1:** 95–99.
21. GOATE, A.M., et al. 1991. Segregation of a missense mutation in the amyloid precursor protein gene with familial Alzheimer's disease. Nature **349:** 704–706.
22. SHERRINGTON, R., et al. 1995. Cloning of a gene bearing missense mutations in early-onset familial Alzheimer's disease. Nature **375:** 754–760.
23. HUTTON, M., et al. 1998. Coding and splice donor site mutations in tau cause autosomal dominant dementia (FTDP-17). Nature **393:** 702–705.
24. BAKER, M., et al. 1999. Association of an extended haplotype in the tau gene with progressive supranuclear palsy. Human Mol. Genet. **4:** 711–715.
25. HOULDEN, H., et al. 2001. Corticobasal degeneration and progressive supranuclear palsy share a common tau haplotype. Neurology **56:** 1702–1706.
26. LEWIS, J., et al. 2000. Neurofibrillary tangles, amyotrophy, and progressive motor disturbance in mice expressing mutant (P301L) tau protein. Nat. Genet. **25:** 402–405.
27. LEWIS, J., et al. 2001. Enhanced neurofibrillary degeneration in transgenic mice expressing mutant tau and APP. Science **293:** 1487–1491.
28. HARDY J. & K. GWINN-HARDY. 1999. Neurodegenerative disease: a different view of diagnosis. Mol. Med. Today **5:** 514–517.
29. DUDA, J.E., et al. 2002. Concurrence of alpha-synuclein and tau brain pathology in the Contursi kindred. Acta Neuropathol. (Berl.) **104:** 7–11.

Transgenic Models of α-Synuclein Pathology

Past, Present, and Future

MAKOTO HASHIMOTO, EDWARD ROCKENSTEIN, AND ELIEZER MASLIAH

Departments of Neurosciences and Pathology, University of California, San Diego, La Jolla, California 92093, USA

ABSTRACT: Accumulation and toxic conversion to protofibrils of α-synuclein has been associated with neurological disorders such as Parkinson's disease (PD), Lewy body disease, multiple system atrophy, neurodegeneration with brain iron accumulation type 1, and Alzheimer's disease. In recent years, modeling these disorders in transgenic (tg) mice and flies has helped improve understanding of the pathogenesis of these diseases and has established the basis for the development of new experimental treatments. Overexpression of α-synuclein in tg mice in a region- and cell-specific manner results in degeneration of selective circuitries accompanied by motor deficits and inclusion formation similar to what is found in PD and related disorders. Furthermore, studies in singly and doubly tg mice have shown that toxic conversion and accumulation can be accelerated by α-synuclein mutations associated with familial parkinsonism, by amyloid β peptide 1–42 (Aβ 1–42), and by oxidative stress. In contrast, molecular chaperones such as Hsp70 and close homologues such as α-synuclein have been shown to suppress toxicity. Similar studies are underway to evaluate the effects of other modifying genes that might play a role in α-synuclein ubiquitination. Among them considerable interest has been placed on the role of molecules associated with familial parkinsonism (*Parkin*, UCHL-1). Furthermore, studying the targeted overexpression of α-synuclein and other modifier genes in the nigrostriatal and limbic system by using regulatable promoters, lentiviral vectors, and siRNA will help improve understanding of the molecular mechanisms involved in selective neuronal vulnerability, and it will aid the development of new treatments.

KEYWORDS: α-synclein; transgenic models

INTRODUCTION

Abnormal accumulation and misfolding (toxic conversion) of synaptic proteins in the nervous system is being extensively explored as a key pathogenic event leading to neurodegeneration in Parkinson's disease (PD), Lewy body disease (LBD), Alzheimer's disease (AD), and other neurological disorders.[1–3] In PD and related conditions, such as LBD, abnormal accumulation of α-synuclein occurs in neuronal cell bodies, axons, and synapses;[4–6] while in AD, misfolded amyloid β peptide 1–42 (Aβ 1–42), a proteolytic product of amyloid precursor protein metabolism, accumu-

Address for correspondence: Dr. E. Masliah, Department of Neurosciences, University of California San Diego, La Jolla, CA 92093-0624. Voice: 858-534-8992; fax 858-534-6232.
emasliah@ucsd.edu

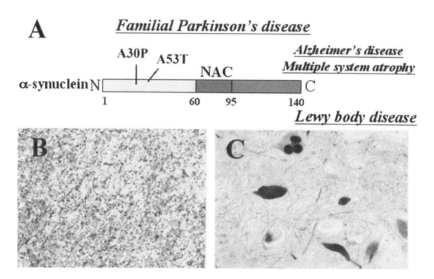

FIGURE 1. α-Synuclein expression in the human nervous system. **(A)** Diagram of α-synuclein structure. **(B)** α-Synuclein synaptic localization in the normal human brain. **(C)** α-Synuclein in Lewy bodies and neurites in Lewy body disease.

lates in the neuronal endoplasmic reticulum and extracellularly.[7–9] In contrast, in disorders with trinucleotide repeat, such as Huntington's disease, accumulation of misfolded proteins occurs in the neuronal cytosol and nuclei.[10,11] The key pathogenic event triggering synaptic loss and selective neuronal cell death in these disorders is still unclear;[12,13] however, recent studies suggest that nerve damage might result from the conversion of normally nontoxic monomers (and small oligomers) to toxic oligomers and protofibrils.[14,15] Larger polymers and fibers that often constitute the intracellular inclusions and extracellular lesions might not be as toxic.[16]

α-Synuclein is a 140–amino acid synaptic molecule (FIG. 1) that was originally identified in human brain as the precursor protein of the non-Aβ component (NAC) of AD amyloid[17–19] and is known to belong to a family that includes β-synuclein (or phosphoneuroprotein 14),[20,21] γ-synuclein (or breast carcinoma–specific factor),[22] and synoretin.[23] In LBD, accumulation of misfolded α-synuclein has been proposed to be centrally involved in the pathogenesis of the disease[24,25] because: (i) this molecule is present in Lewy bodies (LBs)[4,26,27] (FIG. 1); (ii) mutations in the α-synuclein gene are associated with rare familial forms of parkinsonism[28,29] (FIG. 1); and (iii) α-synuclein expression in transgenic (tg) mice[30] (FIG. 2) and *Drososphila*[31] mimics several aspects of PD.

α-Synuclein is capable of self-aggregating to form both oligomers and fibrillar polymers with amyloid-like characteristics[32] (FIGS. 3 and 4). Most recent evidence suggests that there might be both low–molecular weight (MW) nontoxic oligomers that associate with the cell membrane as well as higher-MW toxic oligomers (protofibrils).[32–34] Association of nontoxic oligomers with components of the plasma membrane such as polyunsaturated fatty acids might play a role in synaptic plasticity.[35] In contrast, higher-MW toxic oligomers form protofibrils that can potentially damage the cell membrane.[15,36] The role of fibril formation in PD and related disorders is more controversial, but several studies suggest that fibrils might represent less toxic byproducts or even a cellular strategy to inactivate or isolate more toxic oligomers (Figs. 3 and 4).[32–34] Oligomerization could occur in several stages, including formation of protofibrils, nucleation,[37] and fibril formation.[32,38] For a more detailed description and analysis of this topic, the reader is advised to consult the chapter by Lansbury and colleagues published in these proceedings.

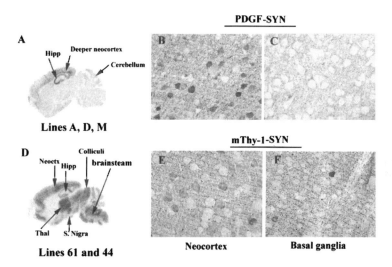

FIGURE 2. α-Synuclein expression in the nervous system of transgenic mice. **(A)** α-Synuclein expression in the mouse brain in under the PDGF promoter (*in situ* hybridization). **(B and C)** α-Synuclein expression and inclusion formation in the neocortex and basal ganglia in the PDGF–α-synuclein tg mouse. **(D)** α-Synuclein expression in the mouse brain in under the mThy1 promoter (*in situ* hybridization). **(E and F)** α-Synuclein expression and neuronal accumulation in the neocortex and basal ganglia in the mThy1-α-synuclein tg mouse.

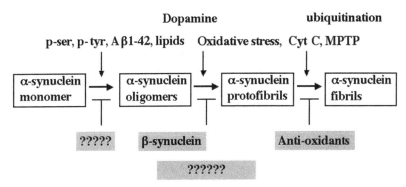

FIGURE 3. A description of the factors promoting or blocking α-synuclein aggregation in Lewy body disease.

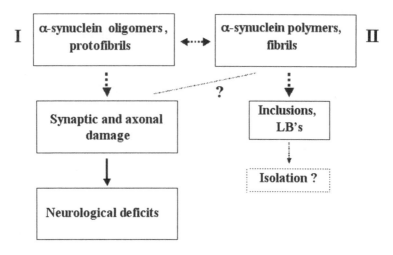

FIGURE 4. Proposed differential action of α-synuclein protofibrils and fibrils in Lewy body disease toxicity and pathogenesis.

Because of the implications for better understanding the disease pathogenesis and development of new treatments, conditions promoting or *blocking* α-synuclein aggregation and toxic conversion are now being extensively studied in tg animals and *in vitro* models. In general terms and for the purposes of this paper, the role of the following factors will be considered: (i) mutations associated with familial parkinsonism;[39,40] (ii) posttranscriptional modifications associated with oxidative stress mediated by neurotoxins 1-methyl-4-phenyl-1,2,3,6-tetrahydropyridine (MPTP, paraquat), iron, cytochrome C, copper (II), and dopamine;[32,41–45] (iii) posttranscriptional modifications associated with signaling events or conjugation (phosphorylation, glycosylation, ubiquitination);[46,47] (iv) binding to lipid membrane vesicles;[35,48,49] and (v) interactions with molecules that promote aggregation (such as NAC and Aβ)[12,50–52] or that block aggregation (such as β-synuclein).[53]

In this context, the main objectives of this paper are to provide a perspective with respect to the following efforts:

(1) the modeling of PD and related disorders in tg mice;
(2) the definition of the *in vivo* role of factors promoting or blocking α-synuclein aggregation in the pathogenesis of PD and related disorders.

Several reviews have been recently published on the subject of tg modeling of PD, and the reader is advised to consult them for additional information.[54–56]

DIFFERENTIAL EFFECTS OF WILD-TYPE AND MUTANT α-SYNUCLEIN IN tg MODELS OF TOXIC CONVERSION

Since progressive intraneuronal aggregation of α-synuclein has been proposed to play a central role in the pathogenesis of PD and related disorders,[9,14,24] most tg

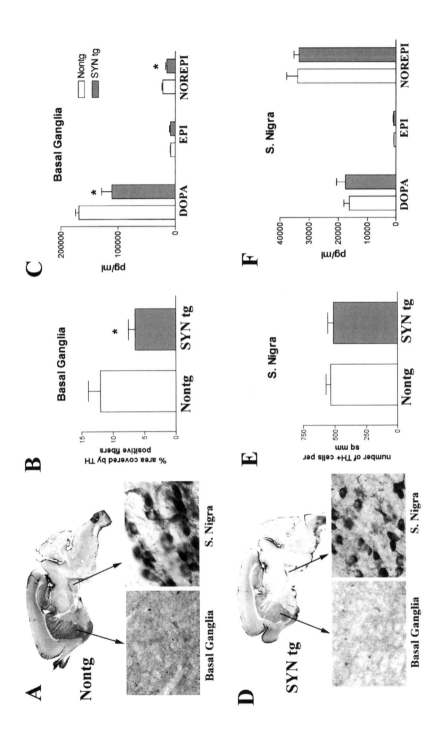

FIGURE 5. Loss of dopaminergic input in the brain of α-synuclein tg mice. (**A**) Tyrosine hydroxylase (TH) immunoreactivity in non-tg mouse. (**B**) Levels of TH immunoreactivity in the basal ganglia. (**C**) Levels of DOPA, EPI, and NOREPI in the basal ganglia. (**D**) TH immunoreactivity in the PDGF–α-synuclein tg mouse. (**E**) TH cell counts in the sustantia nigra (SN). (**F**) Levels of DOPA, EPI, and NOREPI in the SN.

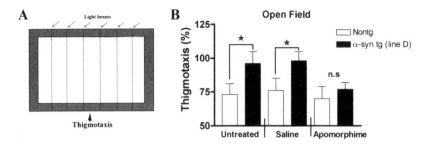

FIGURE 6. Reversal of dopaminergic deficits in α-synuclein tg mice following apomorphine treatment. **(A)** Diagram of the open field. **(B)** Assessment of thigmotaxis (percentage in periphery of cage) before and after apomorphime treatment.

models have been focused on investigating the *in vivo* effects of α-synuclein accumulation using neuronal specific promoters (TABLE 1). Among these models, overexpression of wild-type (wt) α-synuclein under the regulatory control of the platelet-derived growth factor β (PDGFβ) promoter (FIG. 2) has been shown to result in motor deficits, dopaminergic loss, and formation of inclusion bodies.[30] Mice with the highest levels of expression showed (line D) intraneuronal accumulation of α-synuclein that started at 3 months of age and was accompanied by loss of tyrosine hydroxylase (TH) fibers in the caudoputamen region and synapses in the temporal cortex. Although no apparent neuronal loss was detected in the substantia nigra (SN), measurements of dopamine levels in the caudoputamen region showed a 25–50% decrease at 12 months of age (FIG. 5). Analysis of locomotor activity in the open field showed that these tg mice had increased thigmotaxis, a behavior that has been associated with dopaminergic activity. Supporting a role for alterations in the dopaminergic system, this abnormal behavior was ameliorated upon treatment with apomorphine, a compound known to promote dopamine release (FIG. 6). Furthermore, at this age, tg mice showed mild-to-moderate motor deficits in the rotarod, particularly those mice with the greatest loss of dopamine, indicating that more substantial deficits (>75%) of this transmitter might be necessary for more overt deficits to appear.

To determine whether different levels of human (h) α-synuclein expression from distinct promoters might result in neuropathology mimicking other synucleopathies, we also compared patterns of hα-synuclein accumulation in the brains of tg mice expressing this molecule from the murine (m) Thy-1 and PDGFβ promoters[57] (FIG. 2). In mThy-1-hα-synuclein tg mice, this protein accumulated in synapses and neurons throughout the brain, including the thalamus, basal ganglia, SN, and brain stem. Expression of hα-synuclein from the PDGFβ promoter resulted in accumulation in synapses of the neocortex, limbic system, and olfactory regions as well as formation of inclusion bodies in neurons in deeper layers of the neocortex (lines A and D). Furthermore, one of the intermediate expressor lines (line M) displayed hα-synuclein expression in glial cells mimicking some features of multiple system atrophy. These results show a more widespread accumulation of hα-synuclein in tg mouse brains. Taken together, these studies support the contention that hα-synuclein expression in

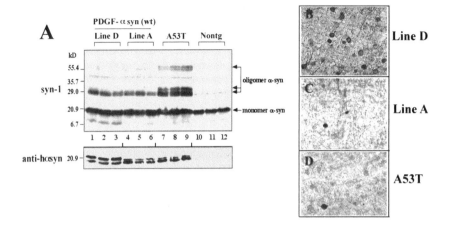

FIGURE 7. Abnormal accumulation of in α-synuclein oligomers in PDGF–α-synuclein (A53T) mutant mice. **(A)** Western blot analysis with 72-10 and syn-1 antibodies against α-synuclein showing increased. **(B–D)** Immunocytochemical analysis with a human specific antibody against α-synuclein (72-10).

tg mice might mimic some neuropathological alterations observed in LBD and other synucleopathies, such as multiple system atrophy.[57]

However, these studies did not clarify the potential relationship among synaptic damage, α-synuclein oligomerization and fibrillation, inclusion formation, and neurological deficits. Because previous studies have shown that mutations associated with familial parkinsonism accelerate α-synuclein aggregation and oligomerization,[39,40] we compared the patterns of neurodegeneration, α-synuclein aggregation, and neurological alterations in tg mice expressing wt or mutant (mut) (A53T) hα-synuclein at comparable levels under the PDGFβ promoter. For this purpose, two tg lines that express moderate levels of α-synuclein in a similar anatomical and cellular distribution were compared (line A, which expresses wt hα-synuclein,[30,57] and a newly developed line 8, which expresses mut hα-synuclein—that is, A53T) (FIG. 7). Additional comparisons were done against our well-described line D, which expresses higher levels of wt hα-synuclein[30,57] (FIG. 7). Lower expresser lines were selected for these experiments to avoid unintended effects of very high levels of expression as observed with other more strong promoters such as Thy-1 and PrP. These mice express about a third of the levels of hα-synuclein, compared to our higher expresser line D, which is approximately equivalent to a 1.5-to-1 ratio with respect to endogenous levels. Remarkably, we found that mice expressing mut α-synuclein developed progressive motor deficits and neurodegeneration, associated with α-synuclein accumulation in synapses and neurons; but very few or no inclusions were found (FIG. 7). In contrast, mice from line A (wt hα-synuclein) did not show neurodegenerative or neurological deficits, but they did display formation of inclusions. Analysis of the patterns of α-synuclein aggregation by Western blot using the Syn-1 antibody showed that in the mut line there was greater formation of α-synuclein oligomers compared to the wt line (FIG. 7). This is consistent with recent studies comparing the neuropathogenic effects of human wt and mut α-synuclein under the control of the PrP promoters (TABLE 1). For example, mice expressing mut, but not wt, α-synuclein developed a severe and complex motor impairment leading to paralysis and death.[58] These animals developed age-dependent intracytoplasmic neuronal α-synuclein inclusions paralleling disease onset, and the α-synuclein inclusions recapitulated features of human counterparts. Moreover, immunoelectron microscopy revealed that the α-synuclein inclusions contained 10–16-nm-wide fibrils similar to human pathological inclusions. These mice demonstrate that A53T α-synuclein leads to the formation of toxic filamentous α-synuclein neuronal inclusions that cause neurodegeneration.[58]

Similarly, other studies have shown that under the PrP promoter, mice expressing the A53T hα-synuclein, but not wt or the A30P variants, develop adult-onset neurodegenerative disease with progressive locomotor dysfunction leading to death[59] (TABLE 1). Pathologically affected mice exhibit neuronal abnormalities (in perikarya and neurites), including pathological accumulations of α-synuclein and ubiquitin. Consistent with abnormal neuronal accumulation of α-synuclein, brain regions with pathology exhibit increases in detergent-insoluble α-synuclein and α-synuclein aggregates.[59]

Under the mThy-1 promoter (TABLE 1), expression of either wt or mut α-synuclein results[60] in extensive α-synuclein accumulation throughout the central nervous system, in some cases including the SN or the motor neurons.[57] In the model developed by van der Putten et al.,[60] mice develop early-onset motor decline, axonal degeneration, and α-synuclein accumulation in the spinal cord but not in the SN. In contrast, in our models, we observed less overt motor deficits, but considerable accumulation of α-synuclein in cortical and subcortical regions.[57] In both models there is accumulation of detergent-insoluble α-synuclein; however, its effects in the nigral system in terms of cell death are not completely clear.

To address the question of selective neuronal vulnerability and involvement of tg mice expressing either wt or mutated (A53T or A30P) forms of hα-synuclein under control of the 9-kb rat TH promoter studies have been developed (TABLE 2).[61] Initial studies in these mice showed accumulation of α-synuclein in the SN neurons but no neurodegeneration or motor deficits. More recent studies in tg mice expressing either wt or doubly mutated forms of hα-synuclein under control of the 9-kb rat TH promoter have shown that the expression of hα-synuclein in nigrostriatal terminals resulted in increased density of the dopamine transporter and enhanced toxicity to the neurotoxin MPTP. Expression of a doubly mutated hα-synuclein reduced locomotor responses to repeated doses of amphetamine and blocked the development of sensitization compared to adult wt hα-synuclein-5 tg mice. Expression of doubly mutated hα-synuclein adversely affects the integrity of dopaminergic terminals and leads to age-related declines in motor coordination and dopaminergic markers.[61]

Further studies to investigate the role of selective neuronal vulnerability in the SN and α-synuclein mutations have been accomplished in rat using lentiviral and adenoassociated viral vectors (TABLE 3).[62–64] In contrast to tg mice models, a selective loss of nigral dopaminergic neurons associated with a dopaminergic denervation of the striatum was observed in animals expressing either wt or mut forms of hα-synuclein. This neuronal degeneration correlates with the appearance of abundant α-synuclein–positive inclusions and extensive neuritic pathology detected with both α-synuclein and silver staining. Rat α-synuclein similarly leads to protein ag-

TABLE 1. Comparison of various α-synuclein transgenic mouse models

Group	Promoter	Construct	Neuropathology	Motor	Biochemistry	Age at onset
Masliah, 2000	PDGFβ	hα-synuclein (wt)	α-synuclein inclusions DOPA loss neocortex limbic system	mild	increased aggregates	3–6 m
Lee, 2002	muPrP	hα-synuclein (wt) hα-synuclein (A53T) hα-synuclein (A30P)	α-synuclein subcortex axonal degeneration gliosis	severe deficits premature death	detergent insoluble	10 m
Giasson, 2002	muPrP	hα-synuclein (wt) hα-synuclein (A53T) homozygous	α-synuclein accumulation spinal cord axonal degeneration gliosis	severe, complex	detergent insoluble	8–12 m
Van de Putten, 2000	muThy-1	hα-synuclein (wt) hα-synuclein (A53T)	α-synuclein motor neuron spinal cord axonal degeneration	early onset	detergent insoluble?	1–2 m
Rockenstein, 2002	muThy-1	hα-synuclein (wt) hα-synuclein (A30P)	accumulation of α-synuclein	NA	increased aggregates	6 m
Kahle, 2002	proteolipid	hα-synuclein (wt)	accumulation of α-synuclein oligonucleotides no myelin loss	NA	detergent insoluble	12 m?

TABLE 2. α-Synuclein models for selective neuronal vulnerability (I)

Group	Promoter	Construct	Neuropathology	Motor	Biochemistry	Age at onset
Richfield, 2002	rat TH	hα-synuclein (wt) hα-synuclein (A53T/A30P)	α-synuclein accumulation MPTP toxicity reduced dopamine	alter motor response to methamphetamine	NA	9–12 m
Matsuoka, 2002	rat TH	hα-synuclein (wt) hα-synuclein (A53T;A30P)	α-synuclein in substantia nigra	none	NA	12 m

TABLE 3. α-Synuclein models for selective neuronal vulnerability (II)

Group	Vector	Construct	Neuropathology	Motor	Age	Age at onset
Kirk, 2002	rAAV	hα-synuclein (wt) A53T	neuron loss DOPA loss α-synuclein accumulation	mild defecits	adult rat substantia nigra	2–3 m
Klein, 2002	rAAV	hα-synuclein (wt) A30P	neuron loss α-synuclein accumulation	no motor deficits	young rat substantia nigra	12 m
Lo Bianco, 2002	lentiviral vector	hα-synuclein (wt) A30P A53T	neuron loss α-synuclein accumulation	?	rat substantia nigra	6 w

gregation but without cell loss, suggesting that inclusions are not the primary cause of cell degeneration in PD.[62]

In summary, under the PDGFβ, both wt and mut α-synuclein tg mice develop behavioral deficits and synaptic alterations following a limbic and cortical pattern; however, mut α-synuclein is more toxic, even though very few inclusions are formed compared to wt α-synuclein tg mice. Under the PrP promoter, mut α-synuclein is more toxic than wt, inclusion-like structures develop, and more widespread involvement of the lower motor system is observed. With the thy-1 construct, both wt and mut α-synuclein are toxic, and inclusion-like structures develop that can affect the cortex, subcortex, or spinal cord. Furthermore, these *in vivo* models support the contention that α-synuclein-dependent neurodegeneration is associated with abnormal accumulation of detergent-insoluble α-synuclein (probably representing oligomeric forms) rather than with inclusion formation representing fibrillar polymeric α-synuclein. The specific accumulation of detergent-insoluble α-synuclein in these tg mice recapitulates a pivotal feature of LBD,[65] and it is of significance in the future development and evaluation of novel treatments.

DIFFERENTIAL EFFECTS OF POSTTRANSCRIPTIONAL MODIFICATIONS IN α-SYNUCLEIN TOXIC CONVERSION

Although characterizing the role of α-synuclein mutations has improved our understanding of the role of protein misfolding in the pathogenesis of PD, these mutations comprehend only a small fraction of the cases. It is estimated that over 95% of the cases of PD and related disorders are sporadic.[66] Thus, complex interactions between environmental and genetic susceptibility factors might be at play. For example, the potential role of factors promoting oxidative stress is under intense investigation (FIG. 3). Factors such as iron, cytochrome C, copper (II), dopamine,[32,41–45,67,68] and neurotoxins have been shown *in vitro* to alter α-synuclein conformation leading to aggregation and toxic protofibril formation. Among such factors, the key discovery by Langston and colleagues of 1-methyl-4-phenylpyridinium ion as a powerful dopaminergic neurotoxin led to the development of acute models of parkinsonism in murine and simian models.[69]

Since the neurotoxin MPTP promotes oxidative stress[70] and degeneration of the dopaminergic system, mimicking some aspects of PD, we seek to determine the effects of chronic MPTP treatment on tg mice overexpressing α-synuclein. For this purpose, tg mice expressing high levels of α-synuclein throughout the cortex and SN under the control of the Thy-1 promoter were treated with low doses of MPTP and analyzed ultrastructurally.[71,72] Electron microscopy analysis demonstrated that compared to control groups, Thy1–α-synuclein tg mice treated with MPTP showed extensive mitochondrial alterations, invagination of the nuclear membrane, and formation of electrodense intracytoplasmic inclusions. Taken together, these studies suggest that oxidative stress and the associated mitochondrial damage might contribute to aggregation of α-synuclein and to the pathogenesis of PD. Further supporting a role of oxidative stress in the pathogenesis of disorders with α-synuclein accumulation, recent studies have shown that this molecule is present in a nitrosylated form that promotes abnormal conformation.[45,68] Consistent with this possibility, we have observed increased 3-NT immunostaining in the α-synuclein tg mice. In neuronal cell lines overexpressing α-synuclein, there is also increased reactivity for markers of oxidative stress that are reversible with antioxidant treatments (for example, vitamin E).[43]

Another factor promoting oxidative damage and abnormal protein conformation that might play a role in α-synucleopathies is amyloid β-protein (FIGS. 3 and 4). This is interesting because AD and PD are associated with the cerebral accumulation of β-amyloid and α-synuclein, respectively.[73] Some patients have clinical and pathological features of both diseases, raising the possibility of overlapping pathogenetic pathways. We refer to this condition as the Lewy body variant (LBV) of AD;[74] however, others prefer different terms such as combined AD+PD, senile dementia of the Lewy body type, or LBD.[75] To better understand the role of amyloid production in α-synucleopathies, we generated tg mice with neuronal expression of human Aβ, α-synuclein, or both.[73] The functional and morphological alterations in doubly tg mice resembled the LBV of AD. These mice had severe deficits in learning and memory, developed motor deficits before α-synuclein singly tg mice did, and showed prominent age-dependent degeneration of cholinergic neurons and presynaptic terminals. They also had more α-synuclein–immunoreactive neuronal inclusions than α-synuclein singly tg mice. Ultrastructurally, some of these inclusions were fibrillar in doubly tg mice, whereas all inclusions were amorphous in α-synuclein singly tg mice. Aβ promoted aggregation of α-synuclein in a cell-free system and intraneuronal accumulation of α-synuclein in cell culture. Aβ may contribute to the development of LBD by promoting the aggregation of α-synuclein and exacerbating α-synuclein–dependent neuronal pathologies. Therefore, treatments that block the production or accumulation of Aβ could benefit a broader spectrum of disorders than previously anticipated.

Other posttranscriptional modifications that might promote α-synuclein aggregation and toxic conversion include phosphorylation and conjugation (FIG. 3). In this regard, recent mass spectrometry analyses and studies with an antibody that specifically recognizes phospho-Ser 129 of α-synuclein have shown that this residue is selectively and extensively phosphorylated in synucleinopathy lesions, including those in patients with PD and related disorders and in α-synuclein tg mice.[47] Furthermore, phosphorylation of α-synuclein at Ser 129 promoted fibril formation in vitro. These results highlight the importance of phosphorylation of filamentous proteins in the pathogenesis of neurodegenerative disorders. In Drosophila, synuclein overexpression results in LB formation and dopaminergic neuronal loss.[31] Furthermore, directed expression of the molecular chaperone Hsp70 prevented dopaminergic neuronal loss associated with α-synuclein in Drosophila, and interference with endogenous chaperone activity accelerated α-synuclein toxicity.[76] The fact that LBs in human postmortem tissue immunostained for molecular chaperones suggests that chaperones may play a role in PD progression. Among them, ubiquitination appears to play an important role. This is significant because mutations in the Parkin gene, also known to be associated with familial PD, have been shown to result in deficient α-synuclein ubiquitination.[77–79] Studies in tg mice are underway in which α-synuclein tg mice are crossed with Parkin or UCHL-1 KO mice. The prediction is that this will result in defective α-synuclein ubiquitination and proteosome degradation, with worsening of the phenotype but probably with no inclusion formation.

ROLE OF ENDOGENOUS INHIBITORS IN PREVENTING AND MODULATING α-SYNUCLEIN TOXIC CONVERSION

Toxic conversion of α-synuclein is not only the result of factors promoting aggregation but might also be the consequence of a failure of factors preventing aggregation (FIG. 3). Thus a critical balance between aggregation and anti-aggregation factors might be at play. Endogenous mechanisms to prevent toxic conversion include clearance, proteolysis, and production of inhibitors of aggregation. Among these, we have characterized β-synuclein, the nonamyloidogenic homologue of α-synuclein, as an inhibitor of aggregation of α-synuclein.[53] For this purpose, doubly tg mice expressing both α- and β-synuclein were generated and analyzed in the rotarod and by confocal microscopy. These studies showed that β-synuclein ameliorated the motor deficits, neurodegenerative alterations, and neuronal accumulation of α-synuclein seen in α-synuclein tg mice. Similarly, cell lines stably transfected with β-synuclein were resistant to accumulating α-synuclein, when this later molecule was expressed under the control of the inducible muristerone A system. α-Synuclein coimmunoprecipitated with β-synuclein both in the brains of doubly tg mice and in the doubly transfected cell lines. Furthermore, β-synuclein has also been shown to reduce Aβ aggregation. Our results raise the intriguing possibility that β-synuclein might be a natural negative regulator of α-synuclein and Aβ aggregation.[53]

The synucleins are natively unfolded proteins.[80] In support of an antiamyloidogenic effect of β-synuclein, we[53] as well as others have shown that β-synuclein, which lacks 11 central hydrophobic residues compared to its homologues, exhibited the properties of a random coil, whereas α- and γ-synucleins were slightly more compact and structured. γ-Synuclein, unlike its homologues, formed a soluble oligomer at relatively low concentrations, which appears to be an off-fibrillation pathway species. Although they have biophysical properties similar to those of α-synuclein, β- and γ-synucleins inhibit α-synuclein fibril formation. Complete inhibition of α-synuclein fibrillation was observed at 4:1 molar excess of β- and γ-synucleins. No significant incorporation of β-synuclein into the fibrils was detected. The lack of fibrils formed by α-synuclein is most readily explained by the absence of a stretch of hydrophobic residues from the middle region of the protein.[81]

The mechanisms by which β-synuclein might block α-synuclein aggregation *in vivo* are under investigation. One possible mechanism is that α-synuclein translocation to the plasma and mitochondrial membranes might be regulated by β-synuclein. In this regard, it was recently described that aggregation of α-synuclein in the membrane fractions was stimulated by mitochondrial dysfunction, suggesting a pathological relevance of α-synuclein in these fractions. Consistent with this view,[82] immunoblot analysis for the tg mice brain using sensitive α-synuclein-1 antibody showed that aggregation of α-synuclein in the particulate fractions in single α-synuclein mice was significantly suppressed in doubly tg mice expressing α and β-synuclein. Thus, pathological aggregation of α-synuclein in the membrane fractions may be negatively regulated by its nonamyloidogenic homologue, β-synuclein (FIG. 4). Interestingly, the 50-kDa immunoreactive band in non-tg mice, which might represent physiological oligomers of α-synuclein,[83] was absent in both singly and doubly tg mice, suggesting that equilibrium of α-synuclein oligomerization under the physiological conditions may be easily affected by different spices of α-synuclein as well as β-synuclein. Currently, it is unknown how interference with this physiological process might interfere with neuroplasticity. However, it may be ideal to design therapeutic drugs that would selectively act on the process of pathological aggregation of α-synuclein. Taken together, these findings suggest that β-synuclein homologues or derivatives might have a therapeutical potential for the treatment of AD, LBD, and PD.

CONCLUSIONS

Several tg mouse models for α-synucleopathy have now been developed. Models employing the PDGFβ promoter display involvement of the neocortex, limbic system, and (to a lesser extent) the nigrostriatal pathways, with α-synuclein accumulation and inclusion formation. Under the mThy-1 and PrP promoters there is more widespread expression of α-synuclein throughout the brain, including the subcortex and spinal cord. In these animals, there is a more dramatic locomotor phenotype and increased lethality with involvement of the neuromuscular junction and motor system. The A53T mut α-synuclein appears to be more toxic, probably because of its increased susceptibility to forming toxic protofibrils. Models selectively targeting the nigral system have been developed using the TH promoter or viral vectors. In tg models, oxidative stress and amyloid β-protein accelerate α-synuclein accumulation, mimicking combined PD and AD. In contrast, molecular chaperones such as Hsp70 and close homologues such as α-synuclein have been shown to suppress toxicity. Similar studies are underway to evaluate the effects of other modifying genes that might play a role in α-synuclein ubiquitination. For example, considerable interest has been focused on the role of molecules associated with familial parkinsonism (*Parkin*, UCHL-1). With the discovery of α-synuclein and the advent of new experimental animal models for PD and related disorders, the potential for the development and discovery of new treatments has been significantly bolstered.

ACKNOWLEDGMENTS

This work was supported by the National Institutes of Health (Grants AG5131, AG10689, and AG18440) and by grants from the M. J. Fox Foundation for Parkinson's Research and the Spencer family.

REFERENCES

1. Koo, E., P.J. Lansbury & J. Kelly. 1999. Amyloid diseases: abnormal protein aggregation in neurodegeneration. Proc. Natl. Acad. Sci. USA **96:** 9989–9990.
2. Ferrigno, P. & P. Silver. 2000. Polyglutamine expansions: proteolysis, chaperones, and the dangers of promiscuity. Neuron **26:** 9–12.
3. Ramassamy, C., et al. 1999. Oxidative damage and protection by antioxidants in the frontal cortex of Alzheimer's disease is related to the apolipoprotein E genotype. Free Rad. Biol. Med. **27:** 544–553.
4. Spillantini, M, et al. 1997. α-Synuclein in Lewy bodies. Nature **388:** 839–840.
5. Takeda, A., et al. 1998. Abnormal accumulation of NACP/α-synuclein in neurodegenerative disorders. Am. J. Pathol. **152:** 367–372.

6. IRIZARRY, M., *et al.* 1998. Nigral and cortical Lewy bodies and dystrophic nigral neurites in Parkinson's disease and cortical Lewy body disease contain alpha-synuclein immunoreactivity. J. Neuropathol. Exp. Neurol. **57**: 334–337.

7. WALSH, D., *et al.* 2000. The oligomerization of amyloid beta-protein begins intracellularly in cells derived from human brain. Biochemistry **39**: 10831–10839.

8. SELKOE, D.J., *et al.* 1996. The role of APP processing and trafficking pathways in the formation of amyloid beta-protein. Ann. N.Y. Acad. Sci. **777**: 57–64.

9. TROJANOWSKI, J.Q. & V.M. LEE. 2000. "Fatal attractions" of proteins: a comprehensive hypothetical mechanism underlying Alzheimer's disease and other neurodegenerative disorders. Ann. N.Y. Acad. Sci. **924**: 62–67.

10. MUCHOWSKI, P.J. 2002. Protein misfolding, amyloid formation, and neurodegeneration: a critical role for molecular chaperones? Neuron **35**: 9–12.

11. CUMMINGS, C.J. & H.Y. ZOGHBI. 2000. Trinucleotide repeats: mechanisms and pathophysiology. Annu. Rev. Genomics Hum. Genet. **1**: 281–328.

12. MASLIAH, E. 2000. The role of synaptic proteins in Alzheimer's disease. Ann. N.Y. Acad. Sci. **924**: 68–75.

13. MASLIAH, E. 2001. Recent advances in the understanding of the role of synaptic proteins in Alzheimer's disease and other neurodegenerative disorders. J. Alz. Dis. **3**: 1–9.

14. VOLLES, M.J. & P.T. LANSBURY, JR. 2002. Vesicle permeabilization by protofibrillar alpha-synuclein is sensitive to Parkinson's disease-linked mutations and occurs by a pore-like mechanism. Biochemistry **41**: 4595–4602.

15. VOLLES, M.J., *et al.* 2001. Vesicle permeabilization by protofibrillar alpha-synuclein: implications for the pathogenesis and treatment of Parkinson's disease. Biochemistry **40**: 7812–7819.

16. LANSBURY, P.T.J. 1999. Evolution of amyloid: what normal protein folding may tell us about fibrillogenesis and disease. Proc. Natl. Acad. Sci. USA **96**: 3342–3344.

17. IWAI, A. 2000. Properties of NACP/alpha-synuclein and its role in Alzheimer's disease. Biochim. Biophys. Acta **1502**: 95–109.

18. MASLIAH, E., *et al.* 1996. Altered presynaptic protein NACP is associated with plaque formation and neurodegeneration in Alzheimer's disease. Am. J. Pathol. **148**: 201–210.

19. UEDA, K., *et al.* 1993. Novel amyloid component (NAC) differentiates Alzheimer's disease from normal aging plaques. Soc. Neurosci. Abstr. **19**: 1254.

20. JAKES, R., M. SPILLANTINI & M. GOEDERT. 1994. Identification of two distinct synucleins from human brain. FEBS Lett. **345**: 27–32.

21. NAKAJO, S., *et al.* 1993. A new brain-specific 14-kDa protein is a phosphoprotein: its complete amino acid sequence and evidence for phosphorylation. Eur. J. Biochem. **217**: 1057–1063.

22. JIA, T., *et al.* 1999. Stimulation of breast cancer invasion and metastasis by synuclein gamma. Cancer Res. **59**: 742–747.

23. SURGUCHOV, A., *et al.* 1999. Synoretin—a new protein belonging to the synuclein family. Mol. Cell. Neurosci. **13**: 95–103.

24. HASHIMOTO, M. & E. MASLIAH. 1999. Alpha-synuclein in Lewy body disease and Alzheimer's disease. Brain Pathol. **9**: 707–720.

25. TROJANOWSKI, J. & V. LEE. 1998. Aggregation of neurofilament and alpha-synuclein proteins in Lewy bodies: implications for pathogenesis of Parkinson disease and Lewy body dementia. Arch. Neurol. **55**: 151–152.

26. TAKEDA, A., *et al.* 1998. Abnormal distribution of the non-Aβ component of Alzheimer's disease amyloid precursor/α-synuclein in Lewy body disease as revealed by proteinase K and formic acid pretreatment. Lab. Invest. **78**: 1169–1177.

27. WAKABAYASHI, K., *et al.* 1997. Neurofibrillary tangles in the dentate granule cells in Alzheimer's disease, Lewy body disease and progressive supranuclear palsy. Acta Neuropathol. **93**: 7–12.

28. KRUGER, R., *et al.* 1998. Ala30Pro mutation in the gene encoding α-synuclein in Parkinsons's disease. Nat. Genet. **18**: 106–108.

29. POLYMEROPOULOS, M., *et al.* 1997. Mutation in the α-synuclein gene identified in families with Parkinson's disease. Science **276**: 2045–2047.

30. MASLIAH, E., *et al.* 2000. Dopaminergic loss and inclusion body formation in alpha-synuclein mice: implications for neurodegenerative disorders. Science **287**: 1265–1269.

31. FEANY, M. & W. BENDER. 2000. A *Drosophila* model of Parkinson's disease. Nature **404:** 394–398.
32. HASHIMOTO, M., *et al.* 1998. Human recombinant NACP/α-synuclein is aggregated and fibrillated in vitro: relevance for Lewy body disease. Brain Res. **799:** 301–306.
33. CONWAY, K.A., *et al.* 2000. Acceleration of oligomerization, not fibrillization, is a shared property of both alpha-synuclein mutations linked to early-onset Parkinson's disease: implications for pathogenesis and therapy. Proc. Natl. Acad. Sci. USA **97:** 571–576.
34. ROCHET, J., K. CONWAY & P.J. LANSBURY. 2000. Inhibition of fibrillization and accumulation of prefibrillar oligomers in mixtures of human and mouse alpha-synuclein. Biochemistry **39:** 10619–10626.
35. PERRIN, R., *et al.* 2000. Interaction of human alpha-synuclein and Parkinson's disease variants with phospholipids: structural analysis using site-directed mutagenesis. J. Biol. Chem. **275:** 34393–34398.
36. NARAYANAN, V. & S. SCARLATA. 2001. Membrane binding and self-association of alpha-synucleins. Biochemistry **40:** 9927–9934.
37. WOOD, S.J., *et al.* 1999. alpha-Synuclein fibrillogenesis is nucleation dependent: implications for the pathogenesis of Parkinson's disease. J. Biol. Chem. **274:** 19509–19512.
38. SERPELL, L., *et al.* 2000. Fiber diffraction of synthetic α–synuclein filaments shows amyloid-like cross-β conformation. Proc. Natl. Acad. Sci. USA **97:** 4897–4902.
39. CONWAY, K., J. HARPER & P. LANSBURY. 1998. Accelerated in vitro fibril formation by a mutant alpha-synuclein linked to early-onset Parkinson disease. Nat. Med. **4:** 1318–1320.
40. NARHI, L., *et al.* 1999. Both familial Parkinson's disease mutations accelerate alpha-synuclein aggregation. J. Biol. Chem. **274:** 9843–9846.
41. HASHIMOTO, M., *et al.* 1999. Oxidative stress induces amyloid-like aggregate formation of NACP/α-synuclein in vitro. Neuroreport **10:** 717–721.
42. HASHIMOTO, M., *et al.* 1999. Role of cytochrome c as a stimulator of α-synuclein aggregation in Lewy body disease. J. Biol. Chem. **274:** 28849–28852.
43. HSU, L.J., *et al.* 2000. α-Synuclein promotes mitochondrial deficiencies and oxidative stress. Am. J. Pathol. **157:** 401–410.
44. PAIK, S.R., *et al.* 1999. Copper(II)-induced self-oligomerization of alpha-synuclein. Biochem. J. **340:** 821–828.
45. SOUZA, J., *et al.* 2000. Dityrosine cross-linking promotes formation of stable alpha-synuclein polymers. J. Biol. Chem. **275:** 18344–18349.
46. OKOCHI, M., *et al.* 2000. Constitutive phosphorylation of the Parkinson's disease associated α-synuclein. J. Biol. Chem. **275:** 390–397.
47. FUJIWARA, H., *et al.* 2002. alpha-Synuclein is phosphorylated in synucleinopathy lesions. Nat. Cell Biol. **4:** 160–164.
48. JO, E., *et al.* 2000. Alpha-synuclein membrane iteractions and lipid specificity. J. Biol. Chem. **275:** 34328–34334.
49. DAVIDSON, W., *et al.* 1998. Stabilization of alpha-synuclein secondary structure upon binding to synthetic membranes. J. Biol. Chem. **273:** 9443–9449.
50. JENSEN, P., *et al.* 1997. Binding of Aβ to α- and β-synucleins: identification of segments in α-synuclein/NAC precursor that bind Aβ and NAC. Biochem. J. **323:** 539–546.
51. PAIK, S., *et al.* 1998. Self-oligomerization of NACP, the precursor protien of the non-amyloid beta/A4 protein (A beta) component of Alzheimer's disease amyloid, observed in the presence of a C-terminal A beta fragment (residues 25–35). FEBS Lett. **421:** 73–76.
52. YOSHIMOTO, M., *et al.* 1995. NACP, the precursor protein of non-amyloid β/A4 protein (Aβ) component of Alzheimer disease amyloid, binds Aβ and stimulates Aβ aggregation. Proc. Natl. Acad. Sci. USA **92:** 9141–9145.
53. HASHIMOTO, M., *et al.* 2001. beta-Synuclein inhibits alpha-synuclein aggregation: a possible role as an anti-parkinsonian factor. Neuron **32:** 213–223.
54. BETARBET, R., T.B. SHERER & J.T. GREENAMYRE. 2002. Animal models of Parkinson's disease. Bioessays **24:** 308–318.

55. BEAL, M.F. 2001. Experimental models of Parkinson's disease. Nat. Rev. Neurosci. **2:** 325–334.
56. DAWSON, T., A. MANDIR & M. LEE. 2002. Animal models of PD: pieces of the same puzzle? Neuron **35:** 219–222.
57. ROCKENSTEIN, E., *et al.* 2002. Differential neuropathological alterations in transgenic mice expressing alpha-synuclein from the platelet-derived growth factor and Thy-1 promoters. J. Neurosci. Res. **68:** 568–578.
58. GIASSON, B.I., *et al.* 2002. Neuronal alpha-synucleinopathy with severe movement disorder in mice expressing A53T human alpha-synuclein. Neuron **34:** 521–533.
59. LEE, M.K., *et al.* 2002. Human alpha-synuclein-harboring familial Parkinson's disease-linked Ala-53→Thr mutation causes neurodegenerative disease with alpha-synuclein aggregation in transgenic mice. Proc. Natl. Acad. Sci. USA **99:** 8968–8973.
60. VAN DER PUTTEN, H., *et al.* 2000. Neuropathology in mice expressing human alpha-synuclein. J. Neurosci. **20:** 6021–6029.
61. RICHFIELD, E.K., *et al.* 2002. Behavioral and neurochemical effects of wild-type and mutated human alpha-synuclein in transgenic mice. Exp. Neurol. **175:** 35–48.
62. LO BIANCO, C., *et al.* 2002. alpha-Synucleinopathy and selective dopaminergic neuron loss in a rat lentiviral-based model of Parkinson's disease. Proc. Natl. Acad. Sci. USA **99:** 10813–10818.
63. KIRIK, D., *et al.* 2002. Parkinson-like neurodegeneration induced by targeted overexpression of alpha-synuclein in the nigrostriatal system. J. Neurosci. **22:** 2780–2791.
64. KLEIN, R.L., *et al.* 2002. Dopaminergic cell loss induced by human A30P alpha-synuclein gene transfer to the rat substantia nigra. Hum. Gene Ther. **13:** 605–612.
65. KAHLE, P.J., *et al.* 2001. Selective insolubility of alpha-synuclein in human Lewy body diseases is recapitulated in a transgenic mouse model. Am. J. Pathol. **159:** 2215–2225.
66. GOEDERT, M. 2001. Alpha-synuclein and neurodegenerative diseases. Nat. Rev. Neurosci. **2:** 492–501.
67. CONWAY, K.A., *et al.* 2001. Kinetic stabilization of the alpha-synuclein protofibril by a dopamine-alpha-synuclein adduct. Science **294:** 1346–1349.
68. GIASSON, B.I., *et al.* 2000. Oxidative damage linked to neurodegeneration by selective alpha-synuclein nitration in synucleinopathy lesions. Science **290:** 985–989.
69. LANGSTON, J.W., E.B. LANGSTON & I. IRWIN. 1984. MPTP-induced parkinsonism in human and non-human primates—clinical and experimental aspects. Acta Neurol. Scand. Suppl. **100:** 49–54.
70. GRUNBLATT, E., S. MANDEL & M.B. YOUDIM. 2000. MPTP and 6-hydroxydopamine-induced neurodegeneration as models for Parkinson's disease: neuroprotective strategies. J. Neurol. **247**(Suppl. 2): 95–102.
71. RATHKE-HARTLIEB, S., *et al.* 2001. Sensitivity to MPTP is not increased in Parkinson's disease-associated mutant alpha-synuclein transgenic mice. J. Neurochem. **77:** 1181–1184.
72. SONG *et al.* 2002. MPTP promotes mitochondrial pathology and aggregation in human α-synuclein transgenic mice. Soc. Neurosci. Abstr. 226.1.
73. MASLIAH, E., *et al.* 2001. beta-Amyloid peptides enhance alpha-synuclein accumulation and neuronal deficits in a transgenic mouse model linking Alzheimer's disease and Parkinson's disease. Proc. Natl. Acad. Sci. USA **98:** 12245–12250.
74. HANSEN, L., *et al.* 1990. The Lewy body variant of Alzheimer's disease: A clinical and pathologic entity. Neurology **40:** 1–7.
75. MCKEITH, I., *et al.* 1996. Clinical and pathological diagnosis of dementia with Lewy bodies (DLB): Report of the CDLB International Workshop. Neurology **47:** 1113–1124.
76. AULUCK, P.K., *et al.* 2002. Chaperone suppression of alpha-synuclein toxicity in a *Drosophila* model for Parkinson's disease. Science **295:** 865–868.
77. HATTORI, N., *et al.* 1998. Point mutations (Thr240Arg and Ala311Stop) in the *Parkin* gene. Biochem. Biophys. Res. Commun. **249:** 754–758.
78. KITADA, T., *et al.* 1998. Mutations in the *Parkin* gene cause autosomal recessive juvenile parkinsonism. Nature **392:** 605–608.

79. SHIMURA, H., *et al.* 2000. Familial Parkinson disease gene product, *Parkin*, is a ubiquitin-protein ligase. Nat. Gen. **25:** 302–305.
80. WEINREB, P., *et al.* 1996. NACP, a protein implicated in Alzheimer's disease and learning, is natively unfolded. Biochemistry **35:** 13709–13715.
81. UVERSKY, V.N., *et al.* 2002. Biophysical properties of the synucleins and their propensities to fibrillate: inhibition of alpha-synuclein assembly by beta- and gamma-synucleins. J. Biol. Chem. **277:** 11970–11978.
82. LEE, H.J., *et al.* 2001. Formation and removal of alpha-synuclein aggregates in cells exposed to mitochondrial inhibitors. J. Biol. Chem. **277:** 5411–5417.
83. LENG, Y., T.N. CHASE & M.C. BENNETT. 2001. Muscarinic receptor stimulation induces translocation of an alpha-synuclein oligomer from plasma membrane to a light vesicle fraction in cytoplasm. J. Biol. Chem. **276:** 28212–28218.

The 1-Methyl-4-Phenyl-1,2,3,6-Tetrahydropyridine Mouse Model

A Tool to Explore the Pathogenesis of Parkinson's Disease

SERGE PRZEDBORSKI[a,b,c] AND MIQUEL VILA[a]

Neuroscience Research Laboratories of the Movement Disorder Division, Departments of [a]Neurology and [b]Pathology and the [c]Center for Neurobiology and Behavior, Columbia University, New York, New York 10032, USA

ABSTRACT: Experimental models of dopaminergic neurodegeneration play a critical role in our quest to elucidate the cause of Parkinson's disease (PD). Despite the recent development of "genetic models" that have followed upon the discovery of mutations causing rare forms of familial PD, toxic models remain at the forefront when it comes to exploring the pathogenesis of sporadic PD. Among these, the model produced by the neurotoxin 1-methyl-4-phenyl-1,2,3,6-tetrahydropyridine (MPTP) has a competitive advantage over all other toxic models because once this neurotoxin causes intoxication, it induces in humans a syndrome virtually identical to PD. For the past two decades, the complex pharmacology of MPTP and the key steps in the MPTP neurotoxic process have been identified. These molecular events can be classified into three groups: First, those implicated in the initiation of toxicity, which include energy failure due to ATP depletion and oxidative stress mediated by superoxide and nitric oxide; second, those recruited subsequently in response to the initial neuronal perturbations, which include elements of the molecular pathways of apoptosis such as Bax; and, third, those amplifying the neurodegenerative insult, which include various proinflammatory factors such as prostaglandins. Herein, these different contributing factors are reviewed, as is the sequence in which it is believed these factors are acting within the cascade of events responsible for the death of dopaminergic neurons in the MPTP model and in PD. How to target these factors to devise effective neuroprotective therapies for PD is also discussed.

KEYWORDS: apoptosis; cell death; nitric oxide; neurotoxicity; neurodegeneration; MPTP; Parkinson's disease (PD); reactive oxygen species; superoxide dismutase

INTRODUCTION

1-Methy-4-phenyl-1,2,3,6-tetrahydropyridine (MPTP) is a byproduct of the chemical synthesis of a meperidine analog with potent heroin-like effects. MPTP can induce a parkinsonian syndrome in humans almost indistinguishable from Par-

Address for correspondence: Dr. Serge Przedborski, BB-307, Columbia University, 650 West 168th Street, New York, New York 10032. Voice: 212-305-1540; fax: 212-305-5450.
SP30@columbia.edu

Ann. N.Y. Acad. Sci. 991: 189–198 (2003). © 2003 New York Academy of Sciences.

kinson's disease (PD).[1] Recognition of MPTP as a neurotoxin occurred early in 1982, when several young drug addicts mysteriously developed a profound parkinsonian syndrome after the intravenous use of street preparations of meperidine analogs that, unknown to anyone, were contaminated with MPTP.[2] In humans and nonhuman primates, depending on the regimen used, MPTP produces an irreversible and severe parkinsonian syndrome that replicates almost all of the features of PD; in nonhuman primates, however, a resting tremor characteristic of PD has been demonstrated convincingly only in the African green monkey.[3] It is believed that in PD the neurodegenerative process occurs over several years, while the most active phase of neurodegeneration is completed within a few days following MPTP administration.[4,5] However, recent data suggest that, following the main phase of neuronal death, MPTP-induced neurodegeneration may continue to progress "silently" over several decades, at least in humans intoxicated with MPTP.[6,7] Except for four cases,[7,8] no human pathological material has been available for study; thus, the comparison between PD and the MPTP model is limited largely to nonhuman primates.[9] Neuropathological data show that MPTP administration causes damage to the nigrostriatal dopaminergic pathway identical to that seen in PD,[10] yet there is a resemblance that goes beyond the loss of substantia nigra pars compacta (SNpc) dopaminergic neurons. Like PD, MPTP causes a greater loss of dopaminergic neurons in the SNpc than in the ventral tegmental area[11,12] and, in monkeys treated with low doses of MPTP (but not in humans), a greater degeneration of dopaminergic nerve terminals in the putamen than in the caudate nucleus.[13,14] However, two typical neuropathologic features of PD have, until now, been lacking in the MPTP model. First, except for the SNpc, pigmented nuclei such as the locus coeruleus have been spared, according to most published reports. Second, the eosinophilic intraneuronal inclusions called Lewy bodies, so characteristic of PD, have not, thus far, been convincingly observed in MPTP-induced parkinsonism;[9] however, in MPTP-injected monkeys, intraneuronal inclusions reminiscent of Lewy bodies have been described.[15] Despite these imperfections, MPTP continues to be regarded as an excellent animal model of sporadic PD, and the belief is that studying MPTP toxic mechanisms will shed light on meaningful pathogenic mechanisms implicated in PD.

Over the years, MPTP has been used in a large variety of animal species, ranging from worms to mammals. To date, the most frequently used animals for MPTP studies have been monkeys, rats, and mice.[16] The administration of MPTP through a number of different routes using different dosing regimens has led to the development of several distinct models, each characterized by some unique behavioral and neuropathological features. Herein, we will restrict our discussion to mice, since they have emerged as the preferred animals to explore cellular and molecular alterations produced by MPTP, in part because lines of engineered animals that are so critical to these types of investigations are available only in mice.[17]

MPTP MODE OF ACTION

As illustrated in FIGURE 1, the metabolism of MPTP is a complex, multistep process.[18] After its systemic administration, MPTP, which is highly lypophilic, rapidly crosses the blood-brain barrier. Once in the brain, the protoxin MPTP is metabolized to 1-methyl-4-phenyl-2,3-dihydropyridinium ($MPDP^+$) by the enzyme monoamine

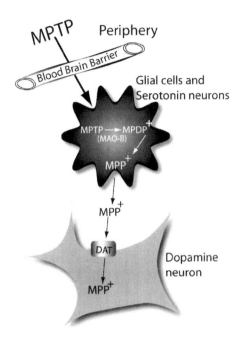

FIGURE 1. Schematic diagram of MPTP metabolism. After its systemic administration, MPTP crosses the blood–brain barrier. Once in the brain, MPTP is converted to MPDP$^+$ by monoamine oxidase B within nondopaminergic cells, and then to MPP$^+$ by an unknown mechanism. Thereafter, MPP$^+$ is released, again by an unknown mechanism, in the extracellular space. From there, MPP$^+$ is taken up by the dopamine transporter and thus enters dopaminergic neurons.

oxidase B within nondopaminergic cells, and then (probably by spontaneous oxidation) to 1-methyl-4-phenylpyridinium (MPP$^+$), the active toxic compound. Thereafter, MPP$^+$ is released (by an unknown mechanism) into the extracellular space. Since MPP$^+$ is a polar molecule, unlike its precursor MPTP, it cannot freely enter cells, but depends on the plasma membrane carriers to gain access to dopaminergic neurons. MPP$^+$ has a high affinity for plasma membrane dopamine transporter (DAT),[19] as well as for norepinephrine and serotonin transporters. The obligatory character of this step in the MPTP neurotoxic process is demonstrated by the fact that blockade of DAT by specific antagonists such as mazindol[20] or ablation of the DAT gene in mutant mice[21] completely prevents MPTP-induced toxicity. Conversely, transgenic mice with increased brain DAT expression are more sensitive to MPTP.[22]

Once inside dopaminergic neurons, MPP$^+$ can follow at least three routes (FIG. 2): (1) it can bind to the vesicular monoamine transporters (VMAT), which will translocate MPP$^+$ into synaptosomal vesicles;[23] (2) it can be concentrated within the mitochondria;[24] and (3) it can remain in the cytosol and interact with different cytosolic enzymes.[25] The fraction of MPP$^+$ destined to each of these routes is probably a function of MPP$^+$ intracellular concentration and affinity for VMAT, mitochondria carriers, and cytosolic enzymes. The importance of the vesicular sequestration of

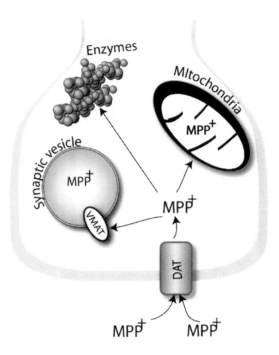

FIGURE 2. Schematic diagram of MPP$^+$ intracellular pathways. Inside dopaminergic neurons, MPP$^+$ can bind to the vesicular monoamine transporters, be translocated into synaptosomal vesicles, be concentrated by an active process within the mitochondria, and remain in the cytosol and interact with different cytosolic enzymes.

MPP$^+$ is demonstrated by the fact that cells transfected to express greater density of VMAT are converted from MPP$^+$-sensitive to MPP$^+$-resistant cells.[23] Conversely, we demonstrated that mutant mice with 50% lower VMAT expression are significantly more sensitive to MPTP-induced dopaminergic neurotoxicity compared to their wild-type littermates.[26] These findings indicate that there is a clear inverse relationship between the capacity of MPP$^+$ sequestration (that is, VMAT density) and the magnitude of MPTP neurotoxicity. Inside dopaminergic neurons, MPP$^+$ can also be concentrated within the mitochondria (FIG. 2),[24] where it impairs mitochondrial respiration by inhibiting complex I of the electron transport chain[27,28] through its binding at or near the site of the mitochondrial poison rotenone.[29,30]

MPTP MECHANISM OF ACTION

Currently, it is believed that the neurotoxic process of MPTP is made up of a cascade of deleterious events, which can be divided into early and late neuronal perturbations and secondary nonneuronal alterations. All of these, to a variable degree and at different stages of the degenerative process, participate in the ultimate demise of dopaminergic neurons.

Early Events

Soon after its entry into dopaminergic neurons, MPP^+ binds to complex I and, by interrupting the flow of electrons, leads to an acute deficit in ATP formation. It appears, however, that complex I activity must be reduced >70% to cause severe ATP depletion in nonsynaptic mitochondria[31] and that, in contrast to *in vitro* MPTP, *in vivo* MPTP causes only a transient 20% reduction in mouse striatal and midbrain ATP levels,[32] raising the question as to whether an MPP^+-related ATP deficit can be the sole factor underlying MPTP-induced dopaminergic neuronal death. Another consequence of complex I inhibition by MPP^+ is an increased production of reactive oxygen species (ROS), especially of superoxide.[33–35] A recent demonstration[36] showed that early ROS production can also occur in this model from the autooxidation of dopamine resulting from an MPP^+-induced massive release of vesicular dopamine to the cytosol. The importance of MPP^+-related ROS production in the dopaminergic toxicity process *in vivo* is demonstrated by the fact that transgenic mice with increased brain activity of copper/zinc superoxide dismutase (SOD1), a key ROS-scavenging enzyme, are significantly more resistant to MPTP-induced dopaminergic toxicity than their nontransgenic littermates.[37] However, several lines of evidence support the concept that ROS exert many or most of their toxic effects in the MPTP model in conjunction with other reactive species such as nitric oxide (NO)[38–41] produced in the brain by both the neuronal and the inducible isoforms of the enzyme NO synthase.[42,43] Comprehensive reviews of the source and the role of NO in the MPTP model can be found in Przedborski and Vila[1] and in Przedborski and Dawson.[44]

Late Events

In response to the variety of functional perturbations caused by the depletion in ATP and the production of ROS, death signals, which can activate the molecular pathways of apoptosis, arise within intoxicated dopaminergic neurons. Although at this time we cannot exclude with certainty the possibility that apoptotic factors are in fact always recruited regardless of MPTP regimen, only prolonged administration of low-to-moderate doses of MPTP is associated with definite morphologically defined apoptotic neurons.[5,45] Supporting the implication of apoptotic molecular factors in the demise of dopaminergic neurons after MPTP administration is the demonstration that the proapoptotic protein Bax is instrumental in this toxic model.[46] Overexpression of the antiapoptotic Bcl-2 also protects dopaminergic cells against MPTP-induced neurodegeneration.[47,48] Similarly, adenovirus-mediated transgenic expression of the X chromosome–linked inhibitor of apoptosis protein (XIAP), an inhibitor of executioner caspases such as caspase-3, also blocks the death of dopaminergic neurons in the SNpc following the administration of MPTP.[49,50] Additional caspases are also activated in MPTP-intoxicated mice such as caspase-8, which is a proximal effector of the tumor necrosis factor receptor (TNFr) family death pathway.[51] Interestingly, however, in the MPTP mouse model it is possible that caspase-8 activation is consequent to the recruitment of the mitochondria-dependent apoptotic pathway and not, as in many other pathological settings, to the ligation of TNFr.[52] Other observations supporting a role of apoptosis in the MPTP neurotoxic process include the demonstration of the resistance to MPTP of the following: mutant mice deficient in p53,[53] a cell cycle control gene involved in programmed cell death; mice with pharmacological or genetic inhibition of c-Jun N terminal kinases;[54–56] or mice that received a striatal adenoassociated virus vector delivery of an Apaf-1–dominant negative inhibitor.[57] Collectively, these data show that during the degenerative process the apoptotic pathways are activated and contribute to the actual death of intoxicated neurons in the MPTP model.

Secondary Events

The loss of dopaminergic neurons in the MPTP mouse model is associated with a glial response composed mainly of activated microglial cells and, to a lesser extent, of reactive astrocytes.[58] From a neuropathological standpoint, microglial activation is indicative of an active, ongoing process of cell death. The presence of activated microglia in postmortem samples from MPTP-intoxicated individuals who came to autopsy several decades after being exposed to the toxin[59] suggests an ongoing degenerative process and thus challenges the notion that MPTP produces a "hit and run" kind of damage. Therefore, this important observation[59] suggests that a single acute insult to the SNpc by MPTP could set in motion a self-sustained cascade of events with long-lasting deleterious effects. With mice injected with MPTP and killed at different time points thereafter, it appears that the time course of reactive astrocyte formation parallels that of dopaminergic structure destruction in both the striatum and the SNpc, and that glial fibrillary acidic protein (GFAP) expression remains upregulated even after the main wave of neuronal death has passed.[60–62] These findings suggest that, in the MPTP mouse model,[63] the astrocyte activation is secondary to the death of neurons and not the reverse. This conclusion is supported by the demonstration that blockade of MPP$^+$ uptake into dopaminergic neurons completely prevents not only SNpc dopaminergic neuronal death but also GFAP upregulation.[64] Remarkably, activation of microglia, which is also quite strong in the MPTP mouse model,[60–62,65] occurs earlier than that of astrocytes and, more important, reaches a maximum before the peak of dopaminergic neurodegeneration.[62] In light of the MPTP data presented above, it can be surmised that the response of both astrocytes and microglial cells in the SNpc clearly occurs within a time frame allowing these glial cells to participate in the demise of dopaminergic neurons in the MPTP mouse model and possibly in PD. Activated microglial cells can produce a variety of noxious compounds, including ROS, reactive nitrogen species (RNS), proinflammatory cytokines, and prostaglandins. Observations showing that blockade of microglial activation mitigates nigrostriatal damage caused by MPTP supports the notion that microglia participate in MPTP-induced neurodegeneration.[66] Among specific deleterious factors, cyclooxygenase type-2 (Cox-2) has emerged as an important determinant of cytotoxicity associated with inflammation.[67,68] In the normal brain, Cox-2 is significantly expressed only in specific subsets of forebrain neurons that are primarily glutamatergic in nature,[69] which suggests a role for Cox-2 in the postsynaptic signaling of excitatory neurons. However, under pathological conditions, especially those associated with a glial response, Cox-2 expression in the brain can increase significantly, as does the level of its products (for example, prostaglandin E$_2$, or PGE$_2$), which are responsible for many of the cytotoxic effects of inflammation. Interestingly, Cox-2 promoter shares many features with inducible nitric oxide synthase (iNOS) promoter;[70] thus, these two enzymes are often coexpressed in disease states associated with gliosis. Therefore, it is not surprising to find Cox-2 and iNOS expressed in SNpc glial cells of postmortem PD samples;[71] PGE_2 content is also elevated in SNpc from PD patients.[72] Of relevance to the potential role of prostaglandin in the pathogenesis of PD is the demonstration that the pharmacological inhibition of both Cox-2 and Cox-1[73] and the genetic ablation of Cox-2 attenuates MPTP neurotoxicity.[74]

ACKNOWLEDGMENTS

The authors wish to thank Brian Jones, for helping to prepare the manuscript, and Kim Tieu, for preparing the illustrations. The authors also wish to acknowledge the support of the NIH/NINDS (Grants R29 NS37345, RO1 NS38586, NS42269, and P50 NS38370); the NIH/NIA (Grant AG13966); the U.S. Department of Defense (Grants DAMD 17-99-1-9471 and DAMD 17-03-1); the Lowenstein Foundation; the Lillian Goldman Charitable Trust; the Parkinson's Disease Foundation; the Muscular Dystrophy Association; the ALS Association; and Project-ALS.

REFERENCES

1. PRZEDBORSKI, S. & M. VILA. 2001. MPTP: a review of its mechanisms of neurotoxicity. Clin. Neurosci. Res. 1: 407–418.
2. LANGSTON, J.W., et al. 1983. Chronic parkinsonism in humans due to a product of meperidine-analog synthesis. Science 219: 979–980.
3. TETRUD, J.W., et al. 1986. MPTP-induced tremor in human and non-human primates. Neurology 36(Suppl. 1): 308.
4. LANGSTON, J.W. 1987. MPTP: the promise of a new neurotoxin. In Movement Disorders 2. C.D. Marsden & S. Fahn, Eds.: 73–90. Butterworths. London.
5. JACKSON-LEWIS, V., et al. 1995. Time course and morphology of dopaminergic neuronal death caused by the neurotoxin 1-methyl-4-phenyl-1,2,3,6-tetrahydropyridine. Neurodegeneration 4: 257–269.
6. VINGERHOETS, F.J., et al. 1994. Positron emission tomographic evidence for progression of human MPTP-induced dopaminergic lesions. Ann. Neurol. 36: 765–770.
7. LANGSTON, J.W., et al. 1999. Evidence of active nerve cell degeneration in the substantia nigra of humans years after 1-methyl-4-phenyl-1,2,3,6-tetrahydropyridine exposure. Ann. Neurol. 46: 598–605.
8. DAVIS, G.C., et al. 1979. Chronic parkinsonism secondary to intravenous injection of meperidine analogs. Psychiatry Res. 1: 249–254.
9. FORNO, L.S., et al. 1993. Similarities and differences between MPTP-induced parkinsonism and Parkinson's disease: neuropathologic considerations. Adv. Neurol. 60: 600–608.
10. PRZEDBORSKI, S., et al. 2002. Dopaminergic system in Parkinson's disease. In Dopamine Receptors and Transporters. A. Sidhu et al., Eds.: 363–402. Marcel Dekker. New York.
11. SENIUK, N.A., et al. 1990. Dose-dependent destruction of the coeruleus-cortical and nigral-striatal projections by MPTP. Brain Res. 527: 7–20.
12. MUTHANE, U., et al. 1994. Differences in nigral neuron number and sensitivity to 1-methyl-4-phenyl-1,2,3,6-tetrahydropyridine in C57/bl and CD-1 mice. Exp. Neurol. 126: 195–204.
13. MORATALLA, R., et al. 1992. Differential vulnerability of primate caudate-putamen and striosome-matrix dopamine systems to the neurotoxic effects of 1-methyl-4-phenyl-1,2,3,6-tetrahydropyridine. Proc. Natl. Acad. Sci. USA 89: 3859–3863.
14. SNOW, B.J., et al. 2000. Pattern of dopaminergic loss in the striatum of humans with MPTP-induced parkinsonism. J. Neurol. Neurosurg. Psychiatry 68: 313–316.

15. FORNO, L.S., et al. 1986. Locus ceruleus lesions and eosinophilic inclusions in MPTP-treated monkeys. Ann. Neurol. **20:** 449–455.
16. PRZEDBORSKI, S., et al. 2001. The parkinsonian toxin 1-methyl-4-phenyl-1,2,3,6-tetrahydropyridine (MPTP): a technical review of its utility and safety. J. Neurochem. **76:** 1265–1274.
17. VILA, M., et al. 2001. Engineered modeling and the secrets of Parkinson's disease. Trends Neurosci. **24:** S49–S55.
18. PRZEDBORSKI, S. & V. JACKSON-LEWIS. 1998. Mechanisms of MPTP toxicity. Mov. Disord. **13**(Suppl. 1): 35–38.
19. MAYER, R.A., et al. 1986. Prevention of the nigrostriatal toxicity of 1-methyl-4-phenyl-1,2,3,6-tetrahydropyridine by inhibitors of 3,4-dihydroxyphenylethylamine transport. J. Neurochem. **47:** 1073–1079.
20. JAVITCH, J.A., et al. 1985. Parkinsonism-inducing neurotoxin, N-methyl-4-phenyl-1,2,3,6-tetrahydropyridine: Uptake of the metabolite N-methyl-4-phenylpyridinium by dopamine neurons explain selective toxicity. Proc. Natl. Acad. Sci. USA **82:** 2173–2177.
21. BEZARD, E., et al. 1999. Absence of MPTP-induced neuronal death in mice lacking the dopamine transporter. Exp. Neurol. **155:** 268–273.
22. DONOVAN, D.M., et al. 1999. Cocaine reward and MPTP toxicity: alteration by regional variant dopamine transporter overexpression. Mol. Brain Res. **73:** 37–49.
23. LIU, Y., et al. 1992. Gene transfer of a reserpine-sensitive mechanism of resistance to N-methyl-4-phenylpyridinium. Proc. Natl. Acad. Sci. USA **89:** 9074–9078.
24. RAMSAY, R.R. & T.P. SINGER. 1986. Energy-dependent uptake of N-methyl-4-phenylpyridinium, the neurotoxic metabolite of 1-methyl-4-phenyl-1,2,3,6-tetrahydropyridine, by mitochondria. J. Biol. Chem. **261:** 7585–7587.
25. KLAIDMAN, L.K., et al. 1993. Redox cycling of MPP$^+$: evidence for a new mechanism involving hydride transfer with xanthine oxidase, aldehyde dehydrogenase, and lipoamide dehydrogenase. Free Radic. Biol. Med. **15:** 169–179.
26. TAKAHASHI, N., et al. 1997. VMAT2 knockout mice: heterozygotes display reduced amphetamine-conditioned reward, enhanced amphetamine locomotion, and enhanced MPTP toxicity. Proc. Natl. Acad. Sci. USA **94:** 9938–9943.
27. NICKLAS, W.J., et al. 1985. Inhibition of NADH-linked oxidation in brain mitochondria by MPP$^+$, a metabolite of the neurotoxin MPTP. Life Sci. **36:** 2503–2508.
28. MIZUNO, Y., et al. 1987. Effects of 1-methyl-4-phenyl-1,2,3,6-tetrahydropyridine and 1-methyl-4-phenylpyridinium ion on activities of the enzymes in the electron transport system in mouse brain. J. Neurochem. **48:** 1787–1793.
29. RAMSAY, R.R., et al. 1991. Interaction of 1-methyl-4-phenylpyridinium ion (MPP$^+$) and its analogs with the rotenone/piericidin binding site of NADH dehydrogenase. J. Neurochem. **56:** 1184–1190.
30. HIGGINS, D.S., JR. & J.T. GREENAMYRE. 1996. [^{3}H]dihydrorotenone binding to NADH: ubiquinone reductase (complex I) of the electron transport chain: an autoradiographic study. J. Neurosci. **16:** 3807–3816.
31. DAVEY, G.P. & J.B. CLARK. 1996. Threshold effects and control of oxidative phosphorylation in nonsynaptic rat brain mitochondria. J. Neurochem. **66:** 1617–1624.
32. CHAN, P., et al. 1991. Rapid ATP loss caused by 1-methyl-4-phenyl-1,2,3,6-tetrahydropyridine in mouse brain. J. Neurochem. **57:** 348–351.
33. ROSSETTI, Z.L., et al. 1988. 1-Methyl-4-phenyl-1,2,3,6-tetrahydropyridine (MPTP) and free radicals in vitro. Biochem. Pharmacol. **37:** 4573–4574.
34. HASEGAWA, E., et al. 1990. 1-Mehtyl-4-phenylpyridinium (MPP$^+$) induces NADH-dependent superoxide formation and enhances NADH-dependent lipid peroxidation in bovine heart submitochondrial particles. Biochem. Biophys. Res. Commun. **170:** 1049–1055.
35. CLEETER, M.W., et al. 1992. Irreversible inhibition of mitochondrial complex I by 1-methyl-4-phenylpyridinium: evidence for free radical involvement. J. Neurochem. **58:** 786–789.
36. LOTHARIUS, J. & K.L. O'MALLEY. 2000. The parkinsonism-inducing drug 1-methyl-4-phenylpyridinium triggers intracellular dopamine oxidation: a novel mechanism of toxicity. J. Biol. Chem. **275:** 38581–38588.

37. PRZEDBORSKI, S., *et al.* 1992. Transgenic mice with increased Cu/Zn-superoxide dismutase activity are resistant to *N*-methyl-4-phenyl-1,2,3,6-tetrahydropyridine-induced neurotoxicity. J. Neurosci. **12:** 1658–1667.

38. SCHULZ, J.B., *et al.* 1995. Inhibition of neuronal nitric oxide synthase by 7-nitroindazole protects against MPTP-induced neurotoxicity in mice. J. Neurochem. **64:** 936–939.

39. PENNATHUR, S., *et al.* 1999. Mass spectrometric quantification of 3-nitrotyrosine, ortho-tyrosine, and o,o'-dityrosine in brain tissue of 1-methyl-4-phenyl-1,2,3,6-tetrahydropyridine-treated mice, a model of oxidative stress in Parkinson's disease. J. Biol. Chem. **274:** 34621–34628.

40. ARA, J., *et al.* 1998. Inactivation of tyrosine hydroxylase by nitration following exposure to peroxynitrite and 1-methyl-4-phenyl-1,2,3,6-tetrahydropyridine (MPTP). Proc. Natl. Acad. Sci. USA **95:** 7659–7663.

41. PRZEDBORSKI, S., *et al.* 2001. Oxidative post-translational modifications of alpha-synuclein in the 1-methyl-4-phenyl-1,2,3,6-tetrahydropyridine (MPTP) mouse model of Parkinson's disease. J. Neurochem. **76:** 637–640.

42. LIBERATORE, G., *et al.* 1999. Inducible nitric oxide synthase stimulates dopaminergic neurodegeneration in the MPTP model of Parkinson's disease. Nat. Med. **5:** 1403–1409.

43. PRZEDBORSKI, S., *et al.* 1996. Role of neuronal nitric oxide in MPTP (1-methyl-4-phenyl-1,2,3,6-tetrahydropyridine)-induced dopaminergic neurotoxicity. Proc. Natl. Acad. Sci. USA **93:** 4565–4571.

44. PRZEDBORSKI, S. & T.M. DAWSON. 2001. The role of nitric oxide in Parkinson's disease. *In* Parkinson's Disease. Methods and Protocols. M.M. Mouradian, Ed.: 113–136. Humana Press. Totowa, NJ.

45. TATTON, N.A. & S.J. KISH. 1997. *In situ* detection of apoptotic nuclei in the substantia nigra compacta of 1-methyl-4-phenyl-1,2,3,6-tetrahydropyridine-treated mice using terminal deoxynucleotidyl transferase labelling and acridine orange staining. Neuroscience **77:** 1037–1048.

46. VILA, M., *et al.* 2001. Bax ablation prevents dopaminergic neurodegeneration in the 1-methyl-4-phenyl-1,2,3,6-tetrahydropyridine mouse model of Parkinson's disease. Proc. Natl. Acad. Sci. USA **98:** 2837–2842.

47. YANG, L., *et al.* 1998. 1-Methyl-4-phenyl-1,2,3,6-tetrahydropyride neurotoxicity is attenuated in mice overexpressing Bcl-2. J. Neurosci. **18:** 8145–8152.

48. OFFEN, D., *et al.* 1998. Transgenic mice expressing human Bcl-2 in their neurons are resistant to 6-hydroxydopamine and 1-methyl-4-phenyl-1,2,3,6-tetrahydropyridine neurotoxicity. Proc. Natl. Acad. Sci. USA **95:** 5789–5794.

49. XU, D., *et al.* 1999. Attenuation of ischemia-induced cellular and behavioral deficits by X chromosome-linked inhibitor of apoptosis protein overexpression in the rat hippocampus. J. Neurosci. **19:** 5026–5033.

50. EBERHARDT, O., *et al.* 2000. Protection by synergistic effects of adenovirus-mediated X-chromosome-linked inhibitor of apoptosis and glial cell line-derived neurotrophic factor gene transfer in the 1-methyl-4-phenyl-1,2,3,6-tetrahydropyridine model of Parkinson's disease. J. Neurosci. **20:** 9126–9134.

51. HARTMANN, A., *et al.* 2001. Caspase-8 is an effector in apoptotic death of dopaminergic neurons in Parkinson's disease, but pathway inhibition results in neuronal necrosis. J Neurosci. **21:** 2247–2255.

52. VISWANATH, V., *et al.* 2001. Caspase-9 activation results in downstream caspase-8 activation and bid cleavage in 1-methyl-4-phenyl-1,2,3,6-tetrahydropyridine-induced Parkinson's disease. J. Neurosci. **21:** 9519–9528.

53. TRIMMER, P.A., *et al.* 1996. Dopamine neurons from transgenic mice with a knockout of the p53 gene resist MPTP neurotoxicity. Neurodegeneration **5:** 233–239.

54. SAPORITO, M.S., *et al.* 2000. MPTP activates c-Jun NH(2)-terminal kinase (JNK) and its upstream regulatory kinase MKK4 in nigrostriatal neurons in vivo. J. Neurochem. **75:** 1200–1208.

55. SAPORITO, M.S., *et al.* 1999. CEP-1347/KT-7515, an inhibitor of c-jun N-terminal kinase activation, attenuates the 1-methyl-4-phenyl tetrahydropyridine-mediated loss of nigrostriatal dopaminergic neurons in vivo. J. Pharmacol. Exp. Ther. **288:** 421–427.

56. XIA, X.G., *et al.* 2001. Gene transfer of the JNK interacting protein-1 protects dopaminergic neurons in the MPTP model of Parkinson's disease. Proc. Natl. Acad. Sci. USA **98:** 10433–10438.
57. MOCHIZUKI, H., *et al.* 2001. An AAV-derived Apaf-1 dominant negative inhibitor prevents MPTP toxicity as antiapoptotic gene therapy for Parkinson's disease. Proc. Natl. Acad. Sci. USA **98:** 10918–10923.
58. VILA, M., *et al.* 2001. The role of glial cells in Parkinson's disease. Curr. Opin. Neurol. **14:** 483–489.
59. LANGSTON, J.W., *et al.* 1999. Evidence of active nerve cell degeneration in the substantia nigra of humans years after 1-methyl-4-phenyl-1,2,3,6-tetrahydropyridine exposure. Ann. Neurol. **46:** 598–605.
60. CZLONKOWSKA, A., *et al.* 1996. Microglial reaction in MPTP (1-methyl-4-phenyl-1,2,3,6-tetrahydropyridine) induced Parkinson's disease mice model. Neurodegeneration **5:** 137–143.
61. KOHUTNICKA, M., *et al.* 1998. Microglial and astrocytic involvement in a murine model of Parkinson's disease induced by 1-methyl-4-phenyl-1,2,3,6-tetrahydropyridine (MPTP). Immunopharmacology **39:** 167–180.
62. LIBERATORE, G.T., *et al.* 1999. Inducible nitric oxide synthase stimulates dopaminergic neurodegeneration in the MPTP model of Parkinson disease. Nat. Med. **5:** 1403–1409.
63. PRZEDBORSKI, S., *et al.* 2000. The parkinsonian toxin MPTP: Action and mechanism. Restor. Neurol. Neurosci. **16:** 135–142.
64. O'CALLAGHAN, J.P., *et al.* 1990. Characterization of the origins of astrocyte response to injury using the dopaminergic neurotoxicant, 1-methyl-4-phenyl-1,2,3,6-tetrahydropyridine. Brain Res. **521:** 73–80.
65. DEHMER, T., *et al.* 2000. Deficiency of inducible nitric oxide synthase protects against MPTP toxicity in vivo. J. Neurochem. **74:** 2213–2216.
66. WU, D.C., *et al.* 2002. Blockade of microglial activation is neuroprotective in the 1-methyl-4-phenyl-1,2,3,6-tetrahydropyridine mouse model of Parkinson disease. J. Neurosci. **22:** 1763–1771.
67. SEIBERT, K., *et al.* 1995. Mediation of inflammation by cyclooxygenase-2. Agents Actions Suppl. **46:** 41–50.
68. O'BANION, M.K. 1999. Cyclooxygenase-2: molecular biology, pharmacology, and neurobiology. Crit. Rev. Neurobiol. **13:** 45–82.
69. KAUFMANN, W.E., *et al.* 1996. COX-2, a synaptically induced enzyme, is expressed by excitatory neurons at postsynaptic sites in rat cerebral cortex. Proc. Natl. Acad. Sci. USA **93:** 2317–2321.
70. NATHAN, C. & Q.W. XIE. 1994. Regulation of biosynthesis of nitric oxide. J. Biol. Chem. **269:** 13725–13728.
71. KNOTT, C., *et al.* 2000. Inflammatory regulators in Parkinson's disease: iNOS, lipocortin-1, and cyclooxygenases-1 and -2. Mol. Cell. Neurosci. **16:** 724–739.
72. MATTAMMAL, M.B., *et al.* 1995. Prostaglandin H synthetase-mediated metabolism of dopamine: Implication for Parkinson's disease. J. Neurochem. **64:** 1645–1654.
73. TEISMANN, P. & B. FERGER. 2001. Inhibition of the cyclooxygenase isoenzymes COX-1 and COX-2 provide neuroprotection in the MPTP-mouse model of Parkinson's disease. Synapse **39:** 167–174.
74. FENG, Z., *et al.* 2002. Cyclooxygenase-2-deficient mice are resistant to 1-methyl-4-phenyl-1,2,3,6-tetrahydropyridine-induced damage of dopaminergic neurons in the substantia nigra. Neurosci. Lett. **329:** 354.

Pathophysiology of Parkinson's Disease: The MPTP Primate Model of the Human Disorder

THOMAS WICHMANN AND MAHLON R. DeLONG

Department of Neurology, Emory University School of Medicine, Atlanta Georgia 30322, USA

ABSTRACT: The striatum is viewed as the principal input structure of the basal ganglia, while the internal pallidal segment (GPi) and the substantia nigra pars reticulata (SNr) are output structures. Input and output structures are linked via a monosynaptic "direct" pathway and a polysynaptic "indirect" pathway involving the external pallidal segment (GPe) and the subthalamic nucleus (STN). According to current schemes, striatal dopamine (DA) enhances transmission along the direct pathway (via D1 receptors), and reduces transmission over the indirect pathway (via D2 receptors). DA also acts on receptors in GPe, GPi, SNr, and STN. Electrophysiologic and other studies in primates rendered parkinsonian by treatment with the dopaminergic neurotoxin MPTP have demonstrated a reduction of neuronal activity of GPe and an increase of neuronal discharge in STN, GPi, and SNr. These findings are compatible with the view that striatal DA loss results in increased activity over the indirect pathway. Prominent bursting, oscillatory discharge patterns, and increased synchronization of neighboring neurons are found throughout the basal ganglia. These may result from changes in the activity of local circuits (e.g., the GPe-STN "pacemaker") or from more global abnormalities of the basal ganglia-thalamocortical network. These findings have been replicated in human patients undergoing microelectrode-guided stereotactic procedures targeted at GPi or STN. PET studies in patients with Parkinson's disease have lent further support to the proposed circuit abnormalities. The current models of basal ganglia function have recently been criticized. For instance, the strict separation of direct and indirect pathways and the segregation of D1 and D2 receptors have been questioned, and the almost complete absence of motor side effects of pallidal or thalamic lesions in human patients and animals is inconsistent. These results suggest that changes in discharge patterns and synchronization between basal ganglia neurons, abnormal network interactions, and compensatory mechanisms are at least as important in the pathopohysiology of parkinsonism as changes in discharge rates in individual basal ganglia nuclei. Lesions of GPi or STN are effective in treating parkinsonism, because they reduce or abolish abnormal basal ganglia output, enabling remaining circuits to function more normally.

KEYWORDS: MPTP; primate; pathophysiology; pallidum; subthalamic nucleus; substantia nigra

Address for correspondence: Thomas Wichmann, M.D., Department of Neurology, Emory University, Suite 6000, Woodruff Memorial Research Building, 1639 Pierce Drive, Atlanta, GA 30322. Voice: 404-727-3818; fax: 404-727-3157.
twichma@emory.edu

Ann. N.Y. Acad. Sci. 991: 199–213 (2003). © 2003 New York Academy of Sciences.

INTRODUCTION

Recent progress in neuroscience research has led to major insights into the structure and function of the basal ganglia and into the pathophysiologic basis of disorders of basal ganglia origin, such as Parkinson's disease.[1-3] The availability of suitable animal models, in particular the MPTP model of primate parkinsonism, has been crucial in this progress.[4,5] In addition, the renaissance of stereotactic surgery for Parkinson's disease and other movement disorders has provided valuable neuronal recording and imaging data from human subjects. In the following, we summarize, from a systems perspective, the pathophysiologic concepts that have arisen from the animal models and from work in patients with Parkinson's disease.

PATHOLOGIC SUBSTRATE IN PARKINSON'S DISEASE

Idiopathic Parkinson's disease is characterized by the cardinal signs of akinesia (impaired movement initiation and poverty of movement), bradykinesia (slowness of movement), muscular rigidity, and tremor at rest. The etiology of the disease is most likely multifactorial, with both genetic and environmental/toxic factors resulting in a relatively selective degeneration of dopaminergic neurons in the substantia nigra pars compacta (SNc), which project to the striatum (e.g., Ref. 6), and, to a lesser extent, to other basal ganglia nuclei such as the external and internal segments of the globus pallidus (GPe, GPi, respectively), the subthalamic nucleus (STN), and the substantia nigra, pars reticulata (SNr).[6] In early phases of the disease, dopamine loss affects particularly the sensorimotor portion of the striatum, the putamen, resulting in the appearance of motor disturbances early in the disease (e.g., Ref. 7). In later stages, more widespread dopamine loss affecting other regions of the basal ganglia (such as the caudate nucleus and the pallidum) and extrabasal ganglia areas (such as cortex, hypothalamus, and thalamus) as well as spread of neuronal degeneration to nondopaminergic systems (such as the locus coeruleus and the raphe nuclei) may cause the development of additional signs and symptoms (such as cognitive disabilities, sleep disorders, and mood disturbances).

ANATOMICAL SUBSTRATE FOR CIRCUIT DYSFUNCTION
IN PARKINSONISM

In order to understand how the loss of dopamine in the basal ganglia leads to the signs and symptoms of parkinsonism, it is necessary first to consider some of the anatomic and physiologic details of the basal ganglia and related structures.

The basal ganglia are a group of functionally related subcortical nuclei that include the neostriatum (comprised of the caudate nucleus and the putamen), ventral striatum, GPe, STN, GPi, SNr and SNc. They are anatomically related to large portions of the cerebral cortex, thalamus, and brain stem. The corticobasal ganglia-thalamocortical circuits appear to be organized in an orderly arrangement of segregated reentrant circuits that is thought to significantly enhance the efficiency and speed of cortical processing (see left half of FIG. 1). Most authors believe, however, that the range of behaviors seen in humans, nonhuman primates, and other species

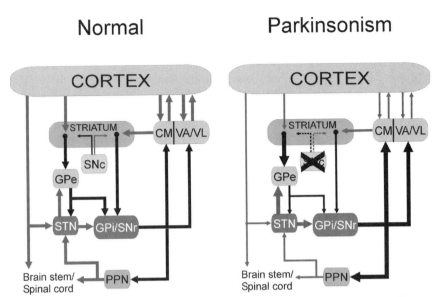

FIGURE 1. Simplified schematic diagram of the basal ganglia–thalamocortical circuitry under normal conditions (**left**) and rate changes in parkinsonism (**right**). Inhibitory connections are shown as *filled arrows*, excitatory connections as *open arrows*. The principal input nuclei of the basal ganglia, the striatum and the STN, are connected to the output nuclei, GPi and SNr. Basal ganglia output is directed at several thalamic nuclei (VA/VL and CM) and at brain stem nuclei (PPN and others). In parkinsonism, dopaminergic neurons in the SNc degenerate, which results, via a cascade of changes in the other basal ganglia nuclei, in increased basal ganglia output from GPi and SNr. This, in turn, is thought to lead to inhibition of related thalamic and cortical neurons. In addition to the changes shown here, there are prominent alterations in discharge patterns (see text). For abbreviations, see text.

requires some intermodular transfer of information. Such cross-talk may occur through interactions of the basal ganglia with some of the brain stem areas or the SNc, which are not as distinctly organized into functional territories.

In primates, projections from the somatosensory, motor, and premotor cortices terminate in the postcommissural putamen, the "motor portion" of the striatum;[8,9] while associative cortical areas project to the caudate nucleus and the precommissural putamen;[10,11] and projections from limbic cortices, amygdala, and hippocampus terminate preferentially in the ventral striatum (e.g., Ref. 12). Cortical inputs also terminate in the STN.[13,14] This projection originates in the primary motor, prefrontal, and premotor cortices.[13,14]

A second major group of inputs to striatum and STN arises from the intralaminar thalamic nuclei, the centromedian nucleus (CM) and the parafascicular nucleus (Pf) (e.g., Refs. 15–17). In primates, CM projects to the motor portions of putamen and STN, whereas Pf projects largely to the associative and limbic territories.[18–20]

Topographically segregated cortical information is conveyed from the striatum to the output nuclei of the basal ganglia (GPi and SNr). Striatofugal projections maintain the striatal organization into motor, limbic, associative, and oculomotor territories.[21] The connections between the striatum and the basal ganglia output nuclei are thought to be organized into a *direct* and an *indirect* pathway.[2,22,23] The direct pathway arises from striatal neurons that project monosynaptically to neurons in GPi and SNr, whereas the indirect pathway arises from a different set of neurons that projects to GPe (see Ref. 24 for a review). Some striatofugal neurons may also collateralize more extensively, reaching GPe, GPi, and SNr.[25] GPe conveys the information it receives either directly to GPi/SNr or via the STN.

The population of striatal neurons that gives rise to the direct pathway can be further characterized by the presence of the neuropeptides substance P and dynorphin, by the preferential expression of the dopamine D1 receptors, and by the fact that these neurons (as well as most striatal interneurons) appear to be the targets of thalamic inputs from the centromedian nucleus.[26,27] The population that gives rise to the indirect pathway expresses preferentially enkephalin and dopamine D2 receptors[28,29] and may be the principal target of cortical inputs.[26,27] The functionally important segregation of D1 and D2 receptors between the direct and indirect pathways has been most clearly demonstrated in dopamine-depleted animals, while several studies in normal animals have supported the existence of a degree of overlap between D1- and D2-positive cell populations (e.g., Refs. 29, 30). However, the D1/D2 dichotomy may still serve to explain the apparent dual action of dopamine, released from the nigrostriatal pathway arising in the substantia nigra pars compacta, on striatal output. Dopamine appears to modulate the activity of the basal ganglia output neurons in GPi and SNr by *facilitation* of transmission over the direct pathway and *inhibition* of transmission over the indirect pathway (e.g., Ref. 31). The net effect of striatal dopamine release appears to be to reduce basal ganglia output. A reduction of dopamine release as is seen in Parkinson's disease will therefore result in a net increase in basal ganglia output.

Basal ganglia output arises from both GPi and SNr. The division of GPi into a caudoventral "motor" portion and rostromedial associative and limbic areas[32] is maintained in the pallidothalamic projections.[33] The motor territory of GPi projects almost exclusively to the posterior part of the ventrolateral nucleus (VLo in macaques), which in turn sends projections towards the supplementary motor area (SMA),[34,35] the primary motor cortex (M1),[35–37] and the premotor (PM) cortical areas.[37] Associative and limbic areas project preferentially to the parvocellular part of the ventral anterior (VA) and the dorsal VL nucleus (VLc in macaques)[33] and may be transmitted in turn to prefrontal cortical areas,[38,39] as well as to motor and supplementary motor regions[35]).

The SNr can be broadly subdivided into a dorsolateral sensorimotor and a ventromedial associative territory (e.g., Refs. 40, 41). Projections from the SNr to the thalamus terminate in the magnocellular division of the ventral anterior nucleus (VAmc) and in the mediodorsal nucleus (MDmc). These nuclei, in turn, innervate anterior regions of the frontal lobe, including the principal sulcus (area 46) and the orbital cortex (area 11),[42] as well as premotor areas and the frontal eye field.[42]

Both GPi and SNr also send projections to the noncholinergic neurons of the PPN[43–45] and the CM/Pf nuclei.[20,33] Additional projections from the SNr reach the superior colliculus; these may play a critical role in the control of saccades and orienting behaviors.[46]

MOVEMENT-RELATED BASAL GANGLIA ACTIVITY IN NORMAL
AND PARKINSONIAN ANIMALS

Voluntary movements appear to be initiated at the cortical level of the motor circuit, with output to brain stem and spinal cord, and to multiple subcortical targets including the thalamus, putamen, and the STN. Cortical activation of an ensemble of striatal motor territory neurons that give rise to the direct pathway leads to a reduction of inhibitory basal ganglia output and subsequent disinhibition of related thalamocortical neurons[47] and facilitation of the movement. In contrast, activation of striatal neurons that give rise to the indirect pathway will lead to increased basal ganglia output and, presumably, to suppression of movement. Since the majority of neurons in GPi increase their firing rate with movement,[48,49] it has been speculated that the main role of the basal ganglia is to inhibit and stabilize the activity of the thalamocortical network. As far as motor function is concerned, the basal ganglia may play a role in the control of specific kinematic parameters, such as amplitude, velocity, and direction (see, e.g., Refs. 47, 50–52) or may "focus" movements,[53] allowing intended movements to proceed and suppressing unintended movement (see discussion in Ref. 1). Besides these elemental functions in motor control, a multitude of other motor functions have been proposed, such as a role in self-initiated (internally generated) movements, in motor (procedural) learning, and in movement sequencing (e.g., Refs. 54–56). The functions of the nonmotor portions of the basal ganglia may be analogous to the motor functions but are less well explored.

Global Activity Changes in the Basal Ganglia

The study of pathophysiologic changes in the basal ganglia that result from loss of dopaminergic transmission has been greatly facilitated by the discovery that primates treated with MPTP develop behavioral and anatomic changes that closely mimic the features of Parkinson's disease in humans.[5,57,58] Early studies in this model suggested that the metabolic activity (as measured with the 2-deoxy-glucose technique) is increased in both pallidal segments (e.g., Refs. 59, 60). This was interpreted as evidence for increased activity of the striatum-GPe connection and the STN-GPi pathway; or, alternatively, as evidence for increased activity via the projections from the STN to both pallidal segments. It was then shown with microelectrode recordings of neuronal activity that MPTP-induced parkinsonism in primates is associated with reduced tonic neuronal discharge in GPe and increased discharge in STN, GPi, and SNr, as compared to normal controls (see example recordings in Fig. 2 and Refs. 61–64). In parkinsonian patients undergoing pallidotomy it has been shown that the average discharge rate in GPe is significantly lower than that in GPi.[65–67]

The changes in discharge rates in the basal ganglia nuclei have been interpreted as indicating that striatal dopamine depletion leads to increased activity of striatal neurons of the indirect pathway, resulting in inhibition of GPe, and subsequent disinhibition of STN and GPi/SNr. In addition, loss of dopamine in the striatum should also lead to reduced activity via the inhibitory direct pathway. Increased basal ganglia output to the thalamus and increased inhibition of thalamocortical neurons have been corroborated by 2-deoxy-glucose studies in which increased (synaptic) activity in the VA and VL nucleus of thalamus was demonstrated.[59,60] PET studies in parkinsonian patients

Normal   Parkinsonism

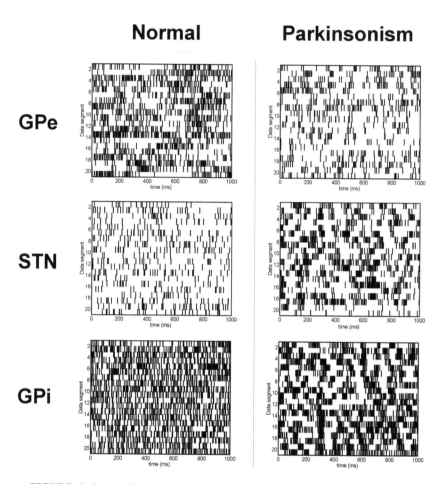

FIGURE 2. Raster displays of spontaneous neuronal activity recorded in different basal ganglia structures within the basal ganglia circuitry in normal and parkinsonian primates.
Shown are 20 consecutive 1000-ms segments of data from GPe, STN, and GPi. The neuronal
activity is reduced in GPe and increased in STN, GPi, and SNr (not shown). In addition to
the rate changes, there are also obvious changes in the firing patterns of neurons in all four
structures, with a marked prominence of burstiness and oscillatory discharge patterns in the
parkinsonian state. For abbreviations and further explanation, see text.

have shown that the activation of motor and premotor areas in parkinsonian patients is
reduced (e.g., Refs. 68, 69) although no changes have been seen in the thalamus. Alterations of cortical activity in motor cortex and supplementary motor areas have also
been demonstrated with single-cell recording in hemiparkinsonian primates.[70] The
proposed pathophysiologic model of changes in the level of activity in the basal ganglia–thalamocortical motor circuit is summarized in FIGURE 1.

The basal ganglia circuitry incorporates multiple negative and positive feedback
loops, which may play a prominent role in the development and maintenance of ab-

normal discharge in the basal ganglia output structures. Some of the primary feedback loops that may directly affect GPi activity involve intrinsic basal ganglia structures such as GPe and STN, or structures outside of the basal ganglia, such as the thalamic nucleus CM, or the pedunculopontine nucleus (PPN).[71,72] Positive feedback loops, for instance those involving PPN and STN and the pathway through CM and the putamen, tend to enhance the abnormalities of discharge in the basal ganglia output nuclei associated with Parkinson's disease; whereas negative feedback circuits, such as a feedback involving CM and STN, will act to normalize neuronal discharge in the basal ganglia output nuclei.

Conceivably, increased tonic inhibition of thalamocortical neurons by excessive output from GPi/SNr may reduce the responsiveness of cortical mechanisms involved in motor control. Increased tonic inhibition of thalamocortical neurons by increased basal ganglia output in parkinsonism may also render precentral motor areas less responsive to other inputs normally involved in initiating movements or may interfere with "set" functions that have been shown to be highly dependent on the integrity of basal ganglia pathways.[22] All of these effects may lead to akinesia.

Brain stem areas such as the PPN may also be involved in the development of akinesia. It has been shown that lesions of this nucleus in normal monkeys can lead to hemiakinesia, possibly by reducing stimulation of SNc neurons by input from the PPN or by a direct influence on descending pathways.[73,74] It remains unclear, however, whether the motor abnormalities seen after PPN inactivation are, in fact, related to parkinsonism, or represent changes in behavioral state or other disturbances that have no direct relation to Parkinson's disease. It is noteworthy that these animals do not manifest rigidity or tremor, which appear to be critically dependent on thalamic circuitry.

Due to the fact that parkinsonism is a *network* or circuit disease, surgical or pharmacologic interventions at a variety of targets within the network could be successful. This can, indeed, be appreciated when considering the results of lesion studies in parkinsonian primates. One of the most important and dramatic in this regard was the demonstration that lesions of the STN in MPTP-treated primates reverse all of the cardinal signs of parkinsonism, presumably by reducing GPi activity.[75,76] Similarly, GPi and SNr inactivation have been shown to be effective against at least some parkinsonian signs in MPTP-treated primates.[77–79]

Over the last decade, these results from animal studies have rekindled interest in functional neurosurgical approaches to the treatment of medically intractable Parkinson's disease. This was first employed in the form of GPi lesions (pallidotomy)[80–84] and, more recently, with STN lesions (see, e.g., Ref. 85). In addition, high-frequency deep-brain stimulation (DBS) of both the STN and GPi have been shown to reverse parkinsonian signs, probably by multiple modes of action—for instance, by inhibition of STN neurons through "depolarization block" or activation of inhibitory afferents, or by true activation of STN efferents to the pallidum. PET studies in pallidotomy and DBS patients performing a motor task have shown that frontal motor areas whose metabolic activity was reduced in the parkinsonian state became active again after the procedure.[81,86]

Altered Discharge Patterns

Several important findings in lesion patients are not compatible with the rate-based model presented in FIGURE 1. For instance, in contrast to the prediction of simple rate-based models, lesions of the "basal ganglia–receiving" areas of the thalamus (VA/VL) do not lead to parkinsonism and are, in fact, beneficial in the treatment of both tremor and rigidity (see, e.g., Ref. 87). Similarly, lesions of GPi in the setting of parkinsonism lead to improvement in all aspects of Parkinson's disease without any obvious detrimental effects. Furthermore, they are effective against both parkinsonism and drug-induced dyskinesias (see, e.g., Refs. 88, 89). Dyskinesias are thought to arise from pathologic *reduction* in basal ganglia outflow[1,90] and should, thus, not respond positively to further reduction of pallidal outflow (see, e.g., Ref. 91). These findings suggest that factors other than changes in the discharge rates may be important in the development of Parkinson's disease.

Alterations in discharge patterns and synchronization between neighboring neurons have been extensively documented in parkinsonian monkeys and patients. For instance, neuronal responses to passive limb manipulations in STN, GPi, and thalamus (e.g., Refs. 61–63, 92) have been shown to occur more often, to be more pronounced, and to have widened receptive fields after treatment with MPTP. There is also a marked change in the synchronization of discharge between neurons in the basal ganglia (see example in FIG. 3). Cross-correlation studies have revealed that a substantial proportion of neighboring neurons in globus pallidus and STN discharge in unison in MPTP-treated primates.[63] This is in contrast to the virtual absence of synchronized discharge of such neurons in normal monkeys (e.g., Ref. 93). Finally, the proportion of cells in STN, GPi, and SNr with discharge in oscillatory or nonoscillatory bursts is greatly increased in the parkinsonian state.[62,63,94,95]

It has been argued that some of these abnormal discharge patterns may develop as a reflection of abnormal, proprioceptive input. This is particularly obvious for tremor, in which proprioceptive input to the basal ganglia would be expected to be oscillatory. However, tremor could also be *caused* by synchronized oscillations in the basal ganglia arising from changes in local pacemaker networks, such as a feedback circuit involving GPe and STN,[96] perhaps through loss of extrastriatal dopamine (see, e.g., Refs. 97, 98). In addition, intrinsic membrane properties of basal ganglia neurons are conducive to the development of oscillatory discharge.[99,100] Increased inhibitory basal ganglia output may also contribute to the generation of oscillatory discharge in the thalamus,[1,101] which may then be transmitted to the cortex. Finally, and perhaps most likely, oscillations throughout the entire basal ganglia-thalamocortical network may be tightly related to each other, so that no one "oscillator" can be identified as their sole source (see, e.g., Ref. 102).

While tremor is perhaps the most obvious example of a parkinsonian sign that may develop as a consequence of abnormally patterned basal ganglia output, certain aspects of akinesia or bradykinesia may also be related to altered neuronal activity. Thus, increased phasic activity in the basal ganglia may erroneously signal excessive movement or velocity to precentral motor areas, leading to a slowing or premature arrest of ongoing movements and to greater reliance upon external clues during movement. Alternatively, phasic alteration of discharge in the basal ganglia may simply introduce noise into thalamic output to the cortex that is detrimental to cortical operations. The polarity and exact nature of the abnormal patterning and overall activity in the basal ganglia–thalamocortical pathways may determine the nature of the resulting movement disorder.

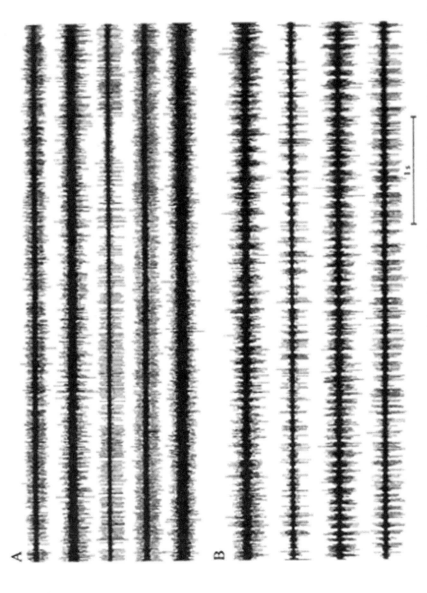

FIGURE 3. Examples of simultaneous recordings of the activity of neurons in the globus pallidus in a monkey before (**A**) and after treatment with MPTP (**B**). (Reprinted from Raz et al.[108] with permission.)

Consistent with the notion that changes in basal ganglia discharge may result in tremor, lesions of the STN or GPi significantly reduce tremor in MPTP-treated African green monkeys and in patients with parkinsonism.[23,80,101]

Besides the skeletomotor abnormalities, parkinsonism is also associated with oculomotor abnormalities, such as hypometric and slow saccades (e.g., Ref. 103), autonomic dysfunction, depression, anxiety, sleep disturbances, impaired visuospatial orientation, and cognitive abnormalities (e.g., Ref. 104). It is likely that at least some of these abnormalities rely on abnormal discharge in nonmotor circuits of the basal ganglia, which may be affected by dopamine loss in much the same way as the motor circuit. This is particularly true for oculomotor abnormalities that may directly result from dopamine depletion in the caudate nucleus (see, e.g., Refs. 105, 106). Similarly, some of the cognitive and psychiatric disturbances seen in parkinsonian patients are reminiscent of syndromes seen after lesions of the dorsolateral prefrontal cortex (problems with executive functions) or of the anterior cingulate (apathy, personality changes) and may be the result of loss of dopamine in the dorsolateral or ventral caudate nucleus, respectively.[107]

CONCLUSIONS

From the considerations above, a complex model of parkinsonism emerges in which relatively selective dopamine depletion in the striatum and other basal ganglia nuclei results in increased and disordered discharge and synchronization in motor areas of the basal ganglia thalamocortical motor loops. In fact, the motor circuit in Parkinson's disease may be "taken hostage" by widespread discharge abnormalities that greatly interfere with its normal functions. Abnormal activity in the basal ganglia feedback loops may contribute to the development of parkinsonism. Individual parkinsonian motor signs appear to be caused by distinct abnormalities in basal ganglia discharge. It is probable that progressive loss of dopamine in nonmotor areas of the striatum and other basal ganglia nuclei may underlie the nonmotor abnormalities of Parkinson's disease. The development of the different signs of movement disorders may be the consequence of changes in the rate, patterns, and degree of synchronization of discharge; of altered proprioceptive feedback; and of the appearance of "noise" in the basal ganglia output signal.

The current models of basal ganglia pathophysiology are incomplete and should be taken as a first draft of basal ganglia dysfunction in the different disease states. Most pertinently, changes in phasic discharge patterns and new anatomical connections need to be better incorporated into any new concept of basal ganglia function, and greater emphasis needs to be placed on the manner in which thalamic, brain stem, and cortical neurons utilize basal ganglia output.

REFERENCES

1. WICHMANN, T. & M.R. DELONG. 1996. Functional and pathophysiological models of the basal ganglia. Curr. Opin. Neurobiol. **6:** 751–758.
2. ALBIN, R.L., *et al.* 1989. The functional anatomy of basal ganglia disorders. Trends Neurosci. **12:** 366–375.
3. GRAYBIEL, A.M. 1996. Basal ganglia: new therapeutic approaches to Parkinson's disease. Curr. Biol. **6:** 368–371.

4. LANGSTON, J.W., *et al.* 1984. Selective nigral toxicity after systemic administration of 1-methyl-4-phenyl-1,2,3,6-tetrahydropyrine (MPTP) in the squirrel monkey. Brain Res. **292**: 390–394.

5. BANKIEWICZ, K.S., *et al.* 1986. Hemiparkinsonism in monkeys after unilateral internal carotid artery infusion of 1-methyl-4-phenyl-1,2,3,6-tetrahydropyridine (MPTP). Life Sciences **39**: 7–16.

6. FORNO, L.S. 1996. Neuropathology of Parkinson's disease. J. Neuropathol. Exp. Neurol. **55**: 259–272.

7. KISH, S.J., *et al.* 1988. Uneven pattern of dopamine loss in the striatum of patients with idiopathic Parkinson's disease. N. Engl. J. Med. **318**: 876–880.

8. KUNZLE, H. 1975. Bilateral projections from precentral motor cortex to the putamen and other parts of the basal ganglia. An autoradiographic study in macaca fascicularis. Brain Res. **88**: 195–209.

9. FLAHERTY, A.W. & A.M. GRAYBIEL. 1991. Corticostriatal transformations in the primate somatosensory sstem. Projections from physiologically mapped body-part representations. J. Neurophysiol. **66**: 1249–1263.

10. SELEMON, L.D. & P.S. GOLDMAN-RAKIC. 1985. Longitudinal topography and interdigitation of cortico-striatal projections in the rhesus monkey. J. Neurosci. **5**: 776–794.

11. YETERIAN, E.H. & D.N. PANDYA. 1998. Corticostriatal connections of the superior temporal region in rhesus monkeys. J. Comp. Neurol. **399**: 384–402.

12. HABER, S.N., *et al.* 1995. The orbital and medial prefrontal circuit through the primate basal ganglia. J. Neurosci. **15**: 4851–4867.

13. HARTMANN-VON MONAKOW, K. *et al.* 1978. Projections of the precentral motor cortex and other cortical areas of the frontal lobe to the subthalamic nucleus in the monkey. Exp. Brain Res. **33**: 395–403.

14. NAMBU, A., *et al.* 1996. Dual somatotopical representations in the primate subthalamic nucleus: evidence for ordered but reversed body-map transformations from the primary motor cortex and the supplementary motor area. J. Neurosci. **16**: 2671–2683.

15. WILSON, C.J., *et al.* 1983. Origins of post synaptic potentials evoked in spiny neostriatal projection neurons by thalamic stimulation in the rat. Exp. Brain Res. **51**: 217–226.

16. SADIKOT, A.F., *et al.* 1992. Efferent connections of the centromedian and parafascicular thalamic nuclei in the squirrel monkey: a light and electron microscopic study of the thalamostriatal projection in relation to striatal heterogeneity. J. Comp. Neurol. **320**: 228–242.

17. FEGER, J., *et al.* 1994. The projections from the parafascicular thalamic nucleus to the subthalamic nucleus and the striatum arise from separate neuronal populations: a comparison with the corticostriatal and corticosubthalamic efferents in a retrograde double-labelling study. Neuroscience **60**: 125–132.

18. SMITH, Y. & A. PARENT. 1986. Differential connections of caudate nucleus and putamen in the squirrel monkey (Saimiri sciureus). Neuroscience **18**: 347–371.

19. NAKANO, K., *et al.* 1990. Topographical projections from the thalamus, subthalamic nucleus and pedunculopontine tegmental nucleus to the striatum in the Japanese monkey, Macaca fuscata. Brain Res. **537**: 54–68.

20. SIDIBE, M., *et al.* 2002. Nigral and pallidal inputs to functionally segregated thalamostriatal neurons in the centromedian/parafascicular intralaminar nuclear complex in monkey. J. Comp. Neurol. **447**: 286–299.

21. ALEXANDER, G.E., *et al.* 1986. Parallel organization of functionally segregated circuits linking basal ganglia and cortex. Ann. Rev. Neurosci. **9**: 357–381.

22. ALEXANDER, G.E. & M.D. CRUTCHER. 1990. Functional architecture of basal ganglia circuits: neural substrates of parallel processing. Trends Neurosci. **13**: 266–271.

23. BERGMAN, H., *et al.* 1990. Amelioration of parkinsonian symptoms by inactivation of the subthalamic nucleus (STN) in MPTP treated green monkeys. Movement Disorders **5**: 79.

24. GERFEN, C.R. & C.J. WILSON. 1996. The basal ganglia. *In* Handbook of Chemical Neuroanatomy, Integrated Systems of the CNS, Part III. A. Björklund, T. Hökfeld & L. Swanson, Eds.: 369. Elsevier. Amsterdam.

25. PARENT, A., *et al.* 1995. Single striatofugal axons arborizing in both pallidal segments and in the substantia nigra in primates. Brain Res. **698**: 280–284.

26. SIDIBE, M. & Y. SMITH. 1996. Differential synaptic innervation of striatofugal neurones projecting to the internal or external segments of the globus pallidus by thalamic afferents in the squirrel monkey. J. Comp. Neurol. **365:** 445–465.
27. PARTHASARATHY, H.B. & A.M. GRAYBIEL. 1997. Cortically driven immediate-early gene expression reflects influence of sensorimotor cortex on identified striatal neurons in the squirrel. J. Neurosci. **17:** 2477–2491.
28. GERFEN, C.R., et al. 1990. D1 and D2 dopamine receptor-regulated gene expression of striatonigral and striatopallidal neurons. Science **250:** 1429–1432.
29. SURMEIER, D.J., et al. 1996. Coordinated expression of dopamine receptors in neostriatal medium spiny neurons. J. Neurosci. **16:** 6579–6591.
30. AIZMAN, O., et al. 2000. Anatomical and physiological evidence for D1 and D2 dopamine receptor colocalization in neostriatal neurons. Nat. Neurosci. **3:** 226–230.
31. GERFEN, C.R. 1995. Dopamine receptor function in the basal ganglia. Clin. Neuropharmacol. **18:** S162–S177.
32. PARENT, A. 1990. Extrinsic connections of the basal ganglia. Trends Neurosci. **13:** 254–258.
33. SIDIBE, M., et al. 1997. Efferent connections of the internal globus pallidus in the squirrel monkey: I. Topography and synaptic organization of the pallidothalamic projection. J. Comp. Neurol. **382:** 323–347.
34. SCHELL, G.R. & P.L. STRICK. 1984. The origin of thalamic inputs to the arcuate premotor and supplementary motor areas. J. Neurosci. **4:** 539–560.
35. INASE, M. & J. TANJI. 1995. Thalamic distribution of projection neurons to the primary motor cortex relative to afferent terminal fields from the globus pallidus in the macaque monkey. J. Comp. Neurol. **353:** 415–426.
36. NAMBU, A., et al. 1988. Projection on the motor cortex of thalamic neurons with pallidal input in the monkey. Exp. Brain Res. **71:** 658–662.
37. HOOVER, J.E. & P.L. STRICK. 1993. Multiple output channels in the basal ganglia. Science **259:** 819–821.
38. GOLDMAN-RAKIC, P.S. & L.J. PORRINO. 1985. The primate mediodorsal (MD) nucleus and its projection to the frontal lobe. J. Comp. Neurol. **242:** 535–560.
39. MIDDLETON, F.A. & P.L. STRICK. 1994. Anatomical evidence for cerebellar and basal ganglia involvement in higher cognitive function. Science **266:** 458–461.
40. HEDREEN, J.C. & M.R. DELONG. 1991. Organization of striatopallidal, striatonigral and nigrostriatal projections in the macaque. J. Comp. Neurol. **304:** 569–595.
41. MIDDLETON, F.A. & P.L. STRICK. 2002. Basal-ganglia "projections" to the prefrontal cortex of the primate. Cerebr. Cortex **12:** 926–935.
42. ILINSKY, I.A., et al. 1985. Organization of the nigrothalamocortical system in the rhesus monkey. J. Comp. Neurol. **236:** 315–330.
43. GROFOVA, I. & M. ZHOU. 1998. Nigral innervation of cholinergic and glutamatergic cells in the rat mesopontine tegmentum: light and electron microscopic anterograde tracing and immunohistochemical studies. J. Comp. Neurol. **395:** 359–379.
44. RYE, D.B., et al. 1988. Medullary and spinal efferents of the pedunculopontine tegmental nucleus and adjacent mesopontine tegmentum in the rat. J. Comp. Neurol. **269:** 315–341.
45. STEININGER, T.L., et al. 1992. Afferent projections to the cholinergic pedunculopontine tegmental nucleus and adjacent midbrain extrapyramidal area in the albino rat. I. Retrograde tracing studies. J. Comp. Neurol. **321:** 515–543.
46. WURTZ, R.H. & O. HIKOSAKA. 1986. Role of the basal ganglia in the initiation of saccadic eye movements. Prog. Brain Res. **64:** 175–190.
47. INASE, M., et al. 1996. Changes in the control of arm position, movement, and thalamic discharge during local inactivation in the globus pallidus of the monkey. J. Neurophysiol. **75:** 1087–1104.
48. GEORGOPOULOS, A.P., et al. 1983. Relations between parameters of step-tracking movements and single cell discharge in the globus pallidus and subthalamic nucleus of the behaving monkey. J. Neurosci. **3:** 1586–1598.
49. MITCHELL, S.J., et al. 1987. The primate globus pallidus: neuronal activity related to direction of movement. Exp. Brain Res. **68:** 491–505.

50. TURNER, R.S., *et al.* 1998. Motor subcircuits mediating the control of movement velocity: a PET study. J. Neurophysiol. **80:** 2162–2176.
51. ANDERSON, M.E. & R.S. TURNER. 1991. A quantitative analysis of pallidal discharge during targeted reaching movement in the monkey. Exp. Brain Res. **86:** 623–632.
52. DELONG, M.R. 1983. The neurophysiologic basis of abnormal movements in basal ganglia disorders. Neurobehav. Toxicol. Teratol. **5:** 611–616.
53. MINK, J.W. & W.T. THACH. 1991. Basal ganglia motor control. III. Pallidal ablation: normal reaction time, muscle cocontraction, and slow movement. J. Neurophysiol. **65:** 330–351.
54. WISE, S.P., *et al.* 1996. The frontal cortex-basal ganglia system in primates. Crit. Rev. Neurobiol. **10:** 317–356.
55. GRAYBIEL, A.M. 1995. Building action repertoires: memory and learning functions of the basal ganglia. Curr. Opin. Neurobiol. **5:** 733–741.
56. SCHULTZ, W. 1998. The phasic reward signal of primate dopamine neurons. Adv. Pharmacol. **42:** 686–690.
57. BURNS, R.S., *et al.* 1983. A primate model of parkinsonism: selective destruction of dopaminergic neurons in the pars compacta of the substantia nigra by N-methyl-4-phenyl-1,2,3,6-tetrahydropyridine. Proc. Natl. Acad. Sci. USA **80:** 4546–4550.
58. LANGSTON, J.W. 1987. MPTP: The promise of a new neurotoxin. *In* Movement Disorders 2. C.D. Marsden & S. Fahn, Eds.: 73–90. Butterworths. London.
59. CROSSMAN, A.R., *et al.* 1985. Regional brain uptake of 2-deoxyglucose in N-methyl-4-phenyl-1,2,3,6-tetrahydropyridine (MPTP)-induced parkinsonism in the macaque monkey. Neuropharmacology **24:** 587–591.
60. SCHWARTZMAN, R.J. & G.M. ALEXANDER. 1985. Changes in the local cerebral metabolic rate for glucose in the 1-methyl-4-phenyl-1,2,3,6-tetrahydropyridine (MPTP) primate model of Parkinson's disease. Brain Res. **358:** 137–143.
61. FILION, M., *et al.* 1988. Abnormal influences of passive limb movement on the activity of globus pallidus neurons in parkinsonian monkeys. Brain Res. **444:** 165–176.
62. MILLER, W.C. & M.R. DELONG. 1987. Altered tonic activity of neurons in the globus pallidus and subthalamic nucleus in the primate MPTP model of parkinsonism. *In* The Basal Ganglia II. M.B. Carpenter & A. Jayaraman, Eds.: 415–427. Plenum. New York.
63. BERGMAN, H., *et al.* 1994. The primate subthalamic nucleus. II. Neuronal activity in the MPTP model of parkinsonism. J. Neurophysiol. **72:** 507–520.
64. WICHMANN, T., *et al.* 1999. Comparison of MPTP-induced changes in spontaneous neuronal discharge in the internal pallidal segment and in the substantia nigra pars reticulata in primates. Exp. Brain Res. **125:** 397–409.
65. DOGALI, M., *et al.* 1994. Anatomic and physiological considerations in pallidotomy for Parkinson's disease. Stereotactic Funct. Neurosurg. **62:** 53–60.
66. LOZANO, A., *et al.* 1996. Methods for microelectrode-guided posteroventral pallidotomy. J. Neurosurg. **84:** 194–202.
67. VITEK, J.L., *et al.* 1993. Neuronal activity in the internal (GPi) and external (GPe) segments of the globus pallidus (GP) of parkinsonian patients is similar to that in the MPTP-treated primate model of parkinsonism. Soc. Neurosci. Abstr. **19:** 1584.
68. BROOKS, D.J. 1991. Detection of preclinical Parkinson's disease with PET. Neurology **41:** 24–27.
69. EIDELBERG, D. & C. EDWARDS. 2000. Functional brain imaging of movement disorders. Neurol. Res. **22:** 305–312.
70. WATTS, R.L. & A.S. MANDIR. 1992. The role of motor cortex in the pathophysiology of voluntary movement deficits associated with parkinsonism. Neurol. Clin. **10:** 451–469.
71. SMITH, Y., *et al.* 1996. Synaptic innervation of midbrain dopaminergic neurons by glutamate-enriched terminals in the squirrel monkey. J. Comp. Neurol. **364:** 231–253.
72. KITAI, S.T. 1998. Afferent control of substantia nigra compacta dopamine neurons: anatomical perspective and role of glutamatergic and cholinergic inputs. Adv. Pharmacol. **42:** 700–702.

73. KOJIMA, J., *et al.* 1997. Excitotoxic lesions of the pedunculopontine tegmental nucleus produce contralateral hemiparkinsonism in the monkey. Neurosci. Lett. **226:** 111–114.
74. MUNRO-DAVIES, L.E., *et al.* 1999. The role of the pedunculopontine region in basal-ganglia mechanisms of akinesia. Exp. Brain Res. **129:** 511-517.
75. BERGMAN, H., *et al.* 1990. Reversal of experimental parkinsonism by lesions of the subthalamic nucleus. Science **249:** 1436–1438.
76. AZIZ, T.Z., *et al.* 1991. Lesion of the subthalamic nucleus for the alleviation of 1-methyl-4-phenyl-1,2,3,6-tetrahydropyridine (MPTP)-induced parkinsonism in the primate. Mov. Disord. **6:** 288–292.
77. WICHMANN, T., *et al.* 1994. Local inactivation of the sensorimotor territories of the internal segment of the globus pallidus and the subthalamic nucleus alleviates parkinsonian motor signs in MPTP treated monkeys. *In* The Basal Ganglia IV: New Ideas and Data on Structure and Function. G. Percheron, J.S. McKenzie & J. Feger, Eds.: 357–363. Plenum. New York.
78. WICHMANN, T., *et al.* 2001. Antiparkinsonian and behavioral effects of inactivation of the substantia nigra pars reticulata in hemiparkinsonian primates. Exp. Neurol. **167:** 410–424.
79. LONSER, R.R., *et al.* 1999. Convection-enhanced selective excitotoxic ablation of the neurons of the globus pallidus internus for treatment of parkinsonism in nonhuman primates [see comments]. J. Neurosurg. **91:** 294–302.
80. BARON, M.S., *et al.* 1996. Treatment of advanced Parkinson's disease by GPi pallidotomy: 1 year pilot-study results. Ann. Neurol. **40:** 355–366.
81. DOGALI, M., *et al.* 1995. Stereotactic ventral pallidotomy for Parkinson's disease. Neurology **45:** 753–761.
82. LAITINEN, L.V., *et al.* 1992. Leksell's posteroventral pallidotomy in the treatment of Parkinson's disease. J. Neurosurg. **76:** 53–61.
83. LOZANO, A.M., *et al.* 1995. Effect of GPi pallidotomy on motor function in Parkinson's disease. Lancet **346:** 1383–1387.
84. VITEK, J.L., *et al.* 1997. Microelectrode-guided pallidotomy for medically intractable Parkinson's disease. Adv. Neurol. **74:** 183–198.
85. GILL, S.S. & P. HEYWOOD. 1998. Bilateral subthalamic nucleotomy can be accomplished safely. Mov. Disord. **13:** 201.
86. CEBALLOS-BAUMAN, A.O. *et al.* 1994. Restoration of thalamocortical activity after posterolateral pallidotomy in Parkinson's disease. Lancet **344:** 814.
87. TASKER, R.R., *et al.* 1997. Pallidal and thalamic surgery for Parkinson's disease. Exp. Neurol. **144:** 35–40.
88. RABEY, J.M., *et al.* 1995. Levodopa-induced dyskinesias are the main feature improved by contralateral pallidotomy in Parkinson's disease. Neurology **45:** A377.
89. OBESO, J.A., *et al.* 2000. Pathophysiology of levodopa-induced dyskinesias in Parkinson's disease: problems with the current model. Ann. Neurol. **47:** S22–32; discussion S32–34.
90. PAPA, S.M., *et al.* 1999. Internal globus pallidus discharge is nearly suppressed during levodopa-induced dyskinesias. Ann. Neurol. **46:** 732–738.
91. MARSDEN, C.D. & J.A. OBESO. 1994. The functions of the basal ganglia and the paradox of stereotaxic surgery in Parkinson's disease. Brain **117:** 877–897.
92. VITEK, J.L., *et al.* 1990. Altered somatosensory response properties of neurons in the "motor" thalamus of MPTP treated parkinsonian monkeys. Soc. Neurosci. Abstr. **16:** 425.
93. WICHMANN, T., *et al.* 1994. The primate subthalamic nucleus. I. Functional properties in intact animals. J. Neurophysiol. **72:** 494–506.
94. WICHMANN, T., *et al.* 1996. Comparison of the effects of experimental parkinsonism on neuronal discharge in motor and non-motor portions of the basal ganglia output nuclei in primates. Soc. Neurosci. Abstr. **22:** 415.
95. FILION, M. & L. TREMBLAY. 1991. Abnormal spontaneous activity of globus pallidus neurons in monkeys with MPTP-induced parkinsonism. Brain Res. **547:** 142–151.
96. PLENZ, D. & S. KITAI. 1999. A basal ganglia pacemaker formed by the subthalamic nucleus and external globus pallidus. Nature **400:** 677–682.

97. BERGMAN, H., *et al.* 1998. Physiology of MPTP tremor. Mov. Disord. **13:** 29–34.
98. BERNHEIMER, H., *et al.* 1973. Brain dopamine and the syndromes of Parkinson and Huntington. J. Neurol. Sci. **20:** 415–455.
99. NAMBU, A. & R. LLINAS. 1990. Electrophysiology of the globus pallidus neurons: an in vitro study in guinea pig brain slices. Soc. Neurosci. Abstr. **16:** 428.
100. BEURRIER, C., *et al.* 1999. Subthalamic nucleus neurons switch from single-spike activity to burst-firing mode. J. Neurosci. **19:** 599–609.
101. WICHMANN, T., *et al.* 1994. The primate subthalamic nucleus. III. Changes in motor behavior and neuronal activity in the internal pallidum induced by subthalamic inactivation in the MPTP model of parkinsonism. J. Neurophysiol. **72:** 521–530.
102. MAGILL, P.J., *et al.* 2000. Relationship of activity in the subthalamic nucleus-globus pallidus network to cortical electroencephalogram. J. Neurosci. **20:** 820–833.
103. VIDAILHET, M., *et al.* 1999. Saccades and antisaccades in parkinsonian syndromes. Adv. Neurol. **80:** 377–382.
104. CUMMINGS, J.L. & D.L. MASTERMAN. 1999. Depression in patients with Parkinson's disease. Int. J. Geriatr. Psychiatry **14:** 711–718.
105. KORI, A., *et al.* 1995. Eye movements in monkeys with local dopamine depletion in the caudate nucleus. II. Deficits in voluntary saccades. J. Neurosci. **15:** 928–941.
106. KATO, M., *et al.* 1995. Eye movements in monkeys with local dopamine depletion in the caudate nucleus. I. Deficits in spontaneous saccades. J. Neurosci. **15:** 912–927.
107. CUMMINGS, J.L. 1993. Frontal-subcortical circuits and human behavior. Arch. Neurol. **50:** 873–880.
108. RAZ, A., *et al.* 2000. Firing patterns and correlations of spontaneous discharge of pallidal neurons in the normal and the tremulous 1-methyl-4-phenyl-1,2,3,6-tetrahydropyridine vervet model of parkinsonism. J. Neurosci. **20:** 8559–8571.

The Role of Glial Reaction and Inflammation in Parkinson's Disease

E. C. HIRSCH, T. BREIDERT, E. ROUSSELET, S. HUNOT,
A. HARTMANN, AND P. P. MICHEL

*INSERM U289, Experimental Neurology and Therapeutics, Hôpital de la Salpêtrière,
75651 Paris Cedex 13, France*

ABSTRACT: The glial reaction is generally considered to be a consequence of
neuronal death in neurodegenerative diseases such as Alzheimer's disease,
Huntington's disease, and Parkinson's disease. In Parkinson's disease, postmortem examination reveals a loss of dopaminergic neurons in the substantia
nigra associated with a massive astrogliosis and the presence of activated
microglial cells. Recent evidence suggests that the disease may progress even
when the initial cause of neuronal degeneration has disappeared, suggesting
that toxic substances released by the glial cells may be involved in the propaga-
tion and perpetuation of neuronal degeneration. Glial cells can release deleterious compounds such as proinflammatory cytokines (TNF-α, Il-1β, IFN-γ),
which may act by stimulating nitric oxide production in glial cells, or which
may exert a more direct deleterious effect on dopaminergic neurons by activating receptors that contain intracytoplasmic death domains involved in apoptosis. In line with this possibility, an activation of proteases such as caspase-3 and
caspase-8, which are known effectors of apoptosis, has been reported in Parkinson's disease. Yet, caspase inhibitors or invalidation of TNF-α receptors
does not protect dopaminergic neurons against degeneration in experimental
models of the disease, suggesting that manipulation of a single signaling pathway may not be sufficient to protect dopaminergic neurons. In contrast, the
antiinflammatory drugs pioglitazone, a PPAR-γ agonist, and the tetracycline
derivative minocycline have been shown to reduce glial activation and protect
the substantia nigra in an animal model of the disease. Inhibition of the glial
reaction and the inflammatory processes may thus represent a therapeutic target to reduce neuronal degeneration in Parkinson's disease.

KEYWORDS: cytokines; neuroprotection; apoptosis; dopamine neuron; substantia nigra

SUBPOPULATIONS OF DOPAMINERGIC NEURONS ARE SELECTIVELY AFFECTED IN PARKINSON'S DISEASE

Parkinson's disease is characterized by a slow and progressive degeneration of
dopaminergic neurons in the mesencephalon. Yet, evidence suggests that the loss of
these neurons is heterogeneous across different catecholaminergic cell groups. In-

Address for correspondence: E.C. Hirsch, INSERM U289, Experimental Neurology and Therapeutics, Hôpital de la Salpêtrière, 47 boulevard de l'Hôpital, 75651 Paris Cedex 13, France.
Voice: +33 (0) 1 42 16 22 02; fax: + 33 (0) 1 44 24 36 58.
hirsch@ccr.jussieu.fr

Ann. N.Y. Acad. Sci. 991: 214–228 (2003). © 2003 New York Academy of Sciences.

deed, neuronal loss is extremely severe in the substantia nigra pars compacta, moderate in the ventral tegmental area and catecholaminergic cell group A8, and almost nil in the central gray substance.[1] Furthermore, within the substantia nigra itself, the most severe loss occurs in the ventrolateral part of the substantia nigra pars compacta.[2,3] More recently, when compartmental patterns of calbindin D28K immunostaining were used to subdivide the substantia nigra with landmarks independent of the degenerative process, zones of very high vulnerability were identified.[4] Dopamine-containing neurons were identified in the calbindin-rich regions (matrix) and in five calbindin-poor pockets (nigrosomes) defined by analysis of the three-dimensional networks formed by the calbindin-poor zones. Within these zones, cell loss followed a strict order, depletion being maximal in the main pocket located in the caudal and mediolateral part of the substantia nigra pars compacta. Furthermore, the degree of loss of dopamine-containing neurons in the substantia nigra pars compacta was related to the duration of the disease, with a pattern of neuronal loss consistent from one parkinsonian substantia nigra to another. The reason for such a differential vulnerability of dopaminergic neurons within the parkinsonian substantia nigra is not known. Yet, the different nigral compartments may differ in terms of their content of growth factor, receptors, compounds related to excitotoxicity, agents involved in oxidative metabolism, and activity of potentially predisposing genes such as those for α-synuclein[5] and parkin.[6]

In addition to their heterogeneity in terms of susceptibility to the as yet unknown agent causing their death, dopaminergic neurons in the parkinsonian substantia nigra may also differ with regard to their individual status. Indeed, at least three types of dopaminergic neurons can be described in the parkinsonian substantia nigra. The first type of dopaminergic neurons, probably located mostly in the matrix, is still unaffected by the pathological process and corresponds to "healthy" surviving neurons. In contrast, the second type of dopaminergic neurons is already engaged in a degenerative process and displays "typical features" of apoptosis or autophagic degeneration.[7] Whether such severely affected neurons can be protected from neurodegeneration using a therapeutic strategy is not known, but *in vitro* experiments using caspase inhibitors suggest this goal will be difficult to attain.[8]

Finally, the last type of dopaminergic neurons in the parkinsonian substantia nigra consists in "suffering" neurons. These neurons may not function adequately and in that respect differ from the still healthy neurons. Yet, unlike apoptotic neurons, they may not be engaged in the irreversible final stage of degeneration. Some of these dopaminergic neurons in the substantia nigra may contain Lewy bodies, which are the histopathological hallmarks of the disease (for review, see Forno[9]). The concept of suffering neurons in the parkinsonian substantia nigra is further supported by the identification of another cell type in the substantia nigra of parkinsonian patients but not in that of normal individuals. These cells contain neuromelanin (the end product in the catabolism of catecholamines by autoxidation) in the absence of tyrosine hydroxylase immunoreactivity.[1] These pigmented tyrosine hydroxylase-negative neurons may represent "wounded" neurons that once contained tyrosine hydroxylase. Within the parkinsonian substantia nigra, these neurons can represent as much as 20% of the surviving melanized neurons, indicating that there are many suffering neurons in the brain of the patients that have ceased to function long before their actual death. If so, it suggests that we should be less concerned about those neurons that are dead, and instead focus our attention more on those in the early stages of degeneration. These neurons may, on the one hand, be a suitable target for neurorestorative and neuroprotective strategies and, on the other hand, be particularly sensitive to a final common pathway of neuronal degeneration. We therefore need to consider the mechanisms involved in the degeneration of these wounded neurons.

IS THE GLIAL REACTION INVOLVED IN THE PROGRESSION OF NEURONAL DEGENERATION IN PARKINSON'S DISEASE?

The mechanism by which dopaminergic neurons degenerate in Parkinson's disease is not yet known. Yet, several lines of evidence suggest that oxidative stress, excitotoxic mechanisms, and altered protein catabolism participate in the cascade of events leading to neuronal degeneration in this disease.[10–12] These cellular and molecular alterations ultimately lead to apoptosis.[7,13,14] In addition, degeneration of dopaminergic neurons is associated with a strong glial reaction, which is generally considered to be a nonspecific consequence of neuronal degeneration. In the following paragraphs, we will review the data suggesting that a subset of reactive glial cells may participate actively in dopaminergic cell demise during Parkinson's disease by virtue of their inflammatory properties.

The astroglial reaction in the substantia nigra of patients with Parkinson's disease is a well-known neuropathological characteristic of the disease. Furthermore, in their seminal study, McGeer and coworkers reported a large number of reactive human leucocyte antigen-DR (HLA-DR)–positive microglial cells in the substantia nigra of patients with Parkinson's disease.[15] Such a glial reaction has also been described in the affected brain regions in other neurological disorders such as Alzheimer's disease and brain infarct (for review, see McGeer and McGeer[16]) as well as in animal models of Parkinson's disease.[17,18] These data suggest that glial activation is not specific to Parkinson's disease and that it likely represents a common phenomenon in neurodegenerative disorders. However, recent evidence supports the notion that a subpopulation of activated glial cells may be deleterious in Parkinson's disease and particularly so for suffering or wounded neurons. Strong support for this hypothesis came from the study of young drug addicts who developed a parkinsonian syndrome after 1-methyl-4-phenyl-1,2,3,6-tetrahydropyridine (MPTP) intoxication.[19] In a recent study, these authors reported a postmortem neuropathological study of three subjects with MPTP-induced parkinsonism.[20] Interestingly, gliosis and clustering of microglial cells around nerve cells were detected despite survival times ranging from 3 to 16 years. These findings not only indicate ongoing nerve cell loss after a time-limited insult, but suggest that activated microglial cells may perpetuate neuronal degeneration. One may thus speculate that after a primary insult of environmental or genetic origin, the glial reaction may enhance the degeneration of dopaminergic neurons. However, this question cannot be resolved by postmortem studies alone. Much insight into the potential involvement of inflammation-mediated nerve cell death in Parkinson's disease has in fact come from experimental models of the disease. Indeed, lipopolysaccharides (LPS), which activate glial cells and induce the expression of proinflammatory cytokines, have been shown to kill dopaminergic neurons in mixed neuron-glial cell cultures but not in pure neuronal cultures.[21] This indicates that the production of a glial factor induced by LPS (very likely cytokines) is able to kill dopaminergic neurons at least *in vitro*. These results were recently confirmed by McNaught and Jenner in experiments in which they showed that LPS-activated astrocytes could cause neuronal death in a time-dependent manner in primary ventral mesencephalic neuronal cultures.[22] Furthermore, these authors extended this finding by showing that the toxicity of agents capable of inducing the death of dopaminergic neurons, such as MPP^+ or 6-hydroxydopamine, was enhanced when the dopaminergic neurons were cultured with LPS-activated astrocytes. *In vivo* models of Parkinson's disease also support the notion that activated glial cells may participate in the degeneration of dopaminergic neurons. Indeed, Herrera and coworkers reported that a single intranigral injection of LPS induces damage to dopaminergic neurons in the substantia nigra with preservation of GABAergic or serotoninergic neurons.[23,24] More recently, the same authors showed that dexamethasone, a potent antiinflammatory drug that interferes with many of the features characterizing proinflammatory glial reaction, prevented the loss of catecholaminergic content, tyrosine hydroxylase activity, and tyrosine-hydroxylase immunostaining induced by LPS injection and also the bulk activation of microglia-macrophages.[25]

Taken together, these data clearly show that activated glial cells can participate in the death of dopaminergic neurons. The mechanism by which microglial cells can amplify injury to the nigral dopaminergic neurons is not yet known. However, the factors involved in this deleterious effect are very likely cytokines, including tumor necrosis factor-α (TNF-α), interleukin-1β (IL-1β), and interferon-γ (IFN-γ).

PROINFLAMMATORY CYTOKINES IN PARKINSON'S DISEASE

Several studies have reported a marked increase of cytokine levels in the brain and cerebrospinal fluid (CSF) of parkinsonian patients.[26] In addition, a higher density of glial cells expressing TNF-α, IL-1β, and IFN-γ was observed in the substantia nigra of patients with Parkinson's disease as compared to age-matched control subjects.[27,28] Some of these cells were sometimes in close proximity to blood vessels and degenerating dopaminergic neurons, suggesting their involvement in the pathophysiology of Parkinson's disease. Two mechanisms that are not mutually exclusive may explain the deleterious role of cytokines in the parkinsonian substantia nigra.

First, proinflammatory cytokines can induce the production of nitric oxide in glial cells.[28] This mechanism involves the induction of a low-affinity receptor for immunoglobulin E (CD23) and its activation by an as yet unknown ligand. Nitric oxide may diffuse towards dopaminergic neurons, where it may play a deleterious role by inducing lipid peroxidation and DNA strand breaks and inhibiting mitochondrial respiration and energy metabolism.[29] In support of this hypothesis, an increased density of glial cells expressing the inducible isoform of nitric oxide synthase and CD23 has been reported in the substantia nigra of patients with Parkinson's disease as compared to age-matched control subjects.[28,30] A role of nitric oxide in cell demise in Parkinson's disease is further supported by the increased nitrite levels observed in the CSF of patients with Parkinson's disease[31] and detectable immunoreactivity for nitrotyrosine in Lewy bodies.[32]

The second mechanism by which proinflammatory cytokines may play a deleterious role in Parkinson's disease may be more direct. Indeed, dopaminergic neurons in the substantia nigra express specific receptors for these molecules. For instance, type 1 TNF-α receptors are expressed on dopaminergic neurons of the human sub-stantia nigra.[27] Two types of TNF-α receptors, type 1 (TNFR1) and type 2 (TNFR2), which are encoded by different genes and are coupled to two distinct transduction pathways, may mediate distinct effects of TNF-α. TNFR1 has the potential to induce apoptotic cytotoxicity,[33] fibroblast proliferation, antiviral activity, NFκB activation, and cell adhesion molecule activation.[34,35] TNFR2 seems to be involved in cellular proliferation processes[36,37] and also to potentiate the effect of TNFR1.[38,39] The transduction pathways coupled to TNFR1 are of great interest in terms of degenera-tion of dopaminergic neurons. Indeed, TNF-α induces trimerization of TNFR1 on binding that leads, through the adaptor molecules TNFR1-associated protein with a death domain (TRADD) and FAS-associated protein with a death domain (FADD), to the autoproteolytical activation of caspase-8.[40] Caspase-8 may in turn either cleave effector caspases, such as caspase-3, directly or amplify the death signal through the translocation of BID, a proapoptotic member of the Bcl-family, to the mitochondria and the subsequent release of cytochrome c from the mitochondrial in-termembrane space into the cytosol.[41] Cytochrome c release also eventually triggers caspase-3 activation, which plays an important role in cell degeneration. Finally, caspase-8 can also be activated downstream of mitochondrial cytochrome c release, possibly to amplify the BID-induced cytochrome c release.[42,43] Such a TNF-α re-ceptor transduction pathway is of particular relevance for Parkinson's disease, as it is very likely to be activated in the neurons most vulnerable to the disease process. Indeed, in a human postmortem study, we showed a significant decrease in the per-centage of FADD-immunoreactive dopaminergic neurons in the substantia nigra pars compacta of patients with Parkinson's disease compared to control subjects.[40] Furthermore, this decrease correlated with the known selective vulnerability of ni-gral dopaminergic neurons in Parkinson's disease, suggesting that this pathway con-tributes to the susceptibility of dopaminergic neurons to TNF-mediated apoptosis in Parkinson's disease. Similar results were obtained for caspase-3. Indeed, we ob-served a positive correlation between the degree of neuronal loss in dopaminergic cell groups affected in the mesencephalon of parkinsonian patients and the percent-age of caspase-3–positive neurons in these cell groups in control subjects. Further-more, we also found a significant decrease of caspase-3-positive pigmented neurons in the substantia nigra pars compacta of parkinsonian patients compared to control subjects.[44] Taken together, these findings suggest that the melanized dopaminergic neurons expressing the TNFR1 transduction pathway are particularly prone to de-generation in Parkinson's disease if this pathway is activated during the course of the disease. A crucial finding in support of the activation of this pathway came from a postmortem study of caspase activation in Parkinson's disease. Using an antibody raised against activated caspase-3, the percentage of active caspase-3–positive neu-rons among dopaminergic neurons was shown to be significantly higher in parkin-sonian patients than in control subjects.[44] Similarly, the proportion of melanized neurons displaying caspase-8 activation in Parkinson's disease was also higher than in control subjects.[8] Interestingly, the proportion of activated caspase-3–positive neurons among neurons containing Lewy bodies was higher than in neurons that did not contain Lewy bodies.[44] In contrast, immunoreactivity for activated caspase-3 was not observed in neurons displaying the typical features of apoptosis. These data suggest that caspase-3 activation occurs in suffering neurons just before degenera-tion by apoptosis. This concept is further supported by experimental models of Parkinson's disease, in which the exact time course of caspase activation and apoptosis could be studied. Thus, in mice intoxicated by MPTP, caspase-3 activation was shown to slightly precede the death of dopaminergic neurons by apoptosis.[45] Taken together, these data suggest that the activation of the TNF-α transduction pathway is very likely involved in the pathophysiology of Parkinson's disease and especially in the induction of apoptosis, which has already been described in this disease (for a review, see Hartmann and Hirsch[46]).

The data reviewed in the preceding paragraph suggest that proinflammatory cytokines may participate in the pathophysiology of Parkinson's disease either by producing nitric oxide, which may subsequently have a deleterious effect on dopaminergic neurons, or by activating specific transduction pathways coupled to receptors for cytokines. Nevertheless, it is very likely that these pathophysiological events are not specific to Parkinson's disease, as similar changes have been described in other neurodegenerative diseases. However, this lack of specificity does not preclude the development of neuroprotective strategies based on inhibition of the inflammatory processes in Parkinson's disease.

ARE INFLAMMATORY PROCESSES A POTENTIAL THERAPEUTIC TARGET IN PARKINSON'S DISEASE?

The use of antiinflammatory drugs to prevent dopaminergic degeneration in Parkinson's disease has not yet been formally tested in patients. The concept that antiinflammatory agents may be beneficial in Parkinson's disease thus relies on preclinical studies of *in vitro* or *in vivo* models of the disease. *In vivo*, various compounds such as nonsteroidal antiinflammatory drugs (NSAIDs) with their targets COX, NFκB, and others, including steroids, immunophilins, thalidomide, and phosphodiesterase IV inhibitors, have been studied with variable results (TABLE 1). Furthermore, gene manipulation in mice has shown that COX2 and iNOS are of particular interest in such strategies (TABLE 2). However, from our own data, it appears that manipulation of a single specific pathway or a downstream pathway involved in the inflammatory processes does not protect dopaminergic neurons against degeneration in models of Parkinson's disease. In contrast, agents with a broader spectrum of action on the inflammatory processes are more likely to protect dopaminergic neurons against degeneration. To analyze the putative role of TNF-α receptor transduction pathways in parkinsonism, we compared the effect of the parkinsonian drug MPTP in mice lacking TNFR1, TNFR2, or both receptors and in wild-type littermates.[47] Postmortem analysis revealed no difference in the number of nigral dopaminergic neurons, whatever the group intoxicated by MPTP. These data suggest that a simple manipulation of the transduction pathway coupled to TNF-α receptors in Parkinson's disease is unlikely to prevent the progressive degeneration of dopaminergic neurons in the disease. Such negative results may be explained by the fact that the other proinflammatory cytokines produced in the parkinsonian substantia nigra and in experimental models of the disease may also participate in the death of dopaminergic neurons. Moreover, experiments in primary dopamine cultures of rat embryo showed that broad-spectrum and specific caspase-8 inhibitors did not result in neuroprotection against MPP+ (the active metabolite of MPTP) intoxication.[8] Not only did the caspase inhibitors not protect dopamine cultures against MPP+ toxicity,

TABLE 1. *In vivo* studies of pharmacological targets involved in the inflammatory response in experimental models of Parkinson's disease

Substance	Action	Dose	Model	Regimen	Parameter	Protection	Ref
salicylate	COX1/2, NFκB, radicals ↓	100 mg/kg ip −1h or +1h	MPTP mouse [1]	1× 15 mg/kg sc † 2ds	ST: DA, metabolites	complete	58
		50 mg/kg ip −0.5h 2×	MPTP mouse (BALB/c)	2×30 mg/kg ip 16h interval † 7ds	ST: DA, metabolites, GSH SN: GSH behavioral study	ST: complete [2] SN: incomplete motor deficit ↓	59
aspirin	COX1/2, NFκB, radicals ↓	100 mg/kg ip −1h or +1h	MPTP mouse	1× 15 mg/kg sc † 2ds	ST: DA, metabolites	complete	58
		100 mg/kg ip −0h	MPTP mouse	1× 30 mg/kg sc † 7ds	ST: DA, metabolites SN: TH, Nissl behavioral study	ST: incomplete [3] SN: complete motor deficit ↓	60
meloxicam	COX2	50 mg/kg ip −0h	MPTP mouse	1× 30 mg/kg ip † 7ds	ST: DA, metabolites SN: TH, Nissl	ST: incomplete [4] SN: near complete	60
paracetamol	COX1/2	100 mg/kg ip −1h	MPTP mouse	1× 15 mg/kg sc † 2ds	ST: DA, metabolites	none	58
diclofenac	COX1/2	100 mg/kg ip −1h	MPTP mouse	1× 15 mg/kg sc † 2ds	ST: DA, metabolites	none	58
ibuprofen	COX1/2, PPAR_/γ	20 mg/kg ip −1h	MPTP mouse	1× 15 mg/kg sc † 2ds	ST: DA, metabolites	none	58
indomethacin	COX1/2, PPAR_/γ	100 mg/kg ip −1h	MPTP mouse	1x 15 mg/kg sc † 2ds	ST: DA, metabolites	none	58
		1 mg/kg [5] ip −24h and 1×/2ds until †	MPTP mouse (age 8-10 ms)	4×10 mg/kg ip at 1h interval † 3/7ds	ST: DA SN: TH, microglial and lymphocytic marker	ST: incomplete at † 7ds [6] SN: incomplete [7], microglia ↓, lymphocytes ↓	61

TABLE 1. *In vivo* studies of pharmacological targets involved in the inflammatory response in experimental models of Parkinson's disease (*Continued*)

Substance	Action	Dose	Model	Regimen	Parameter	Protection	Ref
pioglitazone	PPARγ	20 mg/kg/d po −3d until †	MPTP mouse	4× 15 mg/kg ip at 2h interval † 2/ 5/ 8ds	ST: TH, DA, metabolites, glial marker; SN: TH, glial marker	ST: TH none, DA incomplete[8] SN: complete; glia ↓	52
dexamethasone	SteroidR	30 mg/kg sc −1h	MPTP mouse	1× 15 mg/kg sc † 2ds	ST: DA, metabolites	none	58
		1 mg/kg ip −1h and 1×/d until †	MPTP mouse (age 12 ms)	4×10 mg/kg ip at 1h interval † 3/ 7/ 14ds	SN: TH, microglial and lymphocytic marker	incomplete[9], activated microglia ↓, lymphocytes ↓	62
hydrocortisone	SteroidR	10 mg/kg ip −0.5/ +3h	6-OHDA mouse (ICR)	80 µg icv † 7ds	ST: DA, metabolites	no effect on DA, levels of metabolites partially altered	63
cyclosporin A	N-Immunophilin	20 mg/kg sc −1h/ +3h	6-OHDA mouse (ICR)	80 µg icv † 7ds	ST: DA, metabolites	incomplete[10]	63
		20 mg/kg sc −1d/ −0.5h/ 5h/ 1×/d for 6ds	6-OHDA rat	20 µg iST † 1 and 4ws	ST: DA, metabolites; SN: DA, metabolites, TH, microglial marker	ST: incomplete[11] SN: incomplete,[12] glia unchanged	63
FK-506	N-Immunophilin	10 mg/kg ip −1h/ 1×/d for 5ds	MPTP mouse	25 mg/kg ip 1x/d for 5d † 10ds	ST: DA	incomplete[13]	64
GPI 1046	N-Immunophilin	10 mg/kg po −2ws until +6ws1x/d	MPTP monkey	3 mg intracarotidal unilateral inj. † 6ws	ST and SN: TH behavioral study	none	65
thalidomide	NFκB ↓ via IKK? TNFα ↓	50 mg/kg po −0.5h/ +2.5h each inj.	MPTP mouse	3× 15 mg/kg ip at 2.5h interval † 1d	ST: DA, metabolites	complete[14]	66

TABLE 1. *In vivo* studies of pharmacological targets involved in the inflammatory response in experimental models of Parkinson's disease (*Continued*)

Substance	Action	Dose	Model	Regimen	Parameter	Protection	Ref
NQ-A, XT-A Etc.	microglia ↓ via PD IV	1 mg/kg sc –1h each/ +1h last inj.	MPTP mouse	2–3× 10-20 mg/kg sc † 7ds	ST: DA SN: TH, Nissl	ST + VTA: complete[5] SN: incomplete other PD inhibitors: none	67
minocycline	microglia ↓ via?	120 mg/kg po –3ds until +6ds	MPTP mouse	4× 20 mg/kg ip at 2h interval † 7ds	ST: DA, metabolites SN: TH, iNOS, caspase1	ST: incomplete[16] SN: incomplete[17] iNOS, caspase1 ↓	55
		2×45 mg/kg ip +0.5h/ 1×/d until +4ds	MPTP mouse	4×16 and 18 mg/kg ip at 2h interval † 7ds	SN: TH, microglial marker, iNOS, Il1beta	ST: incomplete[18] SN: incomplete[19]	56
		45 mg/kg ip 1×/d –1d until +14d	6-OHDA mouse (*ICR*)	20 µg iST † 14ds	SN: TH, microglial marker	SN: inomplete[20] microglia ↓	57

[1]Mouse refers to C57/Bl6, 2-4 months, if not stated otherwise. [2]DA complete, GSH in ST+SN: 50% → 75%. [3]DA loss: 50% → 75%. [4]DA loss: 85% → 59%. [5]Neurotoxic effect at higher dose (2.5 mg/kg). [6]DA loss: 52% → 30% at † 7ds. [7]TH neuron loss: 59% → 40% at † 7ds. [8]DA loss: 89% → 79% at † 8ds34% → 0% (VTA). [9]TH neuron loss: 60% → 43%. [10]DA loss: 69% → 59%. [11]DA loss: 76% → 53% at † 4ws. [12]TH neuron loss: 37% → 13%none (18 mg/ kg MPTP). [13]DA loss: 59% → 35%. [14]DA loss: 67% → 26%57% → 39% (18 mg/kg MPTP). [15]TH neuron loss:75% → 38% (SN). [16]DA loss: 80% → 16%. [17]TH neuron loss: 63% → 23%. [18]DA loss: 78% → 49% (16 mg/kg MPTP). [19]TH neuron loss:29% → 9% (16 mg/kg MPTP). [20]TH neuron loss: 41% → 32%.

NOTE TO TABLE 1: Substance: substance tested for protective action in models of Parkinson's dieseas. Action: possible pharmacological targets. Dose: dose of tested substance (the maximal dose used in the study is given) and time of application with reference to the administration of the neurotoxin (– = before; + = after). Parameter: marker used to test for nigrostriatal system and glial activiation. Protection: >95% protection is regarded as "complete."

ABBREVIATIONS IN TABLE 1: †, time until sacrifice; COX, cyclooxygenase; PPAR, peroxisome proliferator–activated receptor; d, day; GSH, glutathione; icv, intraventricular; IKK, I-kappaB kinase; ip, intraperitoneal; iST, intrastriatal; iv, intravenous; MPTP, 1-methyl-4-phenyl-1,2,3,6-tetrahydropyridine; NFκB, nuclear factor-kappaB; 6-OHDA, 6-hydroxydopamine; PD, phosphodiesterase; po, oral; sc, subcutaneous; SN, substantia nigra; ST, striatum; TNF, tumor necrosis factor; TH, tyrosine hydroxylase; VTA, ventral tegmental area; w, week.

TABLE 2. In vivo studies of gene targets involved in the inflammatory response in experimental models of Parkinson's disease

Target	Genotype	Model	Regimen	Parameter	Protection	Ref.
iNOS	-/-	MPTP mouse	4× 20mg/kg ip at 2h interval † 1-7d	ST: DA, metabolites SN: TH, microglial marker	ST: none SN: incomplete[1]	53
	-/-	MPTP mouse	1× 30mg/kg ip at 1×/d for 5d † 7d	ST: DA, metabolites SN: TH, microglial marker	ST: none SN: complete[2]	54
COX-1	-/-	MPTP mouse	1× 20mg/kg sc at 1×/d for 5d † 12d	ST: DA, metabolites SN: TH	ST: none SN: none	68
COX-2	-/- and -/+	MPTP mouse	1× 20mg/kg sc at 1×/d for 5d † 12d	ST: DA, metabolites SN: TH	ST: non SN: incomplete[3]	68
cPLA2	-/- and -/+	MPTP mouse	4× 15mg/kg ip at 2h interval † 1-7d	ST: DA, metabolites SN: TH	ST: -/- incomplete[4], -/+ none SN: -/- complete	69
TNFR1 and 2	-/-, single and double KO	MPTP mouse	1× 12.5 mg/kg	ST: DA, TH, glial marker	double KO: complete	70
	-/-, single and double KO	MPTP mouse	4× 15mg/kg ip † 7d	ST: DA, metabolites, TH SN: TH, behavioral study	no protection but alteration of striatal DA metabolism	47
IL-6	-/-	MPTP mouse	1× 40mg/kg sc	ST: DA	increased DA depletion lethality ↑	71
NFκB p50	-/-	MPTP mouse	1× 30 mg/kg sc	ST: DA, metabolites SN: TH	none	72

[1] TH neuron loss: 71% → 44%.
[2] TH neuron loss: 61% → 4%.
[3] TH neuron loss: 40% → 20% in -/- and -/+.
[4] DA loss: 58% → 34%.

NOTE: Target: gene tested for protective action in models of Parkinson's disease via knockout approach. Parameter: marker used to test for nigrostriatal system and glial activation. Protection: >95% protection is regarded as "complete."

ABBREVIATIONS: -/-, homozygous; -/+, heterozygous; †, time until sacrifice; d, day; DA, dopamine; ip, intraperitoneal; iv, intravenous; KO, knockout; sc, subcutaneous; SN, substantia nigra; ST, striatum; TH, tyrosine hydroxylase.

but they even seemed to enhance the toxic properties of MPP^+. Furthermore, these molecules induced a switch from apoptosis to necrosis. Indeed, apoptotic features could be readily detected in dopaminergic cultures treated with MPP^+ alone, whereas the morphological changes observed in the cultures co-treated with caspase inhibitors were compatible with necrosis with regard to membrane leakage. In contrast, the presence of a high concentration of glucose in the culture medium alone or in conjunction with caspase inhibitors afforded a partial protection of dopamine neuron cultures against MPP^+. Thus, these data indicate that it will be extremely difficult to save neurons with strongly impaired functioning using neuroprotective strategies. The data rather suggest that a cocktail of neuroprotective agents (in our case, caspase inhibitors and glucose) or agents with a broader spectrum of action should be used to protect dopaminergic neurons. We recently tested this hypothesis by activating peroxisome proliferator-activated receptor-γ (PPAR-γ), a member of the nuclear receptor superfamily that has recently been shown to inhibit inflammatory processes (probably by counteracting NFκB activation) in a variety of cell types *in vitro*—including monocytes-macrophages[48,49] and microglial cells[50]—and *in vivo*.[51] We showed that in mice intoxicated by MPTP, orally administered pioglitazone, a selective PPAR-γ agonist currently used in the treatment of diabetes, attenuated the MPTP-induced microglial activation and prevented the dopaminergic cell loss in the substantia nigra.[52] In contrast, pioglitazone did not influence the microglial response in the striatum nor did it affect the loss of striatal tyrosine hydroxylase immunoreactivity induced by MPTP. Similarly, other neuroprotective strategies that efficiently protect dopaminergic neurons in the substantia nigra, such as the invalidation of the inducible form of nitric oxide synthase, have also been shown to have little effect on dopaminergic terminals in the striatum.[53,54] These data suggest that after MPTP intoxication the mechanisms regulating microglial activation may be different in dopaminergic terminals and in dopaminergic cell bodies. Furthermore, they indicate that combined neuroprotective strategies should be developed for dopaminergic cell bodies and terminals. Fulfilling these criteria, minocycline, a tetracycline derivative that inhibits microglial activation, was recently shown to reduce glial activation and protect dopaminergic structures in the entire striatonigral system in the MPTP mouse model[55,56] or 6-hydroxydopamine rat model.[57] The experimental data suggest that the minocycline-induced suppression of microglial activation is essential for its neuroprotective effect. These findings demonstrate the potentially deleterious role of activated glia for the pathogenesis of Parkinson's disease.

In conclusion, the data reviewed here suggest an involvement of the glial reaction and inflammatory processes in the progression of neuronal degeneration in parkinsonian syndromes. Pharmacological manipulation of these pathways affords a relative degree of neuroprotection. Yet, it remains to be determined if such molecules will be neuroprotective in Parkinson's disease. Epidemiological studies concentrating on the effects of nonsteroidal antiinflammatory drugs in Parkinson's disease may help to answer this question before clinical trials are initiated.

REFERENCES

1. HIRSCH, E.C., A.M. GRAYBIEL & Y. AGID. 1988. Melanized dopaminergic neurons are differentially susceptible to degeneration in Parkinson's disease. Nature **334:** 345–348.

2. HASSLER, R. 1938. Zur Pathologie der Paralysis agitans und des postenzephalitischen Parkinsonismus. J. Psychol. Neurol. **48**: 387–476.

3. FEARNLEY, J.M. & A.J. LEES. 1991. Ageing and Parkinson's disease: substantia nigra regional selectivity. Brain **114**: 2283–2301.

4. DAMIER, P., E.C. HIRSCH, Y. AGID, *et al.* 1999. The substantia nigra of the human brain. II. Patterns of loss of dopamine-containing neurons in Parkinson's disease. Brain **122**: 1437–1448.

5. POLYMEROPOULOS, M.H., C. LAVEDAN, E. LEROY, *et al.* 1997. Mutation in the alpha-synuclein gene identified in families with Parkinson's disease. Science **276**: 2045–2047.

6. KITADA, T., S. ASAKAWA, N. HATTORI, *et al.* 1998. Mutations in the parkin gene cause autosomal recessive juvenile parkinsonism. Nature **392**: 605–608.

7. ANGLADE, P., S. VYAS, F. JAVOY-AGID, *et al.* 1997. Apoptosis and autophagy in nigral neurons of patients with Parkinson's disease. Histol. Histopathol. **12**: 25–31.

8. HARTMANN, A., J.-D. TROADEC, S. HUNOT, *et al.* 2001. Caspase-8 is an effector in apoptotic death of dopaminergic neurons in Parkinson's disease, but pathway inhibition results in neuronal necrosis. J. Neurosci. **21**: 2247–2255.

9. FORNO, L.S. 1996. Neuropathology of Parkinson's disease. J. Neuropathol. Exp. Neurol. **55**: 259–272.

10. JENNER, P. & C.W. OLANOW. 1998. Understanding cell death in Parkinson's disease. Ann. Neurol. **44**: S72–S84.

11. OLANOW, C.W. & W.G. TATTON. 1999. Etiology and pathogenesis of Parkinson's disease. Annu. Rev. Neurosci. **22**: 123–144.

12. HIRSCH, E.C., B. FAUCHEUX, P. DAMIER, *et al.* 1997. Neuronal vulnerability in Parkinson's disease. J. Neural Transm. Suppl. **50**: S79–S88.

13. MOCHIZUKI, H., K. GOTO, H. MORI, *et al.* 1996. Histochemical detection of apoptosis in Parkinson's disease. J. Neurol. Sci. **137**: 120–123.

14. TATTON, N.A., A. MACLEAN-FRASER, W.G. TATTON, *et al.* 1998. A fluorescent double-labeling method to detect and confirm apoptotic nuclei in Parkinson's disease. Ann. Neurol. **44**: S142–S148.

15. MCGEER, P.L., S. ITAGAKI, B.E. BOYES, *et al.* 1988. Reactive microglia are positive for HLA-DR in the substantia nigra of Parkinson's and Alzheimer's disease brains. Neurology **38**: 1285–1291.

16. MCGEER, P.L. & E.G. MCGEER. 1998. Mechanisms of cell death in Alzheimer disease-immunopathology. J. Neural Transm. Suppl. **54**: 159–166.

17. HUNOT, S., A. HARTMANN & E.C. HIRSCH. 2001. The inflammatory response in the Parkinson brain. Clin. Neurosci. Res. **1**: 434–443.

18. VILA, M., D.C. WU & S. PRZEDBORSKI. 2001. Engineered modeling and the secrets of Parkinson's disease. Trends Neurosci. **24**: S49–S55.

19. LANGSTON, J.W., J.W. BALLARD, J.W. TETRUD, *et al.* 1983. Chronic parkinsonism in humans due to a product of meperidine-analog synthesis. Science **219**: 979–980.

20. LANGSTON, J.W., L.S. FORNO, J. TETRUD, *et al.* 1999. Evidence of active nerve cell degeneration in the substantia nigra of humans years after 1-methyl-4-phenyl-1,2,3,6-tetrahydropyridine exposure. Ann. Neurol. **46**: 598–605.

21. BRONSTEIN, D.M., I. PEREZ-OTANO, V. SUN, *et al.* 1995. Glia-dependant neurotoxicity and neuroprotection in mesencephalic cultures. Brain Res. **704**: 112–116.

22. MCNAUGHT, K.S. & P. JENNER. 1999. Altered glial function causes neuronal death and increases neuronal susceptibility to 1-methyl-4-phenylpyridinium- and 6-hydroxy-dopamine-induced toxicity in astrocytic/ventral mesencephalic co-cultures. J. Neurochem. **73**: 2469–2476.

23. HERRERA, A.J., A. CASTANO, J.L. VENERO, *et al.* 2000. The single intranigral injection of LPS as a new model for studying the selective effects of inflammatory reactions on dopaminergic system. Neurobiol. Dis. **7**: 429–447.

24. GAO, H.M., J. JIANG, B. WILSON, *et al.* 2002. Microglial activation-mediated delayed and progressive degeneration of rat nigral dopaminergic neurons: relevance to Parkinson's disease. J. Neurochem. **81**: 1285–1297.

25. CASTANO, A., A.J. HERRERA, J. CANO, *et al.* 2002. The degenerative effect of a single intranigral injection of LPS on the dopaminergic system is prevented by dexametha-

sone, and not mimicked by rh-TNF-alpha, IL-1beta and IFN-gamma. J. Neurochem. **81:** 150–157.

26. NAGATSU, T., M. MOGI, H. ICHINOSE, *et al.* 2000. Cytokines in Parkinson's disease. J. Neural Transm. Suppl. **58:** 143–151.

27. BOKA, G., P. ANGLADE, D. WALLACH, *et al.* 1994. Immunocytochemical analysis of tumor necrosis factor and its receptors in Parkinson's disease. Neurosci. Lett. **172:** 151–154.

28. HUNOT, S., N. DUGAS, B. FAUCHEUX, *et al.* 1999. Fc(epsilon)RII/CD23 is expressed in Parkinson's disease and induces, in vitro, production of nitric oxide and tumor necrosis factor-α in glial cells. J. Neurosci. **19:** 3440–3447.

29. VILA, M., V. JACKSON-LEWIS, C. GUEGAN, *et al.* 2001. The role of glial cells in Parkinson's disease. Curr. Opin. Neurol. **14:** 483–489.

30. HUNOT, S., F. BOISSIERE, B. FAUCHEUX, *et al.* 1996. Nitric oxide synthase and neuronal vulnerability in Parkinson's disease. Neuroscience **72:** 355–363.

31. QURESHI, G.A., S. BAIG, I. BEDNAR, *et al.* 1995. Increased cerebrospinal fluid concentration of nitrite in Parkinson's disease. NeuroReport **6:** 1642–1644.

32. GOOD, P.F., A. HSU, P. WERNER, *et al.* 1998. Protein nitration in Parkinson's disease. J. Neuropathol. Exp. Neurol. **57:** 338–342.

33. BAUD, V. & M. KARIN. 2001. Signal transduction by tumor necrosis factor and its relatives. Trends Cell Biol. **11:** 372–377.

34. KRAJCSI, P. & W.S. WOLD. 1998. Inhibition of tumor necrosis factor and interferon triggered responses by DNA viruses. Semin. Cell Dev. Biol. **9:** 351–358.

35. MACKAY, F., J. ROTHE, H. BLUETHMANN, *et al.* 1994. Differential responses of fibroblasts from wild-type and TNF-R55-deficient mice to mouse and human TNF-alpha activation. J. Immunol. **153:** 5274–5284.

36. GRELL, M., F.M. BECKE, H. WAJANT, *et al.* 1998. TNF receptor type 2 mediates thymocyte proliferation independently of TNF receptor type 1. Eur. J. Immunol. **28:** 257–263.

37. TARTAGLIA, L.A., D.V. GOEDDEL, C. REYNOLDS, *et al.* 1993. Stimulation of human T-cell proliferation by specific activation of the 75-kDa tumor necrosis factor receptor. J. Immunol. **151:** 4637–4641.

38. DECLERCQ, W., G. DENECKER, W. FIERS, *et al.* 1998. Cooperation of both TNF receptors in inducing apoptosis: involvement of the TNF receptor-associated factor binding domain of the TNF receptor 75. J. Immunol. **161:** 390–399.

39. LUCAS, R., I. GARCIA, Y.R. DONATI, *et al.* 1998. Both TNF receptors are required for direct TNF-mediated cytotoxicity in microvascular endothelial cells. Eur. J. Immunol. **28:** 3577–3586.

40. HARTMANN, A., A. MOUATT-PRIGENT, B.A. FAUCHEUX, *et al.* 2002. FADD: a link between TNF family receptors and caspases in Parkinson's disease. Neurology **58:** 308–310.

41. GREEN, D.R. 1998. Apoptotic pathways: the roads to ruin. Cell **94:** 695–698.

42. GRANVILLE, D.J., C.M. CARTHY, H. JIANG, *et al.* 1998. Rapid cytochrome c release, activation of caspases 3, 6, 7 and 8 followed by Bap31 cleavage in HeLa cells treated with photodynamic therapy. FEBS Lett. **437:** 5–10.

43. SLEE, E.A., M.T. HARTE, R.M. KLUCK, *et al.* 1999. Ordering the cytochrome c-initiated caspase cascade: hierarchical activation of caspases-2, -3, -6, -7, -8, and -10 in a caspase-9-dependent manner. J. Cell Biol. **144:** 281–292.

44. HARTMANN, A., S. HUNOT, P.P. MICHEL, *et al.* 2000. Caspase-3: a vulnerability factor and final effector in apoptotic death of dopaminergic neurons in Parkinson's disease. Proc. Natl. Acad. Sci. USA **97:** 2875–2880.

45. TURMEL, H., A. HARTMANN, K. PARAIN, *et al.* 2001. Caspase-3 activation in 1-methyl-4-phenyl-1,2,3,6-tetrahydropyridine (MPTP)-treated mice. Mov. Disord. **16:** 185–189.

46. HARTMANN, A. & E.C. HIRSCH. 2001. Parkinson's disease: The apoptosis hypothesis revisited. Adv. Neurol. **86:** 143–153.

47. ROUSSELET, E., J. CALLEBERT, K. PARAIN, *et al.* 2002. Role of TNT-alpha receptors in mice intoxicated with the parkinsonian toxin MPTP. Exp. Neurol. **177:** 183–192.

48. JIANG, C., A.T. TING & B. SEED. 1998. PPAR-gamma agonists inhibit production of monocyte inflammatory cytokines. Nature **391:** 82–86.

49. RICOTE, M., A.C. LI, T.M. WILLSON, *et al.* 1998. The peroxisome proliferator-activated receptor-gamma is a negative regulator of macrophage activation. Nature **391:** 79–82.

50. COMBS, C.K., D.E. JOHNSON, J.C. KARLO, *et al.* 2000. Inflammatory mechanisms in Alzheimer's disease: inhibition of beta-amyloid-stimulated proinflammatory responses and neurotoxicity by PPARgamma agonists. J. Neurosci. **20:** 558–567.

51. HENEKA, M.T., T. KLOCKGETHER & D.L. FEINSTEIN. 2000. Peroxisome proliferator-activated receptor-gamma ligands reduce neuronal inducible nitric oxide synthase expression and cell death in vivo. J. Neurosci. **20:** 6862–6867.

52. BREIDERT, T., J. CALLEBERT, M.T. HENEKA, *et al.* 2002. Protective action of the peroxisome proliferator-activated receptor-gamma agonist pioglitazone in a mouse model of Parkinson's disease. J. Neurochem. **82:** 615–624.

53. LIBERATORE, G.T., V. JACKSON LEWIS, S. VUKOSAVIC, *et al.* 1999. Inducible nitric oxide synthase stimulates dopaminergic neurodegeneration in the MPTP model of Parkinson disease. Nat. Med. **5:** 1403–1409.

54. DEHMER, T., J. LINDENAU, S. HAID, *et al.* 2000. Deficiency of inducible nitric oxide synthase protects against MPTP toxicity *in vivo.* J. Neurochem. **74:** 2213–2216.

55. DU, Y., Z. MA, S. LIN, *et al.* 2001. Minocycline prevents nigrostriatal dopaminergic neurodegeneration in the MPTP model of Parkinson's disease. Proc. Natl. Acad. Sci. USA **98:** 14669–14674.

56. WU, D.C., V. JACKSON-LEWIS, M. VILA, *et al.* 2002. Blockade of microglial activation is neuroprotective in the 1-methyl-4-phenyl-1,2,3,6-tetrahydropyridine mouse model of Parkinson disease. J. Neurosci. **22:** 1763–1771.

57. HE, Y., S. APPEL & W. LE. 2001. Minocycline inhibits microglial activation and protects nigral cells after 6-hydroxydopamine injection into mouse striatum. Brain Res. **909:** 187–193.

58. AUBIN, N., O. CURET, A. DEFFOIS, *et al.* 1998. Aspirin and salicylate protect against MPTP-induced dopamine depletion in mice. J. Neurochem. **74:** 1635–1642.

59. MOHANAKUMAR, K.P., D. MURALIKRISHNAN & B. THOMAS. 2000. Neuroprotection by sodium salicylate against 1-methyl-4-phenyl-1,2,3,6-tetrahydropyridine-induced neurotoxicity. Brain Res. **864:** 281–290.

60. TEISMANN, P. & B. FERGER. 2001. Inhibition of the cyclooxygenase isoenzymes COX-1 and COX-2 provide neuroprotection in the MPTP-mouse model of Parkinson's disease. Synapse **39:** 167–174.

61. KURKOWSKA-JASTRZEBSKA, I., M. BABIUCH, I. JONIEC, *et al.* 2002. Indomethacin protects against neurodegeneration caused by MPTP intoxication in mice. Int. Immunopharmacol. **2:** 1213–1218.

62. KURKOWSKA-JASTRZEBSKA, I., A. WRONSKA, M. KOHUTNICKA, *et al.* 1999. The inflammatory reaction following 1-methyl-4-phenyl-1,2,3,6-tetrahydropyridine intoxication in mouse. Exp. Neurol. **156:** 50–61.

63. MATSUURA, K., H. KABUTO, H. MAKINO, *et al.* 1997. Initial cyclosporin A but not glucocorticoid treatment promotes recovery of striatal dopamine concentration in 6-hydroxydopamine lesioned mice. Neurosci. Lett. **230:** 191–194.

64. KITAMURA, Y., Y. ITANO, T. KUBO, *et al.* 1994. Suppressive effect of FK-506, a novel immunosuppressant, against MPTP-induced dopamine depletion in the striatum of young C57BL/6 mice. J. Neuroimmunol. **50:** 221–224.

65. EMBORG, M.E., P. SHIN, B. ROITBERG, *et al.* 2001. Systemic administration of the immunophilin ligand GPI 1046 in MPTP-treated monkeys. Exp. Neurol. **168:** 171–182.

66. BOIREAU, A., F. BORDIER, P. DUBEDAT, *et al.* 1997. Thalidomide reduces MPTP-induced decrease in striatal dopamine levels in mice. Neurosci. Lett. **234:** 123–126.

67. HULLEY, P., J. HARTIKKA, S. ABDEL'AL, *et al.* 1995. Inhibitors of type IV phosphodiesterases reduce the toxicity of MPTP in substantia nigra neurons in vivo. Eur. J. Neurosci. **7:** 2431–2440.

68. FENG, Z., T. WANG, D. LI, *et al.* 2002. Cyclooxygenase-2-deficient mice are resistant to 1-methyl-4-phenyl-1,2,3,6-tetrahydropyridine-induced damage of dopaminergic neurons in the substantia nigra. Neurosci. Lett. **329:** 354.

69. KLIVENYI, P., M.F. BEAL, R.J. FERRANTE, *et al.* 1998. Mice deficient in group IV cytosolic phospholipase A2 are resistant to MPTP neurotoxicity. J. Neurochem. **71:** 2634–2637.

70. SRIRAM, K., J.M. MATHESON, S.A. BENKOVIC, *et al.* 2002. Mice deficient in TNF receptors are protected against dopaminergic neurotoxicity: implications for Parkinson's disease. FASEB J. **16:** 1474–1476.
71. BOLIN, L.M., I. STRYCHARSKA-ORCZYK, J. SANTOS, *et al.* 2001. Increased vulnerability of dopaminergic neurons in MPTP-lesioned IL-6 K.O. mice. Soc. Neurosci. Abstr. **27:** 194.
72. TEISMANN, P., M. SCHWANINGER, F. WEIH, *et al.* 2001. Nuclear factor-kappaB activation is not involved in a MPTP model of Parkinson's disease. NeuroReport **12:** 1049–1053.

Induction of Adult Neurogenesis

Molecular Manipulation of Neural Precursors *in Situ*

PAOLA ARLOTTA, SANJAY S. MAGAVI, AND JEFFREY D. MACKLIS

MGH-HMS Center for Nervous System Repair, Massachusetts General Hospital Departments of Neurosurgery and Neurology and Program in Neuroscience, Harvard Medical School, Boston, Massachusetts 02114, USA

ABSTRACT: Over most of the past century, it was thought that the adult brain was completely incapable of generating new neurons. However, in the last decade, the development of new techniques has resulted in an explosion of new research showing that (i) neurogenesis, the birth of new neurons, is not restricted to embryonic development, but normally also occurs in two limited regions of the adult mammalian brain (the olfactory bulb and the dentate gyrus of the hippocampus); (ii) that there are significant numbers of multipotent neural precursors in many parts of the adult mammalian brain; and (iii) that it is possible to induce neurogenesis even in regions of the adult mammalian brain, like the neocortex, where it does not normally occur, via manipulation of endogenous multipotent precursors *in situ*. In the neocortex, recruitment of small numbers of new neurons can be induced in a region-specific, layer-specific, and neuronal type-specific manner, and newly recruited neurons can form long-distance connections to appropriate targets. This suggests that elucidation of the relevant molecular controls over adult neurogenesis from endogenous neural precursors/stem cells may allow the development of neuronal replacement therapies for neurodegenerative disease and other central nervous system injuries that may not require transplantation of exogenous cells.

KEYWORDS: neurogenesis; neocortex; neural precursors; neural stem cells; targeted apoptosis; neuronal recruitment

Neural cell replacement therapies are based on the idea that neurological function lost due to injury or neurodegenerative disease can be improved by introducing new cells that can replace the function of lost neurons. Theoretically, the new cells can do this in one of two general ways.[1] New neurons could anatomically integrate into the host brain, becoming localized to the diseased portion of the brain, receiving afferents, expressing neurotransmitters, and forming axonal projections to relevant portions of the brain. Alternatively, newly introduced cells could constitutively secrete neurotransmitters into local central nervous system (CNS) tissue, or they could

Address for correspondence: Jeffrey D. Macklis, MGH-HMS Center for Nervous System Repair, Massachusetts General Hospital, Edwards 4, 55 Fruit Street, Boston, MA 02114. Voice: 617-355-7185; fax: 617-734-1646.
jeffrey.macklis@tch.harvard.edu

Ann. N.Y. Acad. Sci. 991: 229–236 (2003). © 2003 New York Academy of Sciences.

be engineered to produce growth factors to support the survival or regeneration of existing neurons. Growing knowledge about the normal role of endogenous neural precursors, their potential differentiation fates, and their responsiveness to a variety of cellular and molecular controls suggests that neuronal replacement therapies based on manipulation of endogenous precursors either *in situ* or *ex vivo* may be possible.

Neuronal replacement therapies based on the manipulation of endogenous precursors *in situ* may have advantages over transplantation-based approaches, but they may have several limitations as well. The most obvious advantage of manipulating endogenous precursors *in situ* is that there is no need for external sources of cells. Cells for transplantation are generally derived from embryonic tissue, nonhuman species (xenotransplantation), or cells grown in culture. Use of embryo-derived tissue aimed towards human diseases is complicated by limitations in availability and by both political and ethical issues; for example, current transplantation therapies for Parkinson's disease require tissue from several embryos. Xenotransplantation of animal cells carries potential risks of introducing novel diseases into humans and raises questions about how well xenogenic cells will integrate into the human brain. In many cases, cultured cells need to be immortalized by oncogenesis, increasing the risk that the cells may become tumorigenic. In addition, transplantation of cells from many of these sources risks immune rejection and may require immunosuppression.

However, there are also potential limitations to manipulating endogenous precursor cells as a neuronal replacement therapy. First, such an approach may be practically limited to particular regions of the brain, since multipotent neural precursors are densely distributed only in particular subregions of the adult brain (for example, the subventricular zone [SVZ]/subependimal zone [SEZ] and hippocampal subgranular zone). In addition, the potential differentiation fates of endogenous precursors may be too limited to allow their integration into varied portions of the brain. Another potential difficulty is that it may be difficult to provide the precise combination and sequence of molecular signals necessary to induce endogenous precursors to efficiently and precisely proliferate and differentiate into appropriate types of neurons deep in the brain; this will likely be a critical issue to achieve proper integration and function by the newborn neurons.

The substantial amount of prior research regarding constitutively occurring neurogenesis provides insight into the potential and limitations of endogenous precursor based neuronal replacement therapies. In this chapter, we will first review results from several laboratories on the nature and location of endogenous neural precursors and then review some of our experiments demonstrating that endogenous neural precursors can be induced to differentiate into neurons in regions of the adult brain that do not normally undergo neurogenesis, such as the cerebral cortex. Because of space limitations, we refer readers to other review articles that cover the broad field of constitutive adult neurogenesis in more detail.

IDENTITY OF ADULT NEURAL PRECURSORS

The effort to identify the neural precursors that contribute to olfactory bulb neurogenesis has generated a great deal of controversy. Research took an interesting turn with the provocative discovery that "glia-like" cells (for example, cells showing phenotypic and antigenic features of glia, including cytoplasmic glycogen inclusions and expression of the intermediate filament protein GFAP, glial acidic fibrillary protein) from the adult SVZ/SEZ can give rise to neurons and may therefore be neural precursors/stem cells.[2] In a series of elegant experiments, Alvarez-Buylla and colleagues showed that some SVZ astrocytes in the adult mammalian brain are able to form multipotent neurospheres *in vitro* (by many considered a property of neural stem cells) and are the source of new neurons of the olfactory bulb. These data strongly suggest that at least a subset of SVZ astrocyte-like cells are neural precursors. They selectively labeled SVZ astrocytic cells and traced the label via selective viral infection, using a receptor for an avian leukosis virus under the control of the GFAP promoter in transgenic mice, to newly generated neurons of the olfactory bulb.[2] Similarly, GFAP-positive astrocyte-like cells in the subgranular layer (SGL) of the adult hippocampus (the other major site of adult neurogenesis) divide and generate new neurons.[3] These data support the idea that a subset of astrocyte-like cells have the properties of neural precursors and suggests discussion regarding the proper name to assign to these cells. Are they really *bona fide* astrocytes? It appears that only a very small fraction of astrocyte-like cells in the SVZ behave as neural precursors. Could related cells exist in other regions of the postnatal and adult brain? Or rather, is this subset of SVZ astrocytes a unique class of GFAP-expressing precursors that should be considered distinct and potentially given a new name?

In contrast with these results, Frisen's group published experiments reporting that ependymal cells lining the lumenal surface of the adult ventricular zone are adult neural precursors.[4] These results contrast with those of Doetsch *et al.*, who reported that ependymal cells did not divide *in vivo* or under their culture conditions *in vitro*.[5] A parallel report from van der Kooy's lab reported that, while ependymal cells divide as spheres *in vitro*, they do not possess multipotential precursor properties.[6] It remains to be established whether experimental differences between the three groups account for their different results (reviewed in Barres[7]). The idea that some subset of astrocyte-like cells can behave as neural precursors is supported by later studies suggesting that 1–10% of astrocytes isolated from several regions of the early postnatal brain (SVZ, cerebral cortex, cerebellum, spinal cord) and grown as monolayers are able to form "neurospheres" that can give rise to both neurons and glia *in vitro*.[8] Moreover, retrovirally mediated expression of exogenous genes can drive some postnatal astrocyte-like cells to become neurons *in vitro*.[9] Interestingly, there are developmental and spatial constraints to astrocyte-like cells, specifically their multipotency, which is normally restricted to the first two postnatal weeks in mice, with the apparent exception of a subset of astrocyte-like cells from the SVZ that appear to retain their multipotency during adulthood.[5] This could mean that such cells in young animals may still be immature and retain their precursor attributes initially, until approximately P10-11.[8] However, it may be that the neurogenic environment of the SVZ can support and maintain the multipotency of a subset of astrocyte-like precursors, even in the adult brain.

Although the idea that glial cells could be neural precursors may sound unusual, it is supported by previous studies (long ignored) that in lizards and newts a special class of radial ependymoglia that extend from the ventricular zone (VZ) lumen to the pial surface can divide and give rise to both neurons and glia after injury, critical for spinal cord regeneration.[10] In line with these observations, similar radial glial cells are present in the adult brain of the canary in regions of active neurogenesis, suggesting that they may be the progenitors of newly generated neurons.[11] Moreover, results from our laboratory show that adult astrocytes from the cerebral cortex can differentiate into transitional radial glia in response to signals that induce neurogenesis from transplanted immature precursors.[12] In general, the notion that cells of the radial glia lineage may have features of neural precursors during development and thus be able to generate both glia and neurons is not new.[13–15] We may imagine adult astrocyte-like cells as precursors with broad potential in neurogenic regions of the CNS (SVZ and dentate gyrus) and more restricted potential in nonneurogenic regions (cerebral cortex, spinal cord). If this is true, one future challenge will be to understand whether astrocyte-like cells from nonneurogenic regions can be induced to assume multipotential neuronal precursors properties, towards the goal of neuronal repopulation and CNS repair *in situ.*

THE LOCATION OF ADULT MAMMALIAN MULTIPOTENT PRECURSORS

Neurogenesis is normally restricted mainly to two specific regions of the adult mammalian brain: the SVZ or the SEZ, which provides neurons to the olfactory bulb, and the dentate gyrus of the hippocampus. If adult multipotent precursors were limited to these two neurogenic regions of the adult CNS, it would severely limit the potential of neuronal replacement therapies based on *in situ* manipulation of endogenous precursors. However, adult multipotent precursors have been isolated and cultured *in vitro* from several other regions of the adult brain, including caudal portions of the SVZ, spinal cord,[16,17] septum,[18] striatum,[19] neocortex,[18] optic nerve,[18] and retina.[20] The precursors derived from all these regions can self-renew and differentiate into neurons, astroglia, and oligodendroglia (the three main cell types of the brain) *in vitro.* In nonneurogenic regions of the mature brain, it is thought that they normally differentiate only into glia or die. Cells from each region have different requirements for their proliferation and differentiation. Understanding the similarities and differences between the properties of multipotent precursors derived from different regions of the brain will be instrumental in potentially developing neuronal replacement therapies based on manipulation of endogenous precursors.

MANIPULATION OF AN INHIBITORY ENVIRONMENT

The fact that new neurons are born only in very restricted areas of the adult mammalian brain, even though neural precursors are found quite ubiquitously in the adult CNS, suggests that precursors from different regions may have different potential. Alternatively or in addition, local environments may differ in their ability to support/allow neurogenesis from these precursors. Data from several groups have shown that multipotent precursors from several regions of the adult brain have a broad potential and can differentiate into at least the three different broad cell types, astroglia, oligodendroglia, and neurons, given an appropriate *in vitro* or *in vivo* environment. This led us to explore the fate of multipotent precursors in an adult cortical environment, which does not normally support *de novo* neurogenesis.

Our lab has previously shown that cortex undergoing synchronous apoptotic degeneration of projection neurons forms an instructive environment that can guide the differentiation of transplanted immature neurons or neural precursors.[21–25] Immature neurons or multipotent neural precursors transplanted into targeted cortex can migrate selectively to layers of cortex undergoing degeneration of projection neurons, differentiate into projection neurons, receive afferent synapses, express appropriate neurotransmitters and receptors, and reform appropriate long-distance connections to the original contralateral targets of the degenerating neurons in adult murine neocortex.[12,26–30] Together, these results suggested to us that cortex undergoing targeted apoptotic degeneration could direct endogenous multipotent precursors to integrate into adult cortical microcircuitry. In agreement with this hypothesis, we found, for the firs time, that endogenous multipotent precursors, normally located in the adult brain, can be induced to differentiate into neurons in the adult mammalian neocortex, without transplantation.[31] We induced synchronous apoptotic degeneration of corticothalamic neurons in layer 6 of anterior cortex and examined the fates of dividing cells within cortex, using BrdU and markers of progressive neuronal differentiation. BrdU[+] newborn cells expressed NeuN, a mature neuronal marker, and survived at least 28 weeks, while no new neurons were observed in control, intact cortex. Moreover, some newborn neurons displayed typical pyramidal neuron morphology (large, 10–15 μm diameter somata with apical processes) characteristic of neurons that give rise to long-distance projections. Retrograde labeling from thalamus demonstrated that newborn BrdU[+] neurons can form appropriate long-distance corticothalamic connections.[31] Together, these results demonstrate that endogenous neural precursors can be induced *in situ* to differentiate into cortical neurons, survive for many months, and form appropriate long-distance connections in the adult mammalian brain. The same microenvironment that supports the migration, neuronal differentiation, and appropriate axonal extension of transplanted neuroblasts and precursors also supports and instructs the neuronal differentiation and axon extension of endogenous precursors. These results demonstrate that the normal absence of constitutive cortical neurogenesis does not reflect an intrinsic limitation of the endogenous neural precursors' potential, but more likely results from a lack of appropriate microenvironmental signals necessary for neuronal differentiation or survival. Elucidation of these signals could enable CNS repair. Recently, other groups have reported similar and complementary results in hippocampus[32] and striatum,[33] confirming and further supporting this direction of research.

CONCLUSION

Recent research suggests that it may be possible to manipulate endogenous neural precursors *in situ* so that they undergo neurogenesis in the adult brain, towards future neuronal replacement therapy for neurodegenerative disease and other CNS injury. Multipotent precursors, capable of differentiating into astroglia, oligodendroglia, and neurons exist in many portions of the adult brain. These precursors have considerable plasticity; and although they may have limitations in their integration into some host sites, they are, when heterotopically transplanted, capable of differentiation into neurons appropriate to a wide variety of recipient regions. Many adult precursors are capable of migrating long distances, using both tangential and radial forms of migration. Endogenous adult neural precursors are also capable of extending axons significant distances through the adult brain. In addition, *in vitro* and *in vivo* experiments have begun to elucidate the responses of endogenous precursors to both growth factors and behavioral manipulations and are beginning to provide key information towards manipulation of their proliferation and differentiation. Recent experiments from our lab have shown that, under appropriate conditions, endogenous precursors can differentiate into neurons, extend long-distance axonal projections, and survive for long periods of time in regions of the adult brain that do not normally undergo neurogenesis. Other laboratories have recently reported similar results in other systems. These results indicate that there exists a sequence and combination of molecular signals by which neurogenesis can be induced in the adult mammalian cerebral cortex and other regions where it does not normally occur.

Together, these data suggest that neuronal replacement therapies based on manipulation of endogenous precursors may be possible in the future. However, several questions must be answered before neuronal replacement therapies using endogenous precursors become a reality. The multiple signals that are responsible for endogenous precursor division, migration, and differentiation and axon extension and survival will need to be elucidated for such therapies to be developed efficiently.[34] These challenges also exist for neuronal replacement therapies based on transplantation of precursors, since donor cells, whatever their source, must interact with the mature CNS's environment to integrate into the brain. In addition, it remains an open question whether potential therapies manipulating endogenous precursors *in situ* would necessarily be limited to portions of the brain near adult neurogenic regions. However, even if multipotent precursors are not located in very high numbers outside of neurogenic regions of the brain, it may be possible to induce them to proliferate from the smaller numbers that are more widely distributed throughout the neuraxis. Potentially, it may be possible to induce the repopulation of diseased mammalian brain via the specific activation and instructive control over endogenous neural precursors along desired neuronal lineages. However, the field is just beginning to understand the complex interplay between particular neural precursors' potential, their heterogeneity, and how to take advantage of what may be partial cell type restriction, permissive and instructive developmental signals, and modulation of specific aspects of neuronal differentiation and survival. Progress over the past decade has been great, and the coming decades promise to offer significant insight into these and other critical issues for the field.

ACKNOWLEDGMENTS

This work was supported in part by grants from the National Institutes of Health (NS41590, NS45523, HD28478, and MRRC HD18655), the Alzheimer's Association, the Human Frontiers Science Program, and the National Science Foundation to J.D.M. P.A. was supported by a Wills Foundation fellowship. S.S.M. was partially supported by a National Institutes of Health predoctoral training grant and fellowships from the Leopold Schepp Foundation and the Lefler Foundation. Parts of this review were updated and modified from a similar review by the same authors for a different readership.[35]

REFERENCES

1. BJORKLUND, A. & O. LINDVALL. 2000. Cell replacement therapies for central nervous system disorders. Nat. Neurosci. **3:** 537–544.
2. DOETSCH, F., J.M. GARCIA-VERDUGO & A. ALVAREZ-BUYLLA. 1999. Regeneration of a germinal layer in the adult mammalian brain. Proc. Natl. Acad. Sci. USA **96:** 11619–11624.
3. SERI, B., J.M. GARCIA-VERDUGO, B.S. MCEWEN & A. ALVAREZ-BUYLLA. 2001. Astrocytes give rise to new neurons in the adult mammalian hippocampus. J. Neurosci. **21:** 7153–7160.
4. JOHANSSON, C.B. *et al.* 1999. Identification of a neural stem cell in the adult mammalian central nervous system. Cell **96:** 25–34.
5. DOETSCH, F., I. CAILLE, D.A. LIM, *et al.* 1999. Subventricular zone astrocytes are neural stem cells in the adult mammalian brain. Cell **97:** 703–716.
6. CHIASSON, B.J., V. TROPEPE, C.M. MORSHEAD & D. VAN DER KOOY. 1999. Adult mammalian forebrain ependymal and subependymal cells demonstrate proliferative potential, but only subependymal cells have neural stem cell characteristics. J. Neurosci. **19:** 4462–4471.
7. BARRES, B.A. 1999. A new role for glia: generation of neurons! 1999. Cell **97:** 667–670.
8. LAYWELL, E.D., P. RAKIC, V.G. KUKEKOV, *et al.* 2000. Identification of a multipotent astrocytic stem cell in the immature and adult mouse brain. Proc. Natl. Acad. Sci. USA **97:** 13883–13888.
9. HEINS, N. *et al.* 2002. Glial cells generate neurons: the role of the transcription factor Pax6. Nat. Neurosci. **5:** 308–315.
10. CHERNOFF, E.A. 1996. Spinal cord regeneration: a phenomenon unique to urodeles? Int. J. Dev. Biol. **40:** 823–831.
11. ALVAREZ-BUYLLA, A., J.R. KIRN & F. NOTTEBOHM. 1990. Birth of projection neurons in adult avian brain may be related to perceptual or motor learning [published erratum appears in Science 1990 Oct 19;250(4979):360]. Science **249:** 1444–1446.
12. LEAVITT, B.R., C.S. HERNIT-GRANT & J.D. MACKLIS. 1999. Mature astrocytes transform into transitional radial glia within adult mouse neocortex that supports directed migration of transplanted immature neurons. Exp. Neurol. **157:** 43–57.
13. MALATESTA, P., E. HARTFUSS & M. GOTZ. 2000. Isolation of radial glial cells by fluorescent-activated cell sorting reveals a neuronal lineage. Development **127:** 5253–5263.
14. NOCTOR, S.C., A.C. FLINT, T.A. WEISSMAN, *et al.* 2001. Neurons derived from radial glial cells establish radial units in neocortex. Nature **409:** 714–720.
15. NOCTOR, S.C. *et al.* 2002. Dividing precursor cells of the embryonic cortical ventricular zone have morphological and molecular characteristics of radial glia. J. Neurosci. **22:** 3161–3173.
16. SHIHABUDDIN, L.S., J. RAY & F.H. GAGE. 1997. FGF-2 is sufficient to isolate progenitors found in the adult mammalian spinal cord. Exp. Neurol. **148:** 577–586.
17. WEISS, S. *et al.* 1996. Multipotent CNS stem cells are present in the adult mammalian spinal cord and ventricular neuroaxis. J. Neurosci. **16:** 7599–7609.
18. PALMER, T.D., E.A. MARKAKIS, A.R. WILLHOITE, *et al.* 1999. Fibroblast growth factor-2 activates a latent neurogenic program in neural stem cells from diverse regions of the adult CNS. J. Neurosci. **19:** 8487–8497.
19. PALMER, T.D., J. RAY & F.H. GAGE. 1995. FGF-2-responsive neuronal progenitors reside in proliferative and quiescent regions of the adult rodent brain. Mol. Cell. Neurosci. **6:** 474–486.
20. TROPEPE, V. *et al.* 2000. Retinal stem cells in the adult mammalian eye. Science **287:** 2032–2036.
21. MACKLIS, J.D. 1993. Transplanted neocortical neurons migrate selectively into regions of neuronal degeneration produced by chromophore-targeted laser photolysis. J. Neurosci. **13:** 3848–3863.
22. MADISON, R. & J.D. MACKLIS. 1993. Noninvasively induced degeneration of neocortical pyramidal neurons in vivo: selective targeting by laser activation of retrogradely transported photolytic chromophore. Exp. Neurol. **121:** 153–159.

23. SCHARFF, C., J.R. KIRN, M. GROSSMAN, et al. 2000. Targeted neuronal death affects neuronal replacement and vocal behavior in adult songbirds [see comments]. Neuron 25: 481–492.

24. SHEEN, V.L., E.B. DREYER & J.D. MACKLIS. 1992. Calcium-mediated neuronal degeneration following singlet oxygen production. NeuroReport 3: 705–708.

25. SHEEN, V.L. & J.D. MACKLIS. 1994. Apoptotic mechanisms in targeted neuronal cell death by chromophore-activated photolysis. Exp. Neurol. 130: 67–81.

26. HERNIT-GRANT, C.S. & J.D. MACKLIS. 1996. Embryonic neurons transplanted to regions of targeted photolytic cell death in adult mouse somatosensory cortex reform specific callosal projections. Exp. Neurol. 139: 131–142.

27. SHEEN, V.L. & J.D. MACKLIS. 1995. Targeted neocortical cell death in adult mice guides migration and differentiation of transplanted embryonic neurons. J. Neurosci. 15: 8378–8392.

28. SHIN, J.J. et al. 2000. Transplanted neuroblasts differentiate appropriately into projection neurons with correct neurotransmitter and receptor phenotype in neocortex undergoing targeted projection neuron degeneration. J. Neurosci. 20: 7404–7416.

29. SNYDER, E.Y., C. YOON, J.D. FLAX & J.D. MACKLIS. 1997. Multipotent neural precursors can differentiate toward replacement of neurons undergoing targeted apoptotic degeneration in adult mouse neocortex. Proc. Natl. Acad. Sci. USA 94: 11663–11668.

30. FRICKER-GATES, R.A., J.J. SHIN, C.C. TAI, et al. 2002. Late-stage immature neocortical neurons reconstruct interhemispheric connections and form synaptic contacts with increased efficiency in adult mouse cortex undergoing targeted neurodegeneration. J. Neurosci. 22: 4045–4056.

31. MAGAVI, S.S., B.R. LEAVITT & J.D. MACKLIS. 2000. Induction of neurogenesis in the neocortex of adult mice [see comments]. Nature 405: 951–955.

32. NAKATOMI, H., T. KURIU, S. OKABE, et al. 2002. Regeneration of hippocampal pyramidal neurons after ischemic brain injury by recruitment of endogenous neural progenitors. Cell 110: 429–441.

33. CHICHUNG LIE, D., G. DZIEWCZAPOLSKI, A.R. WILLHOITE, et al. 2002. The adult substantia nigra contains progenitor cells with neurogenic potential. J. Neurosci. 22: 6639–6649.

34. CATAPANO, L.A., M.W. ARNOLD, F.A. PEREZ & J.D. MACKLIS. 2001. Specific neurotrophic factors support the survival of cortical projection neurons at distinct stages of development. J. Neurosci. 21: 8863–8872.

35. MAGAVI, S.S. & J.D. MACKLIS. 2001. Manipulation of neural precursors in situ: induction of neurogenesis in the neocortex of adult mice. Neuropsychopharmacology 25: 816–835.

Molecular Mechanisms of Neuronal Cell Death

KIM A. HEIDENREICH

*Department of Pharmacology and Neuroscience Program, University of Colorado
Health Sciences Center, and the Denver Veterans Affairs Medical Center,
Denver, Colorado 80262, USA*

ABSTRACT: Chronic neurodegenerative diseases, including Parkinson's disease,
are characterized by a selective loss of specific subsets of neuronal populations
over a period of years or even decades. While the underlying causes of the various neurodegenerative diseases are not clear, the death of neurons and the loss
of neuronal contacts are key pathological features. Pinpointing molecular
events that control neuronal cell death is critical for the development of new
strategies to prevent and treat neurodegenerative disorders.

KEYWORDS: neuron; cell death; apoptosis

APOPTOTIC DEATH PATHWAYS

Recent data obtained from studies of human postmortem brains, as well as animal
and cell culture models, suggest that apoptosis and other forms of programmed cell
death contribute to neurodegeneration (TABLE 1, Refs. 1–21). Necrosis may also play
a role in neurodegenerative disorders but is probably more important in acute and ex-
treme insults to the brain. Apoptosis is a type of programmed cell death characterized by a cascade of proteolytic events orchestrated by the caspase family of cysteine
proteases (see FIG. 1). There are two principal pathways leading to apoptotic cell
death. These include the "extrinsic" or death receptor–initiated pathway and the "intrinsic" or mitochondrial pathway.[22,23] The extrinsic pathway originates with binding of death-promoting ligands (such as Fas ligand, FasL) to their cognate death
receptors (such as Fas).[24] There is a large family of death ligands and death receptors, and the FasL/Fas system is outlined as a prototype. Ligand binding induces oligomerization of death receptors and promotes their association with adapter
molecules such as Fas-associated death domain protein (FADD).[25] The receptor–
FADD interaction occurs via a protein–protein binding motif known as the death domain.[26] The initiator caspase, procaspase-8, is then recruited to the death-inducing
signaling complex via binding to the death effector domain of FADD.[27] The resulting proximity of multiple procaspase-8 molecules facilitates their autocatalytic
cleavage to the active protease caspase-8.[28]

The intrinsic pathway is initiated by the release of cytochrome c from mitochondria and its subsequent association with apoptosis activating factor-1 and pro-

Address for correspondence: Kim A. Heidenreich, Ph.D., Denver VAMC-111H, 1055 Cler-
mont Street, Denver, Colorado 80220. Voice: 303-399-8020 (3891); fax: 303-393-5271.
kim.heidenreich@uchsc.edu

Ann. N.Y. Acad. Sci. 991: 237–250 (2003). © 2003 New York Academy of Sciences.

TABLE 1. Evidence that programmed cell death contributes to neurodegenerative diseases

Disease	Type of neuron	Reference
Parkinson's disease	dopamine	1–4
Alzheimer's disease	hippocampal/cortical	5–9
Huntington's disease	striatal/cortical	1–13
Amyotrophic lateral sclerosis	motor	14–18
Spinocerebellar ataxias	cerebellar	19–21

caspase-9.[29] This large protein complex (the apoptosome) promotes the activation of caspase-9.[30] Each of the above initiator caspases, 8 and 9, cleave downstream executioner caspases, such as caspase-3, from the pro-form to the active protease. Activation of the executioner caspases then results in the cleavage of critical cellular proteins and apoptosis.[31,32]

The intrinsic death pathway is regulated by both pro- and antiapoptotic members of the Bcl-2 family.[33] Bax and Bak are pro-apoptotic members of the Bcl-2 family that appear to serve a redundant function in making the mitochondrial membrane permeable to cytochrome c.[34] Cytochrome c release from mitochondria occurs by formation of a Bax- or Bak-containing "pore" in the outer mitochondrial membrane that permits passage of small proteins.[35] The proapoptotic function of Bax is attenuated by antiapoptotic members of the Bcl-2 family (Bcl-2, Bcl-X_L) that heterodimerize with Bax and sequester it away from mitochondria.[36] Conversely, BH3 domain-only Bcl-2 family members, including Bim, Bid, Dp5/Hrk, and Bad, promote the proapoptotic effects of Bax by binding to Bcl-2, thus freeing Bax to incorporate into the mitochondrial membrane.[37]

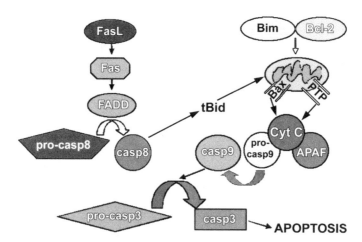

FIGURE 1. Extrinsic and intrinsic death signaling cascades.

Besides the sequestration of Bcl-2 away from Bax by BH3-only proteins, another critical step required for initiation of cytochrome c release is the active translocation of Bax from the cytoplasm to mitochondria. The factors regulating this process are unclear at present, but recent data indicate that opening of the mitochondrial permeability transition pore (mitoPTP) stimulates Bax movement to mitochondria.[38] The mitoPTP is a heteromeric protein complex that includes the voltage-dependent anion channel, the adenine nucleotide translocator, and cyclophilin D, as well as several other proteins.[39] The mitoPTP is localized at contact sites between the inner and outer mitochondrial membranes. Some apoptotic stimuli are capable of opening the mitoPTP, resulting in disruption of the mitochondrial membrane potential (depolarization), a decline in ATP production, and entry of solutes and water into the mitochondrial matrix. Ultimately, mitochondrial swelling and rupture of the outer mitochondrial membrane can occur. Precisely how opening of the mitoPTP induces Bax translocation to mitochondria is unknown, but an inhibitor of the pore, cyclosporin A (which binds to cyclophilin D in the pore), blocks Bax localization to mitochondria.[40] Thus, cytochrome c release is regulated by multiple signals that involve Bcl-2 family members: (1) opening of the mitoPTP stimulates Bax translocation to mitochondria; (2) increased expression of BH3-only proteins, such as Bim, results in sequestration of Bcl-2 away from Bax; and 3) Bax, once free from Bcl-2, inserts into the mitochondrial outer membrane to form a pore for cytochrome c release.

In some cells, the extrinsic death pathway plays the major role in the execution of apoptosis. The death-inducing signaling complex (DISC) forms very efficiently, generating large amounts of active caspase-8, which directly activates caspase-3. In other cells, small amounts of caspase-8 are generated because of insufficient DISC formation, requiring a mitochondrial contribution to the execution of apoptosis. The extrinsic pathway can activate the mitochondrial pathway by the cleavage of Bid by active caspase-8. Truncated Bid (tBid) sequesters Bcl-2 and promotes cytochrome c release and caspase-9 activation. Still, in other cell types, the mitochondrial pathway appears to be the dominant mechanism for executing apoptosis. The signaling events that regulate activation of the mitochondrial death pathway are poorly understood.

APOPTOSIS AND NEURODEGENERATION

Aberrant apoptotic mechanisms are thought to contribute significantly to many neurodegenerative disorders, including Parkinson's disease and Alzheimer's disease.[1–9] Recent findings indicate that components of both the extrinsic (death receptors or their ligands) and intrinsic (Bcl-2 family members) death pathways are regulated at the level of expression during neurodegeneration or neuronal injury *in vivo*.[41,42] Moreover, transgenic animal models or spontaneously occurring mutants of specific death receptor signaling molecules or Bcl-2 family members provide further evidence that these pathways are involved in neuronal injury.[43,44]

In vitro studies using cultured neurons have shown that the BH3-only protein Bim is upregulated following either nerve growth factor (NGF) withdrawal from primary sympathetic neurons[45] or serum and potassium withdrawal from primary cerebellar granule neurons.[46] Moreover, overexpression of Bim or related BH3-only family members promotes neuronal apoptosis in a Bax-dependent manner,[47] and neurons isolated from Bim knock-out mice show increased resistance to apoptosis.[48] These observations support a general mechanism by which BH3-only proteins, such as Bim, block the Bcl-2-mediated repression of Bax-dependent cytochrome c release, thus initiating the intrinsic or mitochondrial death pathway in some neurons.

In contrast to the above findings implicating a role of the intrinsic death pathway in neurodegenerative conditions, there have been fewer *in vitro* studies examining the involvement of the extrinsic death pathway in promoting neuronal apoptosis. Le-Niculescu *et al.* showed that FasL mRNA is induced following trophic factor withdrawal in cerebellar granule neurons; and furthermore, sequestration of FasL with FasFc attenuates granule neuron apoptosis.[49] However, additional data supporting a role for the extrinsic death pathway in neuronal apoptosis have not been forthcoming. Recently, our laboratory has investigated the role of both extrinsic and intrinsic signaling pathways in regulating neuronal death in an *in vitro* model system, which is described in the text that follows. We have learned two general features from our studies: (1) Some types of neurons die using the classic apoptotic machinery described in the preceding text; whereas other neurons die by programmed mechanisms distinct from apoptosis. (2) Multiple signaling pathways are either activated or interrupted during neuronal death, but interruption of a single pathway is sometimes sufficient to block apoptosis.

MODEL SYSTEM FOR STUDYING NEURONAL CELL DEATH

We have investigated signaling pathways that control neuronal death using primary cerebellar neuronal cultures. These cultures, derived from the cerebella of early postnatal rats, survive and differentiate when maintained in media containing 10% serum and 25 mM potassium.[50] Granule neurons, which constitute ~95% of the cell population, undergo apoptosis when they are switched to serum-free medium containing 5 mM potassium. Purkinje neurons, which make up ~3% of the culture, undergo delayed cell death when serum factors are removed from their culture media.

INVOLVEMENT OF EXTRINSIC PATHWAYS IN
NEURONAL CELL DEATH

To investigate whether death receptor signaling is involved in the apoptotic cell death of cerebellar granule neurons subjected to trophic factor withdrawal, we used adenoviral gene transfer to introduce a gene encoding a mutant protein that blocks death receptor signaling. The gene encoded ΔFADD, a truncated protein that lacks the death effector domain, and therefore inhibits coupling of liganded death receptors to the initiator caspase-8.[51,52] Cerebellar cell cultures were infected with increasing titers of adenoviral, AU1-tagged, dominant-negative FADD (Ad-AU1-ΔFADD). Forty-eight hours following infection, cells were switched from control medium containing serum and 25 mM potassium to apoptotic medium lacking serum and containing 5 mM potassium. After an additional 24-h incubation, cells were fixed and nuclei were stained with Hoechst dye. Granule neurons containing condensed and/or fragmented nuclei were scored as apoptotic. In most experiments, apoptosis increased from about 6% in control medium to approximately 70% after

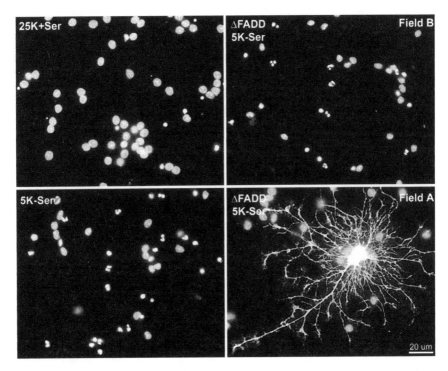

FIGURE 2. Granule neurons in proximity to ΔFADD-expressing Purkinje cells demonstrate increased survival. Uninfected granule neurons **(left panels)** or granule neurons infected with Ad-AU1-ΔFADD at an m.o.i. = 50 **(right panels)** were incubated in either control (25K + Ser) or apoptotic (5K − Ser) medium for 24 hr and then stained with DAPI and anti-AU1. Condensed and/or fragmented nuclei were abundant in uninfected granule neurons incubated in 5K − Ser medium. Apoptotic granule neurons were also plentiful in fields infected with ΔFADD that did not contain any ΔFADD-expressing Purkinje cells **(Field A)**. In contrast, fields infected with ΔFADD that contained one or more ΔFADD-positive Purkinje cells displayed a significant decrease in the number of apoptotic granule neurons following trophic factor withdrawal **(Field B)**. *Scale bar* = 20 microns.

24 h of trophic factor withdrawal. Infection with a control adenovirus had no effect on granule neuron apoptosis, whereas infection with ΔFADD adenovirus resulted in a significant reduction in granule neuron apoptosis.[53] Initially, this result suggested that death receptor signaling may play a direct role in cerebellar granule neuron apoptosis. However, immunocytochemical analysis revealed that adenoviral ΔFADD was not efficiently expressed in granule neurons, but instead showed marked expression in the small number of Purkinje neurons found in these cerebellar cell cultures (FIG. 2). Moreover, the ability of adenoviral ΔFADD to rescue granule neurons from apoptosis was dependent on their proximity to ΔFADD-expressing Purkinje cells. Experiments using IGF-I receptor blocking antibodies indicated that ΔFADD-mediated survival of cerebellar granule neurons requires local action of Purkinje cell–derived IGF-I. Two major conclusions were drawn from these results. First, although the data did not support a direct role for the extrinsic death pathway in cerebellar

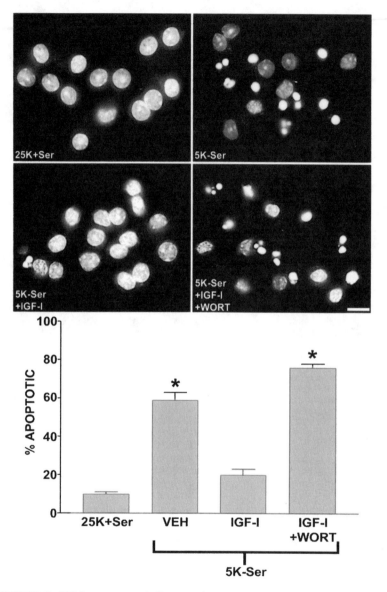

FIGURE 3. IGF-I protects cerebellar granule neurons from apoptosis in a PI3K-dependent manner. **Top panel:** Cerebellar granule neurons were incubated for 24 hr in either control (25K + Ser) or apoptotic (5K − Ser) medium containing either PBS vehicle (VEH) or IGF-I (200 ng/mL) in the absence or presence of wortmannin (WORT, 100 nM). Following incubation, cerebeller granule neurons were fixed and nuclei were stained with DAPI. *Scale bar* = 10 microns. **Bottom panel:** The percentages of apoptotic cerebellar granule neurons observed under the conditions described in images were quantified by counting approximately 500 granule neurons per field in two fields per condition.

granule neuron apoptosis, the results were the first to demonstrate that death receptor signaling in Purkinje neurons indirectly influences the survival of granule neurons. Second, selective suppression of the extrinsic death pathway in Purkinje cells is sufficient to rescue neighboring granule neurons that depend on Purkinje cell–derived trophic support including IGF-I.

INTRINSIC DEATH PATHWAYS AND NEURONAL DEATH

Recent data from a number of laboratories indicate that the intrinsic death pathway plays an important role in executing apoptosis of granule neurons.[54,55] To determine if IGF-I protected granule neurons from apoptosis by blocking components of the intrinsic pathway, we examined the effects of IGF-I on the various components of the intrinsic pathway working from the executioner caspases backward to the initiator caspases and mitochondrial regulators (see FIG. 1). Apoptosis was induced in the cerebellar granule neurons by removing serum from the medium and lowering the potassium concentration from 25 mM to 5 mM. FIGURE 3 demonstrates the neuroprotective effects of IGF-I in granule neurons. Apoptosis was quantified by counting the percentage of Hoesht-stained nuclei that were condensed or fragmented. In culture medium containing 25 mM potassium and serum, less than 10% of the granule neurons are apoptotic. When the extracellular potassium is reduced to 5 mM and serum is removed from the medium, about 80% of the neurons are apoptotic by 24 h. IGF-I markedly blocks apoptosis in a PI3-kinase (PI3K)–dependent manner. Using Western blotting techniques with antibodies against activated caspase 3, we detected caspase 3 activation within 6 h of serum and potassium deprivation. IGF-I totally inhibited caspase-3 activation in a PI3K-dependent manner. Immediately upstream of caspase-3 cleavage in the intrinsic pathway is the activation of the initiator caspase-9. Recently, caspase-9 activation was shown to be required for caspase-3 cleavage in cerebellar granule neurons deprived of serum and depolarizing potassium.[56] Consistent with this finding, we observed marked cleavage of caspase-9 indicative of its activation in granule neurons deprived of trophic support. As was observed for caspase-3 cleavage, activation of caspase-9 was significantly inhibited by IGF-I in a PI3K-dependent manner, demonstrating that IGF-I suppresses a key component of the intrinsic death pathway in granule neurons.

Caspase-9 is activated following its association with Apaf-1 and cytochrome c, which assemble into a large oligomeric complex known as the apoptosome.[30] Formation of the apoptosome occurs after release of the mitochondrial protein cytochrome c into the cytoplasm. Our studies showed that in granule neurons maintained in the presence of serum and depolarizing potassium, cytochrome c was localized predominantly in mitochondria, with only diffuse staining observed in neuronal processes. Removal of serum and depolarizing potassium for 4 h resulted in a rapid redistribution of cytochrome c from mitochondria to a diffuse staining throughout the cytoplasm (FIG. 4). This redistribution was accompanied by the formation of many pronounced punctate areas of cytochrome c staining. The latter were observed primarily, although not exclusively, in distinct focal complexes localized to neuronal processes. In contrast to cytochrome c staining, no detectable redistribution of the mitochondrial marker Mitotracker Green was observed in neuronal processes under apoptotic conditions, indicating that the punctate areas of cytochrome c staining

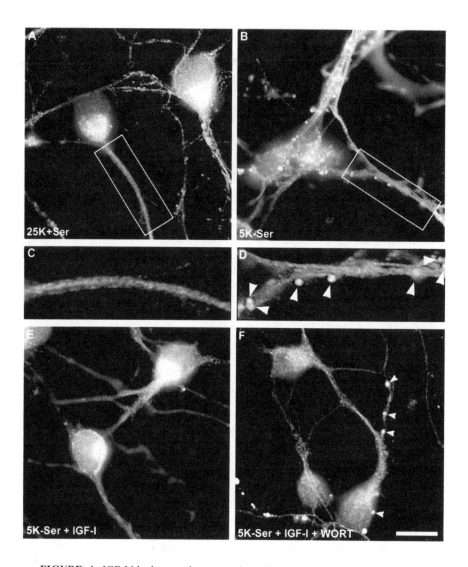

FIGURE 4. IGF-I blocks cytochrome c release from mitochondria and prevents its redistribution to focal complexes localized in neuronal processes. Cerebellar granule neurons were incubated for 4 h in control (25K + Ser) or apoptotic (5K – Ser) medium containing either PBS vehicle or IGF-I (200 ng/mL) in the absence or presence of wortmannin (WORT, 100 nM). Following incubation, neurons were fixed in 4% paraformaldehyde, permeabilized with 0.2% Triton-X-100, and blocked with 5% BSA. Cytochrome c was localized by incubating the cells with a polyclonal antibody to cytochrome c and a Cy3-conjugated secondary antibody. Digitally deconvolved images were then captured using a 63× oil objective. *Scale bar* = 10 microns. **(A)** Cerebellar granule neuron incubated in control medium demonstrated intense cytochrome C staining in the perinuclear region consistent with localization to mitochondria. Very diffuse staining was observed in neuronal processes. **(B)** Granule neurons incubated in apoptotic medium for 4 h showed a marked redistribution of cytochrome c. Note the overall diffuse staining throughout the cytoplasm accompanied by the formation of dis-

were not associated with intact mitochondria. Inclusion of IGF-I during trophic factor withdrawal prevented the release and redistribution of cytochrome c from mitochondria. Addition of wortmannin in combination with IGF-I restored the release of cytochrome c from mitochondria and its redistribution to focal complexes in neuronal processes, indicating that the effects of IGF-I on cytochrome c release were PI3K-dependent (FIG. 4). Thus, IGF-I inhibits the release of cytochrome c from mitochondria, and in this manner blocks the subsequent activation of the intrinsic initiator caspase-9.

A potential mechanism by which cytochrome c release is regulated involves the formation of a Bax- or Bak-containing "pore" in the outer mitochondrial membrane that permits passage of proteins.[34,57] The BH3-only Bcl-2 family members, including Bad, Bid, Dp5/Hrk, and Bim, promote the proapoptotic effects of Bax and Bak, while concomitantly suppressing the prosurvival function of Bcl-2.[37,58] Recently, Bim has been shown to be upregulated following both nerve growth factor (NGF) withdrawal from primary sympathetic neurons, and serum and potassium withdrawal from granule neurons.[45,59] Moreover, overexpression of Bim has been shown to promote apoptosis of cerebellar granule neurons.[47] Our laboratory examined whether IGF-I was capable of regulating Bim induction in cerebellar granule neurons. Immunoblotting for Bim following acute trophic factor withdrawal in granule neurons (FIG. 5) demonstrated a marked increase in the expression of Bim short, the most proapoptotic splice variant of this protein family.[60] IGF-I completely blunted the induction of Bim, indicating that suppression of Bim is one mechanism by which IGF-I inhibits cytochrome c release from mitochondria.

Bim expression is regulated by multiple transcription factors. In NGF-deprived sympathetic neurons, dominant-negative c-Jun partially attenuated the induction of Bim mRNA and Bim_{EL} protein, inhibited cytochrome c release, and rescued sympathetic neurons from apoptosis.[45] c-Jun has also been implicated in the apoptosis of cerebellar granule neurons,[61] and an inhibitor of the JNK signaling pathway (CEP-1347) was recently shown to partially blunt the induction of Bim mRNA in cerebellar granule neurons subjected to trophic factor withdrawal.[47] In agreement with these findings, we found that the p38/JNK inhibitor SB203580 significantly attenuated both the activation of c-Jun and the increase in Bim_S expression in cerebellar granule neurons deprived of trophic support. However, IGF-I failed to inhibit c-Jun activation under conditions where it significantly blocked induction of Bim_S. These results indicated that c-Jun plays a role in the regulation of Bim expression during granule neuron apoptosis, but IGF-I suppresses the induction of Bim via a mecha-

tinct, brightly fluorescent focal complexes on the cell bodies and processes. (**C**) The area demarcated by the *box* in **A** is enlarged to show the diffuse cytochrome c staining in a control neuronal process. (**D**) The area demarcated by the *box* in **B** is enlarged to show the intense cytochrome c staining localized to discrete focal complexes (indicated by *arrowheads*) in neuronal processes. (**E**) Granule neurons incubated in apoptotic medium containing exogenous IGF-I displayed cytochrome c localization to mitochondria similar to controls. (**F**) Granule neurons incubated in apoptotic medium containing both IGF-I and wortmannin showed cytochrome c staining similar to granule neurons incubated in apoptotic medium alone. Focal complexes of cytochrome c staining are indicated by *arrowheads*.

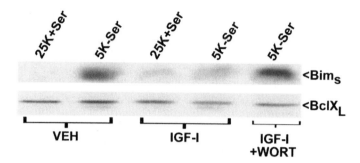

FIGURE 5. IGF-I inhibits induction of the BH3-only Bcl-2 family member Bim in a PI3K-dependent manner. Cerebellar granule neurons were incubated for 6 h in either control (25K + Ser) or apoptotic (5K − Ser) medium containing either PBS vehicle (VEH) or IGF-I (200 ng/mL) ± wortmannin (WORT, 100 nM). Following incubation, cell lysates were subjected to SDS-PAGE on 15% polyacrylamide gels and proteins were transferred to PVDF membranes. Bim expression was assessed by immunoblotting with a polyclonal antibody to Bim that specifically recognized an approximately 15-kDa protein, consistent with the apparent molecular weight of Bim short (Bim_S). To affirm equal protein loading, the blot was then stripped and reprobed for the antiapoptotic Bcl-2 family member $BclX_L$, which did not demonstrate any significant change in expression under the conditions of this experiment.

nism that does not involve modulation of JNK/c-Jun signaling. This conclusion was in agreement with the work of Whitfield *et al.*,[45] who proposed that JNK/c-Jun signaling cooperates with a distinct JNK/c-Jun–independent pathway to stimulate the expression of Bim in sympathetic neurons deprived of NGF.

In this context, the forkhead transcription factor, FKHRL1 had recently been shown to regulate Bim expression in hematopoietic cells.[62] Cytokine withdrawal from a pro-B cell line induced activation (dephosphorylation) of FKHRL1, induction of Bim, and apoptosis.[62] Moreover, expression of a constitutively active mutant of FKHRL1, in which three putative AKT phosphorylation sites are mutated to alanine, induced Bim expression, cytochrome c release, and apoptosis in hematopoietic cells.[62] Given that FKHRL1 is a known substrate for AKT in neurons,[63] we questioned whether the AKT-mediated inactivation of FKHRL1 may be one mechanism by which IGF-I inhibits apoptosis. Indeed, overexpression of a constitutively active, FKHRL1 triple phosphorylation site mutant had been shown to induce apoptosis of cerebellar granule neurons.[64] In our studies, we showed that trophic factor withdrawal from cerebellar granule neurons led to an inactivation of AKT, a corresponding activation of FKHRL1, and translocation of FKHRL1 to the nucleus. All of these effects, along with the induction of Bim, were prevented by IGF-I in a PI3K-dependent manner. In addition, adenoviral expression of a dominant-negative mutant of AKT was sufficient to activate FKHRL1 and induce Bim expression in granule neurons maintained in the presence of serum and depolarizing potassium. Taken together, our data suggest that IGF-I attenuates the induction of Bim in trophic factor–deprived granule neurons via a PI3K/AKT-mediated inactivation of the FKHRL1 transcription factor. Overall, our results demonstrated that suppression of the intrinsic death signaling cascade is a principal mechanism underlying the neuroprotective effects of IGF-I in granule neurons. IGF-I blocks Bim induction, cytochrome cre-lease, and activation of the intrinsic initiator caspase-9 and the executioner caspase-3 in granule neurons deprived of trophic support. Moreover, IGF-I inhibits the actions of FKHRL1, a transcriptional regulator of Bim, suggesting a novel c-Jun–in-dependent mechanism for the modulation of Bim in neurons.

PROGRAMMED CELL DEATH DISTINCT FROM APOPTOSIS

The data discussed above indicate that cerebellar granule neurons, when deprived of trophic support, die by classic apoptotic mechanisms involving the mitochondrial death pathway. The extrinsic or death receptor pathway indirectly regulates the survival of granule neurons by its effects on Purkinje cells that provide trophic support such as IGF-I to the granule neurons. Ongoing studies in our laboratory indicate that Purkinje neurons, in contrast to the granule neurons, die by a cell death program that is caspase independent and morphologically distinct from apoptosis (manuscript in preparation). Death is not characterized by nuclear condensation but rather by extensive autophagic-lysosomal vacuolation. Thus, even under the same culture conditions with the same apoptotic stimulus, some neurons die using the classic apoptotic machinery described above; whereas other types of neurons die by programmed mechanisms distinct from apoptosis. Recent data from other laboratories support the notion that, in addition to apoptosis, other forms of programmed cell death may participate in neurodegeneration. In light of numerous unique mechanisms of neuronal cell death, care must be taken in making broad general conclusions about mechanisms of neuronal cell death as they relate to specific disease pathology. It will be necessary to investigate the molecular mechanisms of cell death in specific neuronal subtypes to define better therapeutic strategies for the various neurodegenerative disorders.

ACKNOWLEDGMENTS

The author would like to thank Dr. Daniel Linseman, Maria McClure, Reid Phelps, and Ron Bouchard for their contributions to this manuscript. This research was supported by grants from the U.S. Army Medical Research Command (DAMD17-99-1-9481), the National Institutes of Health (NS38619-01A1), and the Department of Veterans Affairs (Merit Award and REAP Award) to K.A.H.

REFERENCES

1. MOCHIZUKI, H., et al. 1996. Histochemical detection of apoptosis in Parkinson's disease. J. Neurol. Sci. **137:** 120–123.
2. ANGLADE, P., et al. 1997. Apoptosis and autophagy in nigral neurons of patients with Parkinson's disease. Histol. Histopathol. **12:** 25–31.
3. TATTON, N.A., et al. 1998. A fluorescent double-labling method to detect and confirm apoptotic nuclei in Parkinson's disease. Ann. Neurol. **44:** S142–S148.
4. HIRSCH, E.C., et al. 1999. Dopaminergic neurons degenerate by apoptosis in Parkinson's disease. Mov. Disord. **14:** 383–385.

5. SMALE, G., *et al.* 1995. Evidence for apoptotic cell death in Alzheimer's disease. Exp. Neurol. **133:** 225–230.
6. LASSMANN, H., *et al.* 1995. Cell death in Alzheimer's disease evaluated by DNA fragmentation in situ. Acta Neuropathol. (Berlin) **89:** 35–41.
7. ANDERSON, A.J., J.H. SU & C.W. COTMAN. 1996. DNA damage and apoptosis in Alzheimer's disease: colocalization with c-Jun immunoreactivity, relationship to brain area, and effect of postmortem delay. J. Neurosci. **16:** 1710–1719.
8. TRONCOSO, J.C., *et al.* 1996. In situ labeling of dying cortical neurons in normal aging and in Alzheimer's disease: correlations with senile plaques and disease progression. J. Neuropathol. Exp. Neurol. **55:** 1134–1142.
9. SU, J.H., G. DENG & C.W. COTMAN. 1997. Bax protein expression is increased in Alzheimer's brain: Correlations with DNA damage, Bcl-2 expression, and brain pathology. J. Neuropathol. Exp. Neurol. **56:** 86–93.
10. DRAGUNOW, M., *et al.* 1995. In situ evidence for DNA fragmentation in Huntington's disease striatum and Alzheimer's disease temporal lobes. Neuroreport **6:** 1053–1057.
11. THOMAS, L.B., *et al.* 1995. DNA end labeling (TUNEL) in Huntington's disease and other neuropathological conditions. Exp. Neurol. **133:** 265–272.
12. ZEITLIN, S., *et al.* Increased apoptosis and early embryonic lethality in mice nullizygous for the Huntington's disease gene homologue. Nat. Genet. **11:** 155–163.
13. GOLDBERG, Y.P., *et al.* 1996. Cleavage of huntingtin by apopain, a proapoptotic cysteine protease, is modulated by the polyglutamine tract. Nat. Genet. **13:** 442–449.
14. TROOST, D., *et al.* 1995. Apoptosis in amyotrophic lateral sclerosis is not restricted to motor neurons. Bcl-2 expression is increased in unaffected post-central gyrus. Neuropathol. Appl. Neurobiol. **21:** 498–504.
15. RABIZADEH, S., *et al.* 1995. Mutations associated with amyotrophic lateral sclerosis convert superoxide dismutase from an antiapoptotic gene to a proapoptotic gene: studies in yeast and neural cells. Proc. Natl. Acad. Sci. USA **92:** 3024–3028.
16. MU, X., *et al.* 1996. Altered expression of bcl-2 and bax mRNA in amyotrophic lateral sclerosis spinal chord motor neurons. Ann. Neurol. **40:** 379–386.
17. GHADGE, G.D., *et al.* 1997. Mutant superoxide dismutase-1-linked familial amyotrophic lateral sclerosis: molecular mechanisms of neuronal death and protection. J. Neurosci. **17:** 8756–8766.
18. PASINELLI, P., *et al.* 1998. Caspase-1 is activated in neural cells and tissue with amyotrophic lateral sclerosis-associated mutations in copper-zinc superoxide dismutase. Proc. Natl. Acad. Sci. USA **95:** 15763–15768.
19. IKEDA, H., *et al.* 1996. Expanded polyglutamine in the Machado-Joseph disease protein induces cell death in vitro and in vivo. Nat. Genet. **13:** 196–202.
20. WELLINGTON, C.L., *et al.* 1998. Caspase cleavage of gene products associated with triplet expansion disorders generates truncated fragments containing the polyglutamine tract. J. Biol. Chem. **273:** 9158–9167.
21. WARRICK, J.M., *et al.* 1998. Expanded polyglutamine protein forms nuclear inclusions and causes neural degeneration in Drosophila. Cell. **93:** 939–949.
22. STRASSER, A., L. O'CONNOR & V.M. DIXIT. 2000. Apoptosis signaling. Annu. Rev. Biochem. **69:** 217–245.
23. GREEN, D.R. 1998. Apoptotic pathways: the roads to ruin. Cell **94:** 695–698.
24. PINKOSKI, M.J. & D.R. GREEN. 1999. Fas ligand, death gene. Cell Death Differ. **6:** 1174–1181.
25. CHINNAIYAN, A.M., *et al.* 1996. FADD/MORT1 is a common mediator of CD95 (Fas/APO-1) and tumor necrosis factor receptor-induced apoptosis. J. Biol. Chem. **271:** 4961–4965.
26. FEINSTEIN, E., *et al.* 1995. The death domain: a module shared by proteins with diverse cellular functions. Trends Biochem. Sci. **20:** 342–344.
27. MUZIO, M., *et al.* 1996. FLICE, a novel FADD-homologous ICE/CED-3-like protease, is recruited to the CD95 (Fas/APO-1) death-inducing signaling complex. Cell **85:** 817–827.
28. MUZIO, M., *et al.* 1998. An induced proximity model for caspase-8 activation. J. Biol. Chem. **273:** 2926–2930.
29. CAI, J., J. YANG & D.P. JONES. 1998. Mitochondrial control of apoptosis: the role of cytochrome c. Biochim. Biophys. Acta **1366:** 139–149.

30. Zou, H., *et al.* 1999 An APAF-1/cytochrome c multimeric complex is a functional apoptosome that activates caspase-9. J. Biol. Chem. **274:** 11549–11556.
31. Stennicke, H.R. 1998. Pro-caspase-3 is a major physiologic target of caspase-8. J. Biol. Chem. **273:** 27084–27090.
32. Pan, G., E.W. Humke & V.W. Dixit. 1998. Activation of caspases triggered by cytochrome c in vitro. FEBS Lett. **426:** 151–154.
33. Tsujimoto, Y. 1998. Role of Bcl-2 family proteins in apoptosis: apoptosomes or mitochondria? Genes Cells **3:** 697–707.
34. Wei, M.C., *et al.* 2001. Proapoptotic BAX and BAK: a requisite gateway to mitochondrial dysfunction and death. Science **292:** 727–730.
35. Polster, B.M., K.W. Kinally & G. Fiskum. 2001. BH3 death domain peptide induces cell type-selective mitochondrial outer membrane permeability. J. Biol. Chem. **276:** 37887–37894.
36. Otter, I., *et al.* 1998. The binding properties and biological activities of Bcl-2 and Bax in cells exposed to apoptotic stimuli. J. Biol. Chem. **273:** 6110–6120.
37. Zong, W.X., *et al.* 2001. BH3-only proteins that bind pro-survival Bcl-2 family members fail to induce apoptosis in the absence of Bax and Bak. Genes Dev. **15:** 1481–1486.
38. De Giorgi, F., *et al.* 2002. The permeability transition pore signals apoptosis by directing Bax translocation and multimerization. FASEB J. **16:** 607–609.
39. Halestrap, A.P., G.P. McStay & S.J. Clark. 2002. The permeability transition pore complex: another view. Biochimie **84:**153–166.
40. Waldmeier, P. C., *et al.* 2002. Inhibition of the mitochondrial permeability transition by the nonimmunosuppressive cyclosporin derivative NIM811. Mol. Pharmacol. **62:** 22–29.
41. Kitamura, Y., *et al.* 1998. Alteration of proteins regulating apoptosis, Bcl-2, Bcl-x, Bax, Bak, Bad, ICH-1 and CPP32, in Alzheimer's disease. Brain Res. **780:** 260–269.
42. Felderhoff-Mueser, U., *et al.* 2000. Fas/CD95/APO-1 can function as a death receptor for neuronal cells in vitro and in vivo and is upregulated following cerebral hypoxic-ischemic injury to the developing rat brain. Brain Pathol. **10:** 17–29.
43. Martin-Villalba, A., *et al.* 1999. CD95 ligand (Fas-L/APO-1L) and tumor necrosis factor-related apoptosis-inducing ligand mediate ischemia-induced apoptosis in neurons. J. Neurosci. **19:** 3809–3817.
44. Parsadanian, A.S., *et al.* 1998. Bcl-xL is an antiapoptotic regulator for postnatal CNS neurons. J. Neurosci. **18:** 1009–1019.
45. Whitfield, J., *et al.* 2001. Dominant-negative c-Jun promotes neuronal survival by reducing BIM expression and inhibiting mitochondrial cytochrome c release. Neuron **29:** 629–643.
46. Linseman, D.A., *et al.* 2002. Insulin-like growth factor-I blocks Bcl-2 interacting mediator of cell death (Bim) induction and intrinsic death signaling in cerebellar granule neurons. J. Neurosci. **22:** 9287–9297.
47. Harris C.A. & E.M. Johnson, Jr. 2001. BH3-only Bcl-2 family members are coordinately regulated by the JNK pathway and require Bax to induce apoptosis in neurons. J. Biol. Chem. **276:** 37754–37760.
48. Bouillet, P., *et al.* 2001. Degenerative disorders caused by Bcl-2 deficiency prevented by loss of its BH3-only antagonist Bim. Dev. Cell. **5:** 645–653.
49. Le-Niculescu, H., *et al.* 1999. Withdrawal of survival factors results in activation of the JNK pathway in neuronal cells leading to Fas ligand induction and cell death. Mol. Cell. Biol. **19:** 751–763.
50. D'Mello, S.R., *et al.* 1993. Induction of apoptosis in cerebellar granule neurons by low potassium: inhibition of death by insulin-like growth factor I and cAMP. Proc. Natl. Acad. Sci. USA **90:** 10989–10993.
51. Streetz, K., *et al.* 2000. Tumor necrosis factor alpha in the pathogenesis of human and murine fulminant hepatic failure. Gastroenterology **119:** 446–460.
52. Bradham, C.A., *et al.* 1998. The mitochondrial permeability transition is required for tumor necrosis factor alpha-mediated apoptosis and cytochrome c release. Mol. Cell. Biol. **18:** 6353–6364.
53. Linseman, D.A., *et al.* 2002. Suppression of death receptor signaling in cerebellar Purkinje neurons protects neighboring granule neurons from apoptosis via an insulin-like growth factor-I dependent mechanism. J. Biol. Chem. **277:** 24546–24553.

54. MILLER, T.M., *et al.* 1997. Bax deletion further orders the cell death pathway in cerebellar granule cells and suggests a caspase-independent pathway to cell death. J. Cell. Biol. **139:** 205–217.
55. SELIMI, F., *et al.* 2000. Target-related and intrinsic neuronal death in Lurcher mutant mice are both mediated by caspase-3 activation. J. Neurosci. **20:** 992–1000.
56. GERHARDT, E., *et al.* 2001. Cascade of caspase activation in potassium-deprived cerebellar granule neurons: targets for treatment with peptide and protein inhibitors of apoptosis. Mol. Cell. Neurosci. **17:** 717–731.
57. KORSMEYER, S.J. 2000. Pro-apoptotic cascade activates BID, which oligomerizes BAK or BAX into pores that result in the release of cytochrome c. Cell Death Differ. **7:** 1166–1173.
58. DESAGHER, S., *et al.* 1999. Bid-induced conformational change of Bax is responsible for mitochondrial cytochrome c release during apoptosis. J. Cell. Biol. **144:** 891–901.
59. PUTCHA, G.V., *et al.* 2001. Induction of BIM, a proapoptotic BH3-only BCL-2 family member, is critical for neuronal apoptosis. Neuron **29:** 615–628.
60. O'CONNOR, L., *et al.* 1998. Bim: A novel member of the Bcl-2 family that promotes apoptosis. EMBO J. **17:** 384–395.
61. WATSON, A., *et al.* 1998. Phosphorylation of c-Jun is necessary for apoptosis induced by survival signal withdrawal in cerebellar granule neurons. J. Neurosci. **18:** 751–762.
62. DIJKERS, P.F., *et al.* 2002. FKHR-L1 can act as a critical effector of cell death induced by cytokine withdrawal: protein kinase B-enhanced cell survival through maintenance of mitochondrial integrity. J. Cell. Biol. **156:** 531–542.
63. ZHENG, W.H., S. KAR & R. QUIRION. 2000. Insulin-like growth factor-1-induced phosphorylation of the forkhead family transcription factor FKHRL1 is mediated by Akt kinase in PC12 cells. J. Biol. Chem. **275:** 39152–39158.
64. BRUNET, A., *et al.* 1999. Akt promotes cell survival by phosphorylating and inhibiting a Forkhead transcription factor. Cell **96:** 857–868.

Redox State as a Central Modulator of Precursor Cell Function

MARK NOBLE,[a] JOEL SMITH,[b] JENNIFER POWER,[c]
AND MARGOT MAYER-PRÖSCHEL[a]

[a]Department of Biomedical Genetics, University of Rochester School of Medicine,
Rochester, New York 14642, USA

[b]Memorial Sloan-Kettering Hospital, Laboratory of Developmental Hematopoiesis,
New York, New York 10021, USA

[c]Columbia University, Center for Neurobiology and Behavior,
New York, New York 10032, USA

ABSTRACT: In our attempts to understand how the balance between self-renewal and differentiation is regulated in dividing precursor cells, we have discovered that intracellular redox state appears to be a critical modulator of this balance in oligodendrocyte–type-2 astrocyte (O-2A) progenitor cells. The intracellular redox state of freshly isolated progenitor cells allows prospective isolation of cells with different self-renewal characteristics, which can be further modulated in opposite directions by prooxidants and antioxidants. Redox state is itself modulated by cell-extrinsic signaling molecules that alter the balance between self-renewal and differentiation: growth factors that promote self-renewal cause progenitors to become more reduced, while exposure to signaling molecules that promote differentiation causes progenitors to become more oxidized. Moreover, pharmacological antagonists of the redox effects of these cell-extrinsic signaling molecules antagonize their effects on self-renewal and differentiation, further suggesting that cell-extrinsic signaling molecules that modulate this balance converge on redox modulation as a critical component of their effector mechanism. A further example of the potential relevance of intracellular redox state to development processes emerges from our attempts to understand why different central nervous system (CNS) regions exhibit different temporal patterns of oligodendrocyte generation and myelinogenesis. Characterization of O-2A progenitor cells (O-2A/OPCs) isolated from different regions indicates that these developmental patterns are consistent with properties of the specific O-2A/OPCs resident in each region. Marked differences were seen in self-renewal and differentiation characteristics of O-2A/OPCs isolated from cortex, optic nerve, and optic chiasm. In conditions where optic nerve-derived O-2A/OPCs generated oligodendrocytes within 2 days, oligodendrocytes arose from chiasm-derived cells after 5 days and from cortical O-2A/OPCs after only 7–10 days. These differences, which appear to be cell intrinsic, were manifested both in reduced percentages of clones producing oligodendrocytes and in a lesser representation of oligodendrocytes in individual clones. In addition, responsiveness of optic nerve–, chi-

Address for correspondence: Mark Noble, Department of Biomedical Genetics, University of Rochester School of Medicine, 601 Elmwood Avenue, Box 633, Rochester, New York 14642. Voice: 716-273-1448; fax: 716-273-1450.
mark_noble@urmc.rochester.edu

Ann. N.Y. Acad. Sci. 991: 251–271 (2003). © 2003 New York Academy of Sciences.

asm-, and cortex-derived O-2A/OPCs to thyroid hormone (TH) and ciliary neurotrophic factor (CNTF), well-characterized inducers of oligodendrocyte generation, was inversely related to the extent of self-renewal observed in basal division conditions. These results demonstrate hitherto unrecognized complexities among the precursor cells thought to be the immediate ancestors of oligodendrocytes and suggest that the properties of these different populations may contribute to the diverse time courses of myelination in different CNS regions. Strikingly, O-2A/OPCs isolated from cortex and analyzed immediately upon isolation were more reduced in their redox state than were optic nerve–derived cells, precisely as would be predicted from our analysis of the role of redox state in modulating the balance between self-renewal and differentiation. Chiasm-derived cells, which exhibited self-renewal properties intermediate between cortex- and optic nerve–derived cells, were more reduced than optic nerve cells but more oxidized that cortical O-2A/OPCs.

KEYWORDS: myelination; development; oligodendrocyte-type-2 astrocyte progenitor; oligodendrocyte precursor cell; oligodendrocyte; self-renewal; precursor cell

INTRODUCTION

Modulation of the balance between self-renewing divisions and differentiation is at the heart of precursor cell function in development, tissue repair, and tissue homeostasis, yet relatively little is known about physiological mechanisms central to such modulation. For example, on a biochemical level, one of the only properties reported to be predictive of self-renewal characteristics in precursor cells of different lineages (i.e., hematopoietic stem cells and hepatic precursor cells, as described, e.g., in Refs. 1–3) was that cells with a greater tendency to undergo self-renewing divisions showed a lesser extent of labeling with such mitochondrial dyes as rhodamine-123. This reduced labeling was originally thought to be due to expression of P-glycoprotein by cells with a greater self-renewal potential, but subsequent studies on hematopoietic stem cells raised the possibility that it may instead be reflective of mitochondrial activity and intracellular redox state.[4] Such a correlation of such an important physiological state with self-renewal characteristics is potentially of great interest. It is not known, however, whether this correlation is coincidental or whether it provides an important clue to understanding this critical feature of precursor cell biology.

To examine the possibility that intracellular redox regulation plays an important functional role in modulating the self-renewal characteristics of precursor cells, we studied the correlation between redox state and the balance between self-renewal and differentiation in dividing oligodendrocyte–type-2 astrocyte (O-2A) progenitor cells (also referred to has oligodendrocyte precursor cells, or OPCs, and here abbreviated as O-2A/OPCs).[5] This population, which gives rise to the myelin-forming oligodendrocytes of the central nervous system (CNS) (see, e.g., Refs. 6–8), provides one of the most extensively characterized and tractable precursor cell systems available for such studies. It is possible to obtain pure populations of O-2A/OPCs that can be induced to undergo division and differentiation by growth in simple chemically defined medium supplemented with platelet-derived growth factor (PDGF, the best characterized O-2A/OPC mitogen; see, e.g., Refs. 9 and 10).

O-2A/OPCs obtained from the optic nerves of 7-day-old (P7) rat pups and grown in the presence of saturating levels of PDGF, one of the important mitogens for these cells[9,11] exhibit an approximately equal probability of undergoing a self-renewing division or exiting the cell cycle and differentiating into an oligodendrocyte.[12] The tendency of dividing O-2A/OPCs to generate oligodendrocytes is enhanced if cells are coexposed to such signaling molecules as thyroid hormone, ciliary neurotrophic factor, or retinoic acid (see, e.g., Refs. 13–15). Signaling molecules of the bone morphogenetic protein family induce differentiation along oligodendrocyte and astrocyte pathways, respectively.[13,15,16] In contrast, coexposure to neurotrophin-3 or basic fibroblast growth factor (bFGF) inhibits differentiation and is associated with increased precursor cell division and self-renewal.[15,17,18]

Previous studies have shown that the degree to which exposure to signaling molecules alters the balance between self-renewal and differentiation in dividing O-2A/OPCs is very extensive. It is possible to induce nearly synchronous differentiation of all clonally related cells into oligodendrocytes when cells are exposed to thyroid hormone (TH) and type-1 astrocytes;[19,20] varying degrees of asymmetric division and differentiation are seen in the presence of other combinations of factors;[15] and almost complete suppression of differentiation with continuous promotion of self-renewal occurs when cells are grown in the presence of both PDGF and bFGF.[17] At least a subset of these signaling molecules is also known to be of importance *in vivo*. For example, hypothyroid animals show reduced oligodendrocyte generation,[15,21] and animals in which neurotrophin-3 (NT-3) levels are artificially increased show increases in O-2A/OPC proliferation.[18] Both of these results are consistent with the outcomes of *in vitro* studies on the effects of TH and NT-3 on O-2A/OPC division and differentiation.[13,15,18]

In a consideration of situations in which plasticity of precursor cell behavior might play a role, one possibility is seen in the striking phenomenon that different regions of the CNS develop according to different schedules, with great variations seen in the timing of both neurogenesis and gliogenesis.[22] For example, neuron production in the rat spinal cord is largely complete by the time of birth, is still ongoing in the rat cerebellum for at least several days after birth, and continues in the olfactory system and in some regions of the hippocampus of multiple species throughout life. Similarly, myelination has long been known to progress in a rostral-caudal direction, beginning in the spinal cord significantly earlier than in the brain (see, e.g., Refs. 23–25). Even within a single CNS region, myelination is not synchronous. In the rat optic nerve, for example, myelinogenesis occurs with a retinal-to-chiasmal gradient, with regions of the nerve nearest the retina becoming myelinated first.[25,26] The cortex itself shows the widest range of timing for myelination, both initiating later than many other CNS regions (see, e.g., Refs. 23–25) and exhibiting an ongoing myelinogenesis that can extend over long periods of time. This latter characteristic is seen perhaps most dramatically in the human brain, for which it has been suggested that myelination may not be complete until after several decades of life.[27,28]

Variant time courses of development in different CNS regions could be due to two fundamentally different reasons. One possibility is precursor cells are sufficiently plastic in their developmental programs that local differences in exposure to modulators of division and differentiation may account for these variances. Alternatively, it may be that the precursor cells resident in particular tissues express differing biological properties related to the timing of development in the tissue to which they contribute.

Taken together, all of the above observations lead to a series of potentially related questions:

(1) The balance between self-renewal and differentiation in dividing O-2A/OPCs can be modified by a wide range of signaling molecules, acting through diverse receptor systems. Is it possible to identify points at which these differing pathways converge, at least to the extent of identifying common elements by which different kinds of signaling molecules can promote self-renewing division, with perhaps other elements common to factors that induce differentiation? Or is it possible that there are biochemical or molecular pathways within the cell at which all these influences converge?

(2) Are the diverse signaling molecules that have been found to modulate the balance between self-renewal and differentiation in dividing O-2A/OPCs of importance in understanding the different timing of oligodendrocyte generation in diverse CNS regions *in vivo*? Knowledge of the role of these molecules may help in identifying means of modifying precursor cell function *in vivo*.

(3) To what extent do previously unrecognized differences in precursor cell behavior contribute to the variability in oligodendrocyte generation *in vivo*? If precursor cells themselves exhibit substantial regional heterogeneity in their function, this would indicate a hitherto unsuspected complexity in precursor cell biology. Moreover, different populations might express properties of greater or lesser value in the context of using them to repair damaged tissue following cell transplantation.

(4) Do the observations that hematopoietic stem cells and liver precursor cells that show less labeling with rhodamine-123—and thus may be more reduced—provide an important clue to understanding the above problems?

THE ROLE OF REDOX STATE IN MODULATING SELF-RENEWAL CHARACTERISTICS OF O-2A/OPCs DERIVED FROM THE OPTIC NERVE OF P7 RATS

Cellular Redox State Allows Prospective Isolation of Cells with Different Self-Renewal Characteristics

To determine whether intracellular redox state might be associated with the self-renewal potential of O-2A/OPCs developing *in vivo*, we determined whether low levels of labeling with redox-sensitive dyes were indicative of enhanced self-renewal capacity in freshly isolated O-2A/OPCs.[5] Different dyes provide information on different aspects of redox state, which ultimately reflects the balance between reducing and oxidative equivalents within the cell. Redox state, however, is influenced in many ways, including by the state of mitochondrial activation, levels of reduced glutathione and other thiols, levels of NADH and NADPH, and levels of thioredoxin and other factors. In our experiments, cells were labeled with JC-1, rhodamine-123, or dihydrotetramethylrosamine (reduced rosamine), and FACS sorting was used to provide enriched populations of the upper and lower quintiles of labeled cells. Cells from each group were then plated at clonal density in the presence of PDGF, and basal self-renewal characteristics were determined. All dyes gave similar results, but rosamine was consistently associated with the best postsort viability. As rosamine fluorescence is most directly related to the balance between oxidative and reducing equivalents, this dye also provides one of the broadest measures of redox state.[29]

Results obtained using this purification procedure were striking. rosamine[low] cells grown in the presence of 10 ng/mL PDGF generated clones in which self-renewing divisions were prevalent. Five days after plating, $70 \pm 4.3\%$ of these consisted only of dividing progenitor cells, and the average number of cells per clone was 11.1 ± 0.9. In contrast, rosamine[high] cells, which would have had a higher intracellular level of oxidizing equivalents *in vivo*, underwent very little division in these same conditions. With rare exceptions, the largest clones consisted of four cells (mean = 2.5 ± 0.4 cells/clone). rosamine[high] cells also demonstrated a greatly increased tendency to generate oligodendrocytes. At day 5, $47 \pm 4.6\%$ of clones derived from rosamine[high] cells consisted of one oligodendrocyte and no progenitor cells, and only $29 \pm 5.4\%$ of clones contained any progenitors at all. Thus, in agreement with results obtained for hematopoietic stem cells and hepatic precursor cells (see, e.g., Refs. 1–4), rosamine[low] O-2A/OPCs appeared better able to undergo self-renewing divisions than rosamine[high] cells. It is important to note that the viability of all populations was identical, and both rosamine[low] and rosamine[high] cells were able to undergo division and differentiation without undergoing any extensive cell death for at least a week after isolation. Cell morphology and antigenic phenotype were as seen in several previous publications.

Antioxidant and Prooxidant Drugs Modulate Self-Renewal and Differentiation Characteristics in Opposite Directions

Despite their low frequency of division, rosamine[high] O-2A/OPCs had not already irreversibly committed to differentiation *in vivo*. This was demonstrated by altering intracellular redox state through exposure to *N*-acetyl-L-cysteine (NAC), a potent antioxidant that also acts as a cysteine prodrug, thus enhancing production of glutathione, which is the most prevalent reduced thiol within cells and is crucial for maintaining a reduced intracellular environment.[30,31] Self-renewal of rosamine[high] cells was markedly enhanced in these conditions. The percentage of progenitor cell–containing clones at day 5 increased from $29 \pm 5.4\%$ to $65 \pm 3.4\%$, and the average clone size increased almost threefold, from 2.5 ± 0.4 cells to 7.0 ± 1.2 cells per clone. These results suggest that alteration of intracellular redox state is a dynamic modulator of the balance between self-renewal and differentiation rather than merely being a secondary consequence of an irrevocable fate determination.

Further studies confirmed that the balance between self-renewal and differentiation in dividing O-2A/OPCs could be modulated by manipulation of intracellular redox state. In these experiments, clonal O-2A/OPCs were grown in the presence of PDGF with or without compounds known to alter intracellular redox state. To increase oxidative levels, we used *tert*-butylhydroperoxide (*t*-BuOOH) and buthionine sulfoximine (BSO). *t*-BuOOH is a potent prooxidant,[32] while BSO inhibits synthesis of glutathione.[33] To render cells more reduced, the medium of dividing cells was supplemented with NAC. We also examined the effects of three polyhydroxyalkyl thiazolidine carboxylic acid drugs (GlcCys, ProCys, and RibCys). These procysteine drugs contribute to glutathione biosynthesis when they are taken up by cells and their thilozolidine ring is opened enzymatically.[34] Thus, the antioxidant activity of these compounds, unlike NAC, is targeted to intracellular thiol pools.

Treatment of dividing O-2A/OPCs with PDGF plus 1 mM BSO or 50 nM t-BuOOH was associated with diminished progenitor cell division and increased oligodendrocyte generation. In the presence of either BSO or t-BuOOH, approximately half of the founder cells differentiated in the absence of division, with the rest undergoing one to two divisions and yielding clones containing two to seven cells after 5 days. Average clone sizes at this time point, in either condition, were 2.1 ± 0.4 cells per clone, less than half that seen in basal division conditions (5.7 ± 0.8 cells/clone). Exposure to BSO or t-BuOOH also was associated with both a reduction in the number of clones containing only progenitor cells and an increase in the proportion of clones containing only oligodendrocytes. For example, when clones were grown in the presence of PDGF for 5 days, 43 ± 3.0% of the clones consisted wholly of progenitor cells. In contrast, in cultures exposed to PDGF plus BSO or t-BuOOH for 5 days, only 5 ± 2.4% and 7 ± 3.7% of clones consisted solely of progenitor cells, respectively. Complementary changes were seen in the proportion of clones consisting solely of oligodendrocytes. After 5 days, 88 ± 8.3% of clones exposed to BSO or 83 ± 6.0% of clones exposed to t-BuOOH consisted wholly of oligodendrocytes, as compared with complete differentiation of only 35 ± 6.6% of clones in basal division conditions.

In contrast with the effects of exposure to prooxidants, clones of O-2A/OPCs cultured in PDGF plus 1 mM NAC exhibited enhanced self-renewal and a marked reduction in oligodendrocyte generation. After 5 days in culture, clones growing in medium supplemented with NAC contained an average of 11.3 ± 2.2 cells per clone, almost twice the value seen in clones growing in the presence of PDGF alone, with many clones containing more than 15 cells. In cultures grown in the presence of NAC for 3 days, 80 ± 2.7% of clones contained only progenitor cells. Even after 5 days, 60 ± 2.8% of clones contained only progenitor cells in these conditions. In contrast, when cells were grown in basal division conditions for 3 days, 47 ± 1.1% of clones consisted only of progenitor cells, with similar values (43 ± 3.0%) observed after 5 days. Cells exposed to NAC alone (i.e., no PDGF present) differentiated into oligodendrocytes without undergoing division.

Enhanced self-renewal of O-2A/OPCs grown in the presence of NAC continued for at least 7 days. Clones examined at this time were on average six times larger than clones exposed to PDGF alone. Moreover, in cultures exposed to PDGF plus NAC for 7 days, 40 ± 5.9% of clones still contained only progenitors. In contrast, only 5 ± 2.6% of PDGF-stimulated clones consisted solely of progenitor cells after 7 days. It is important to note that in cultures exposed to PDGF plus NAC for this time, in those clones in which division occurred, 49 ± 8.5% contained one or more oligodendrocytes. Moreover, absolute numbers of oligodendrocytes in either condition were similar (151 ± 21 and 116 ± 38 for control and NAC-treated cultures, respectively), demonstrating that exposure to NAC did not preclude eventual differentiation. Supplementation of basal division medium with the cysteine prodrugs GlcCys, ProCys, or RibCys had virtually identical effects to NAC, thus suggesting that the capacity of NAC to modify intracellular thiol balance was more important to its activity than its ability to function as an extracellular antioxidant. All of the prooxidants and cysteine prodrugs examined caused the expected direction of change in intracellular redox state, as determined by rosamine fluorescence.

Signaling Molecules That Promote Differentiation Cause Greater Intracellular Oxidative Turnover, While Signaling Molecules Which Promote Self-Renewal Cause More Reduced Intracellular States

While it is possible that differences in intracellular redox state *in vivo* might be due to cell-intrinsic properties or to direct exposure to pro- or antioxidants, it is also possible that the cell-extrinsic signaling molecules that have been previously found to modulate the balance between self-renewal and differentiation have as part of their activity the modulation of redox state. We therefore next determined whether redox modulation might be of any relevance in the action of cell-extrinsic signaling molecules upon O-2A/OPCs.

Growth of cells in the presence of PDGF supplemented with factors that promote self-renewal was associated with a more reduced intracellular redox state, as indicated by rosamine fluorescence; while supplementation with inducers of differentiation was associated with increased rosamine fluorescence, indicating an increase in oxidative levels. Such effects were seen within 18 h, well before it is possible to observe any differences in progenitor or oligodendrocyte numbers. For example, after exposure of cells to NT-3 plus PDGF for 12 h, aggregate rosamine fluorescence was 15 ± 6% lower than in the presence of PDGF alone. This compares to treatment with either 1 mM NAC or 1 mM ProCys, which after 6 h in culture led to a decrease in rosamine fluorescence by 12 ± 4% and 18 ± 7%, respectively, relative to control values ($P < 0.05$). By 18 h after exposure to NT-3, relative fluorescence was 29 ± 3% lower than for control cells ($P = 0.0075$). Similarly, O-2A/OPCs exposed to PDGF plus bFGF exhibited a 23 ± 8% reduction in aggregate fluorescence values ($P < 0.05$; 18-h time point) as compared with cells exposed only to PDGF. The effect of NT-3 on redox levels was inhibited by simultaneous treatment with BSO. After exposure of cells to 1 mM BSO plus NT-3 plus PDGF for 12 h, mean rosamine fluorescence was increased by 6 ± 7% relative to growth in PDGF alone, a difference that was not significant.

Exposure to TH, which induces oligodendrocyte generation, had the opposite effect with respect to NT-3 and was associated with greater rosamine fluorescence, indicating an increase in oxidative levels. Exposure of cells to TH was associated with an 11 ± 4% increase in fluorescence after 3 h and a statistically significant (23 ± 4%; $P < 0.01$) increase in fluorescence by 12 h after initiation of treatment. This effect was significantly diminished with simultaneous exposure to 1 mM NAC: after 12 h in the presence of NAC plus TH plus PDGF, cells displayed mean rosamine fluorescence 4 ± 13% greater than control compared with the 23 ± 4% increase observed for cells grown in just TH plus PDGF ($P < 0.01$). By comparison, cells treated with either 1 mM BSO or 50 nM *t*-BuOOH for 6 h displayed an increase in rosamine fluorescence of 6 ± 3% ($P = 0.0723$) and 9 ± 2% ($P < 0.05$) over control cells, respectively (data not shown). An effect of increased oxidative activation of rosamine was also associated with exposure to bone morphogenetic protein-4 (BMP-4), even though this protein causes O-2A/OPCs to differentiate into type-2 astrocytes[16] and is thought to act through receptor and signaling systems very different from those relevant to TH action. O-2A/OPCs exposed to PDGF plus BMP-4 exhibited a significant increase in fluorescence by 12 h (25 ± 11%; $P < 0.05$), and a highly significant increase (38 ± 13%; $P = 0.004$) after 18 h. Thus, exposure to inducers of differentiation caused an increase in rosamine fluorescence, indicative of an increase in oxidative levels, independent of whether oligodendrocyte or astrocyte differentiation was being stimulated.

We also noted that the changes in geometric means of rosamine fluorescence values were associated with a redistribution of cells within the normal range of redox values, rather than an alteration of the range itself. A lower mean is associated with more cells exhibiting low levels of rosamine fluorescence, while a higher value is associated with a redistribution of cells to a more oxidatively active portion of the range. Thus, exposure to NT-3, bFGF, TH, and BMP-4 appears to alter intracellular redox profiles within a distribution that is otherwise tightly regulated as to its upper and lower boundaries.

Further demonstration of the effects on redox state of NT-3 and TH, the two signaling molecules for which the best evidence for an *in vivo* role has been provided,[15,18,21] was obtained by analysis of cells with the JC-1 dye, which provides information on mitochondrial inner membrane potential ($\Delta\Psi$). Treatment with TH for 18 h resulted in a $18 \pm 11\%$ decrease in $\Delta\Psi$ (aggregate red:green fluorescence ratio; $P < 0.05$), indicative of a more oxidative state within the cells.[35] In contrast, treatment with NT-3 for 18 h was associated with a $16 \pm 11\%$ increase in $\Delta\Psi$ ($P < 0.05$), indicative of a more reduced state within the cells.

Pharmacological Agents That Antagonize the Redox Effects of NT-3 and TH Also Antagonize Their Effects on Self-Renewal and Differentiation

We next asked whether the effects of cell-extrinsic signaling molecules on self-renewal and differentiation could be blocked by pharmacological manipulation of redox state in the opposite direction to that induced by the signaling molecule itself. As the best evidence for an *in vivo* role of such compounds in O-2A/OPC development has been provided for NT-3 and TH,[15,18,21] we specifically studied the action of these agents.

Cells grown in the presence of PDGF supplemented with TH and NAC exhibited a similar profile of self-renewal to cells grown in the presence of PDGF alone, indicating that NAC countered the effects of TH. After 5 days, $60 \pm 4.8\%$ of clones consisted of only progenitor cells in cultures exposed to TH plus NAC, a proportion even greater than that observed in clones exposed only to PDGF (i.e., $43 \pm 3.0\%$). In contrast, only $10 \pm 1.4\%$ of clones consisted entirely of progenitor cells when cells were exposed to PDGF plus TH alone. Progenitor cells were able to undergo more self-renewal when exposed to TH plus NAC, and the average clone size was 4.7 ± 1.1 cells after 5 days (as compared with 2.1 ± 0.4 cells per clone in cultures exposed to PDGF plus TH). Just under half of the clones differentiated without division when TH was present, and $81 \pm 10.8\%$ of the clones in which at least one division occurred contained one or more oligodendrocytes. When NAC was also present, in contrast, only $30 \pm 4.0\%$ of clones consisted wholly of oligodendrocytes (and most of these clones consisted of a single oligodendrocyte), and only $17 \pm 4.2\%$ of clones in which at least one division occurred contained at least one oligodendrocyte.

In complementary experiments, exposure of cells to PDGF plus 1 μM BSO inhibited the ability of NT-3 to enhance self-renewal, in agreement with our observations that BSO antagonizes the NT-3–associated alterations in redox state. Clones grown in the presence of PDGF plus NT-3 showed an increase in self-renewing divisions as determined by average clonal size (9.7 ± 1.2 cells), a 70% increase over control values. In contrast, in cultures treated also with 1 μM BSO, mean clone size after 5 days was 2.2 ± 0.4 cells, and half of the clones were single cells that differentiated into oligodendrocytes in the absence of division. NT-3 exposure also was associated with a decrease in the proportion of clones containing at least one oligodendrocyte (36 ± 2.6% by day 5, as compared with 57 ± 3.0% in basal division medium). BSO inhibited this effect, and 74 ± 5.7% of clones contained at least one oligodendrocyte in cultures treated with NT-3 plus BSO.

The above results indicate strongly that the redox alterations caused by NT-3 and TH are essential to the mechanism by which these cell-signaling molecules modulate the balance between self-renewal and differentiation. Because BSO inhibits glutathione production, thus making cells more oxidized, our results suggest that the ability of NT-3 to render cells more reduced is necessary for this signaling molecule to promote self-renewal. Similarly, the ability of NAC to protect against oxidative agents suggests that the increased intracellular oxidation associated with exposure to TH may be a necessary aspect of the mechanism by which TH enhances oligodendrocyte generation.

BALANCE BETWEEN SELF-RENEWAL AND DIFFERENTION IN O-2A/ OPCs FROM DIVERSE CNS REGIONS REVEALS REDOX-ASSOCIATED, CELL-INTRINSIC DIFFERENCES IN TIMING OF MYELINATION

A2B5+ Precursor Cells Isolated from P7 Rat Cortex, Optic Chiasm, and Optic Nerve Exhibit Identical Patterns of Response to Inducers of Astrocyte Generation

One of the most critical means by which a precursor cell population is defined is by determining what kind of differentiated progeny it may generate. In particular, in respect to glial precursor cells of the CNS, the characterization of a novel A2B5+ tripotential glial-restricted progenitor (GRP) cell from embryonic spinal cord has demonstrated the importance of identifying the kinds of astrocytes to which a precursor cell may give rise. GRP cells and O-2A/OPCs differ markedly in their response to inducers of astrocyte generation. Specifically, GRP cells exposed to either fetal calf serum or bone morphogenetic proteins give rise predominantly to A2B5− astrocytes with a flattened fibroblast-like morphology (i.e., type-1 astrocytes) while O-2A/OPCs exposed to these same inducers of differentiation give rise exclusively to A2B5+ stellate (i.e., type-2) astrocytes.[36,37]

Examination of the response of A2B5+ cells purified from cortex (CX), optic chiasm (OC), and optic nerve (ON) of P7 rats to 3 days of exposure to FCS or BMP-4 confirmed that all of these populations were O-2A/OPCs. All astrocytes generated expressed the stellate A2B5+GFAP+ phenotype of type-2 astrocytes (as described previously for ON[36,37]) with no generation of type-1 astrocytes. All of these populations also give rise to oligodendrocytes.

Optic Chasm O-2A/OPCs and Cortex O-2A/OPCs Differ from Optic Nerve O-2A/OPCs in Their Capacity to Undergo Self-Renewal When Grown in the Presence of Platelet-Derived Growth Factor

Examination of the *in vitro* development of purified O-2A/OPCs (ON), O-2A/OPCs (OC), and O-2A/OPCs (CX) progenitor cells in cultures exposed to PDGF revealed that although all populations were responsive to this mitogen, strikingly different patterns of differentiation were seen.[22] Both O-2A/OPCs (OC) and O-2A/OPCs (CX) displayed much greater tendencies than O-2A/OPCs (ON) to undergo self-renewing divisions (in contrast to generating nondividing oligodendrocytes).

O-2A/OPCs (ON) grown in the basal growth conditions that we have previously described to promote cell division and allow oligodendrocyte generation for these cells (i.e., DMEM-BS/PDGF$^+$, TH$^-$, as described in Ref. 15) yielded results similar to those seen previously. In addition, $57 \pm 11\%$ (mean $\pm$ SEM) of clones of O-2A/OPCs (ON) contained at least one oligodendrocyte after 3 days of *in vitro* growth in these conditions, and this proportion increased to $86 \pm 8\%$ after 6 days of *in vitro* growth and $94 \pm 4\%$ after 7 days of *in vitro* growth. The percentage of oligodendrocytes in these cultures was $21 \pm 11\%$ on day 3, $53 \pm 15\%$ on day 6, and $56 \pm 15\%$ on day 7.

O-2A/OPCs (OC) exhibited markedly reduced generation of oligodendrocytes as compared with O-2A/OPCs (ON). After 3 days of *in vitro* growth, $25 \pm 8\%$ of clones of O-2A/OPCs (OC) contained oligodendrocytes, less than half the value obtained for O-2A/OPCs (ON). Even after 6 days of *in vitro* growth, only $36 \pm 13\%$ of clones of O-2A/OPCs (OC) contained oligodendrocytes. Indeed, if we specifically excluded those cells that differentiated in the absence of any division (and those yielded clones consisting of one oligodendrocyte), only $2 \pm 1\%$ of the clones of O-2A/OPCs (OC) contained oligodendrocytes at this time point. The relative absence of oligodendrocyte generation at the clonal level was associated with a greatly reduced contribution of oligodendrocytes to the total culture of O-2A/OPCs (OC) as compared with O-2A/OPCs (ON) .

Self-renewal was even more enhanced, and generation of oligodendrocytes even more reduced, in populations of O-2A/OPCs (CX) than in cells derived from the optic nerve or optic chiasm. In clones of O-2A/OPCs (CX) grown in DMEM-BS/TH$^-$, only $3 \pm 2\%$ of clones contained at least one oligodendrocyte after 3 days of *in vitro* growth, and this proportion increased only to $6 \pm 6\%$ after 7 days of *in vitro* growth. Even after 10 days of *in vitro* growth, less than $20 \pm 1\%$ of O-2A/OPC (CX) clones grown in PDGF contained one or more oligodendrocytes. Similarly, the overall percentage of oligodendrocytes in O-2A/OPC (CX) cultures was markedly lower in O-2A/OPC (CX) clones than in clones of O-2A/OPCs (ON) at all time points analyzed. The percentage of oligodendrocytes seen in clonal cultures of O-2A/OPCs (CX) was $<2\%$ on days 3, 7, and 10 in these basal division conditions. Even in those clones that did contain oligodendrocytes, the proportion of oligodendrocytes in these clones was still low: these clones rarely contained more than one to two oligodendrocytes regardless of the number of O-2A/OPCs found within the clone.

The ability of O-2A/OPCs (CX) to undergo extended self-renewal when exposed to PDGF was associated with the generation of large clonal sizes and with division that continued for several weeks of *in vitro* growth. O-2A/OPCs (CX) isolated as single cells and grown in the presence of PDGF for 10 days generated clones with average sizes of 100 ± 16 cells/clone, a threefold expansion in clonal size over that observed on day 7. In contrast, clones derived from ON did not exhibit significant expansion in their numbers after day 7, at which time point the average clonal size was 7 ± 4 cells. Moreover, O-2A/OPCs (CX) cells were capable of dividing for more than 6 weeks when exposed continuously to PDGF.

The Differing Self-Renewal Potentials of O-2A/OPCs (CX) and O-2A/OPCs (OC) as Compared with O-2A/OPCs (ON) Cells Appear to Be Due to Cell-Intrinsic Differences

One possible explanation for the differing behaviors of O-2A/OPCs from the different CNS regions examined could be that cells that undergo more self-renewal secrete a factor(s) that promotes this process and/or that precursor cell populations more likely to differentiate secrete a factor(s) that curtails self-renewal and promotes differentiation. To examine these possibilities, we first tested whether O-2A/OPCs (CX) were secreting soluble factors that promoted self-renewal by growing O-2A/OPCs (ON) in the presence of O-2A/OPCs (CX) and examining the generation of oligodendrocytes by the O-2A/OPCs (ON). In converse experiments, we determined whether soluble factor(s) secreted by O-2A/OPCs (ON) could enhance oligodendrocyte generation by O-2A/OPCs (CX). Cells were plated in ratios of 1:20, with the population to be examined in a smaller dot surrounded by a larger ring of the putative producers of a modulatory factor(s). (Cells in the dot numbered 800–1000; in the ring, 10,000–30,000.) As controls, we cultured both the O-2A/OPCs (CX) and the O-2A/OPCs (ON) in the presence of other cells of the same type. To determine whether co-culture might alter the ability of one population to influence the behavior of the other population, we also grew the cells in medium conditioned by either progenitor population in the absence of coculture.

We found that the likelihood of O-2A/OPCs (CX) and O-2A/OPCs (ON) undergoing either self-renewal or differentiation into oligodendrocytes was unchanged by exposure to medium conditioned by the other cell type. Whether O-2A/OPCs (CX) were grown in the presence of O-2A/OPCs (ON), or in the two control conditions of either no additional cells or additional cortical cells, $<2\%$ of the cells differentiated into oligodendrocytes over 5 days of growth in DMEM-BS/TH$^-$, PDGF$^+$. Control cultures of ON-derived O-2A/OPCs had a >10-fold higher representation of oligodendrocytes than was seen in comparable cultures of O-2A/OPCs (CX). Although growth in the presence of a larger number of either O-2A/OPCs (CX) or O-2A/OPCs (ON) was associated with a slightly lower representation of oligodendrocytes than occurred in noncoculture controls, the differences were not significant.

Similar results to those in the above coculture experiments were obtained when O-2A/OPCs (ON) or O-2A/OPCs (OC) were exposed to conditioned medium from either cells from the same or the comparative tissue. Cells derived from the ON exhibited extensive differentiation, while cells derived from chiasm exhibited extensive self-renewal.

O-2A/OPCs (OC) and O-2A/OPCs (CX) Differ from O-2A/OPCs (ON) in Their Responsiveness to TH and to Ciliary Neurotrophic Factor as Inducers of Differentiation

We next examined the responsiveness of O-2A/OPCs (OC) and O-2A/OPCs (CX) to two well-characterized inducers of oligodendrocyte generation, TH and ciliary neurotrophic factor (CNTF),[13-15] to determine whether these cells also differed from their ON-derived counterparts in their responsiveness to these signaling molecules.

Both O-2A/OPCs (OC) and O-2A/OPCs (CX) were induced to generate oligo-dendrocytes by exposure to TH, but the extent of induction was markedly less than was observed in cultures of ON-derived cells. In OC-derived cells, TH exposure was associated with a marked reduction in the proportion of clones consisting only of O-2A/OPCs after 6 days of *in vitro* growth (22 ± 9% in the presence of TH, 64 ± 13% without), as well as with a marked increase in the number of clones containing only oligodendrocytes (49 ± 9% in the presence of TH, 28 ± 5% without). The extent of oligodendrocyte generation that occurred in these cultures was less than that ob-served in ON-derived cultures, in which 14 ± 8% of the clones consisted only of pre-cursor cells at this time point in the absence of TH, and 6 ± 5% when TH was present.

O-2A/OPCs (CX) were even less responsive to TH exposure than were O-2A/OPCs (OC), although the cortical cells did exhibit some TH responsiveness. Expo-sure of O-2A/OPCs (CX) to TH for 7 days was associated with a marked increase in the generation of oligodendrocytes, with an eightfold increase in the percentage of clones containing only oligodendrocytes (2% vs. 16%) and a 3.5-fold increase in the number of clones containing at least one oligodendrocyte (16% vs. 58%). Still fur-ther increases in the proportion of clones containing at least one oligodendrocyte were seen after 10 days of *in vitro* growth in the presence of TH. At this time point, 93 ± 2% of the clones contained at least one oligodendrocyte, thus confirming that the overwhelming majority of these clones were capable of generating oligodendro-cytes. Nonetheless, when compared directly with the extent of differentiation seen in cultures of O-2A/OPCs (ON) grown in these conditions, it was apparent that even when grown in the presence of TH, cultures of O-2A/OPCs (CX) were far less likely to exhibit extensive differentiation than was seen in the ON-derived cultures. For ex-ample, after 7 days of growth in the presence of TH, only 5 ± 2% of the total O-2A/OPC lineage cells in O-2A/OPC (CX) cultures were oligodendrocytes, as compared with >80% of cells in O-2A/OPC (ON) cultures.

CNTF also was able to induce oligodendrocyte generation in cultures of O-2A/OPCs (OC), but to a lesser extent than was seen in cultures of O-2A/OPCs (ON). Af-ter 3 days of *in vitro* growth in the presence of PDGF, 25 ± 8% of O-2A/OPC (OC) clones contained oligodendrocytes. When CNTF was present in the cultures, 34 ± 5% of the clones contained oligodendrocytes. When grown in minimal division me-dium supplemented with CNTF for 6 days, 73 ± 8% of O-2A/OPC (OC) clones con-tained oligodendrocytes in the presence of CNTF, as compared to only 36 ± 13% of clones containing oligodendrocytes at this time point in the absence of CNTF. The proportionate representation of oligodendrocytes in these cultures was similarly modulated, such that 86 ± 6% of O-2A/OPCs (ON) were oligodendrocytes after 6 days of growth in the presence of CNTF, as compared with a 34 ± 11% representa-tion of oligodendrocytes in cultures of O-2A/OPC (OC). Similarly, on day 6, 36 ±

13% of clones contained oligodendrocytes in the absence of CNTF, and $73 \pm 18\%$ of clones contained oligodendrocytes in the presence of CNTF.

In contrast with effects on O-2A/OPC (ON) and O-2A/OPC (OC) populations, CNTF was far less effective at inducing oligodendrocyte generation in O-2A/OPC (CX) cultures. When these cells were grown in the presence of CNTF for 7 days, ~2 $\pm 1\%$ differentiated into oligodendrocytes, as compared with a figure of $\leq 1 \pm 0\%$ in cultures exposed to PDGF alone. The proportion of clones containing oligodendrocytes in the absence and presence of CNTF was also approximately the same after 7 days in culture ($6 \pm 6\%$ in the absence of CNTF, and $7 \pm 1\%$ when CNTF was present). However, CNTF did have an effect on 0-2A/OPC (CX) cultures by reducing cell numbers within a clone, presumably by slowing the rate of cell division. The average clone size in the presence of CNTF was 8 ± 2 cells, as compared with 31 ± 9 cells in its absence. CNTF also seemed slightly to enhance differentiation induction by TH. As mentioned above, the percentage of oligodendrocytes generated by O-2A/OPC (CX) after 7 days *in vitro* growth was $5 \pm 2\%$ in the presence of TH and $2 \pm 1\%$ in the presence of CNTF. In contrast, exposure to both factors induced $12 \pm 4\%$ of O-2A/OPC (CX) progenitors to become oligodendrocytes, a very marked increase over the value of $0.2 \pm 0.2\%$ observed in cultures growing in the presence of PDGF alone.

Freshly Isolated O-2A/OPCs (ON), O-2A/OPCs (OC), and O-2A/OPCs (CX) Exhibit Differences in Their Intracellular Redox States, with the Degree of Oxidation Correlating Inversely with the Capacity for Self-Renewal

The differences between O-2A/OPCs from ON, OC, and CX bear a striking resemblance to the differences we found to be associated with the redox balance of ON-derived O-2A/OPCs. As discussed earlier, in our studies on ON-derived cells, we found that freshly isolated O-2A/OPCs that possessed a relatively reduced intracellular environment were most likely to undergo continued self-renewing divisions when grown in the presence of PDGF. In contrast, when grown in precisely the same conditions, cells that were more oxidized were more likely to differentiate into oligodendrocytes in the absence of extensive *in vitro* division. Moreover, we found that pharmacological manipulation to make cells more reduced antagonized the differentiation-inducing abilities of TH. Thus, in several respects, the behavior of O-2A/OPCs (OC) and, to an even greater degree O-2A/OPCs (CX), resembled the behavior of O-2A/OPCs (ON) with a more reduced intracellular redox state. Therefore, to determine whether O-2A/OPCs isolated from ON, OC, or CX differed in their intracellular redox state in a manner consistent with their self-renewal characteristics, we labeled freshly isolated cells with rosamine and analyzed them by flow cytometry.

O-2A/OPCs (CX) progenitors displayed significantly lower levels of oxidative equivalents (as determined by rosamine fluorescence) than either O-2A/OPCs (ON) or O-2A/OPCs (OC) ($P < 0.05$), indicating a more reducing intracellular environment in O-2A/OPCs (CX). Data from six independent trials were compiled and standardized so that the fluorescence level of O-2A/OPCs (CX) was set equal to 100 units (± 21 units SEM). In comparison, average fluorescence of O-2A/OPCs (ON) progenitors was 207 ± 41 units, indicating greater oxidative turnover of the fluorescent probe. O-2A/OPCs (OC) had an intermediate level of mean fluorescence at 180 ± 39 units, significantly higher than the mean fluorescence of O-2A/OPCs (CX).

This value was, in addition, lower than that for O-2A/OPCs (ON), though not significantly ($P = 0.212$). Thus, these results point to a trend in intracellular redox state between freshly isolated O-2A/OPCs (CX), O-2A/OPCs (OC), and O-2A/OPCs (ON), such that those cells that undergo the most self-renewal (i.e., O-2A/OPCs [CX]) were the most reduced, those that undergo the least self-renewal (i.e., O-2A/OPCs [ON]) were the most oxidized, and O-2A/OPCs (OC) were intermediate both in respect to self-renewal and intracellular redox state.

DISCUSSION

The results presented point to a remarkable association between redox regulation and precursor cell function. In the first portion of these studies,[5] we discovered that intracellular redox state modulation appears to be a central biochemical/molecular regulator of the balance between self-renewal and differentiation. In particular, redox state modulation satisfies all of the following criteria required to support such a conclusion:

(1) The proposed regulator should be altered in its level and/or function by cell-extrinsic signaling molecules that modulate the balance between self-renewal and differentiation, with signaling molecules that have opposite effects on self-renewal and differentiation exerting opposite effects on the proposed regulator.

(2) Alterations like those caused by exposure to these signaling molecules should have the same effect as the signaling molecules themselves.

(3) Substances that antagonize the alterations in the regulator caused by the cell-extrinsic signaling molecules should block their effects on this balance.

(4) Progenitor cell populations isolated from developing animals on the basis of the state of the proposed regulator should exhibit predictably different self-renewal characteristics consistent with the outcome of the other analyses.

Identification of a biochemical/molecular regulator that meets all of the above criteria is a strikingly different outcome from past efforts to understand how the balance between self-renewal and differentiation is controlled. For example, the strongest evidence for a protein that might represent such a regulator has been reported for the cyclin-dependent kinase inhibitor p27^{Kip1}. P27 levels progressively accumulate as O-2A/OPCs proliferate,[38] and O-2A/OPCs isolated from p27$^{-/-}$ mice undergo more division than do wild-type cells.[39,40] Ectopic p27 expression, however, causes O-2A/OPCs to undergo cell cycle arrest in the absence of differentiation,[41] a different outcome from that of rendering dividing O-2A/OPCs slightly more oxidized by exposure to TH or pharmacological prooxidants. Moreover, no data has been provided that p27 levels are predictive of self-renewal potential or that experimental alterations in p27 levels yield the characteristic outcomes caused by TH, NT-3, or redox manipulation. Thus, while p27 may be a part of the mechanism that modulates the balance between self-renewal and differentiation, the evidence for intracellular redox state as a central modulator appears to be more comprehensive.

The second portion of these studies[22] initially were focused on what appeared to be a quite separate issue, that of whether differing times of myelination in different regions of the CNS might in any way be associated with the properties of the resident precursor cell populations. Characterization of precursor cells for oligodendrocytes isolated from ON, OC, and CX of P7 rats has revealed that each of these populations expresses distinct biological properties. In particular, cells isolated from ON, OC, and CX of identically aged rats show marked differences in their tendency to undergo self-renewing division and in their sensitivity to known inducers of oligodendrocyte generation. Precursor cells isolated from the CX, a CNS region where myelination is a more protracted process than in the ON, appear to be intrinsically more likely to begin generating oligodendrocytes at a later stage and over a longer time period than cells isolated from the ON, raising the possibility that the different time courses of myelination in these CNS regions may reflect different biological properties of the resident precursor cell population.

It was striking that the redox state of O-2A/OPCs from different CNS regions showed an excellent correlation with the properties expressed by cells of the ON in which redox state was experimentally manipulated. In particular, those cells with the greatest self-renewal potential (i.e., cortical O-2A/OPCs), and the least response to inducers of oligodendrocyte generation, exhibited the most reduced redox state when examined as freshly isolated cells.

Previous studies had already demonstrated that O-2A/OPCs isolated from animals of different ages can have different properties.[42–45] The results described here extend such observations on heterogeneity to demonstrate that the CNS of early postnatal rats contains multiple O-2A/OPCs that exhibit markedly different properties, both in respect to their intrinsic tendency to undergo self-renewing divisions and in their response to inducers of oligodendrocyte generation. These differences, which appear to be cell intrinsic and also appear to be correlated with intracellular redox state, indicate a previously unanticipated complexity of phenotypes among precursor cells that give rise to the same differentiated cell type. The characteristics of these populations are such as to be consistent with the hypothesis that differences in the timing of myelinogenesis may be due, at least in part, to the local utilization of oligodendrocyte precursor cell populations with fundamentally different properties.

One of the surprising findings to emerge from our studies was the extent to which self-renewal characteristics and response to inducers of differentiation differed in precursor cells that all give rise to oligodendrocytes and are isolated from postnatal animals of a single age. For example, O-2A/OPCs isolated even from adjoining CNS regions, the ON and the OC, exhibited marked differences in their probability of undergoing differentiation when grown in the presence of PDGF sans inducers of differentation (such as TH and CNTF). Still more different from ON-derived cells were O-2A/OPCs (CX), which were able to undergo continuous self-renewal for many days when grown in basal division conditions, generating large clones of up to 300 cells that consisted predominantly of O-2A/OPCs and containing very few oligodendrocytes. Even after 10 days of *in vitro* growth in these conditions, the average clonal composition in O-2A/OPC (CX) cultures consisted of 99.5% progenitors and 0.5% oligodendrocytes. The average clonal composition in O-2A/OPC (ON) cultures at this time point, in contrast, was 37% O-2A/OPCs and 63% oligodendrocytes. Indeed, OPCs (CX) derived from P7 rats could be maintained as dividing cells in basal division medium for at least 6 weeks (unpublished observations), a continuation of division that we have never observed in cultures of O-2A/OPCs (ON) grown in these conditions.

The varied properties we have observed in different O-2A/OPC populations could theoretically represent a developmental progression, for which the phenotype of O-2A/OPC (ON) cells represents the most mature pattern of behavior. While it is difficult to rule out this possibility, some observations suggest that, at least for O-2A/OPC (CX) cells, this may not be true. As all cells were isolated from animals of the same age, invoking a developmental progression would require positing a different timing of this progression in each tissue, which would still make these populations biologically different from one another. Indeed, the fact that O-2A/OPCs (CX) continue to express their characteristic potential for continuous and extended self-renewal even after 6 weeks of *in vitro* growth suggests that if such a transition occurs, it may occur over quite a long time frame. In addition, O-2A/OPCs (CX) derived from P13 CX remain far more prone to undergoing self-renewal than O-2A/OPCs (ON) isolated from P7 animals (unpublished observations). For example, <20% of O-2A/OPC (CX) clones derived from P13 rats contained one or more oligodendrocytes after 7 days of *in vitro* growth in the basal division conditions of DMEM-BS/ TH$^-$, PDGF$^+$, as compared with a value of 94% for O-2A/OPC (ON) clones from P7 rats. The proportion of P13-derived O-2A/OPC (CX) clones containing at least one oligodendrocyte was increased to 67% in the presence of TH, but even in these conditions only 25% of the cells in the cultures actually differentiated into oligodendrocytes after 7 days (as compared with a value of 56% for O-2A/OPC (ON) cells from P7 rats). Thus, it is possible that the CX-derived cells are continuously different from their counterparts isolated from other regions of the CNS. Considering prior suggestions that O-2A/OPCs of the ON migrate into this tissue from the OC,[46,47] however, we suspect it is more likely that the nerve and chiasm populations will be found to represent a developmental continuum.

We suggest that our present results may be analogous with our earlier discovery that O-2A/OPCs isolated from postnatal and adult ON express properties consistent with the physiological requirements of the tissue of origin.[42–44,48,49] O-2A/OPCs isolated from perinatal and adult ON (originally termed O-2A^{perinatal} and O-2A^{adult} progenitor cells, respectively, in our earlier studies on these populations) differ in a number of characteristics. In contrast with the rapid cell cycle times (18 ± 4 h) and migration (21.4 ± 1.6 µm h^{-1}) of O-2A/OPCs^{perinatal} progenitor cells, O-2A/OPC-^{adult} progenitor cells exposed to identical growth conditions divide *in vitro* with cell cycle times of 65 ± 18 h and migrate at rates of 4.3 ± 0.7 µm h^{-1}. Moreover, when grown in conditions that promote the differentiation into oligodendrocytes of all members of clonal families of O-2A/OPC^{perinatal} progenitor cells, O-2A/OPC^{adult} progenitor cells exhibit extensive asymmetric behavior and continuously generate both oligodendrocytes and more progenitor cells.[49] In short, O-2A/OPC^{perinatal} progenitor cells express properties that might reasonably be expected to be required during early CNS development (e.g., rapid division and migration, and the ability to rapidly generate large numbers of oligodendrocytes). In contrast, O-2A/OPC^{adult} progenitor cells express stem cell-like properties that appear to be more consistent with the requirements for maintenance of a largely stable oligodendrocyte population and the ability to enter rapid division, as might be required for repair of demyelinated lesions.[42,48,49]

If it is correct that distinctive physiological requirements of tissues of dissimilar developmental ages are associated with different biological properties of their resident precursor cells, then similar principles might apply also at a single physiological age. In analogy with our proposal that the differences between O-2A/OPC^{adult} and O-2A/OPC^{perinatal} progenitor cells of the rat ON are reflective of the differing physiological requirements of tissue development and tissue homeostasis, we propose that the differences that distinguish O-2A/OPCs (ON), O-2A/OPCs (OC), and O-2A/OPCs (CX) reflect differing physiological requirements of the tissues to which these cell contribute. For example, a variety of experiments have indicated that the O-2A/OPC population of the ON arises from a germinal zone located in or near the OC and enters the nerve by migration.[46,50] Thus, it would not be surprising if progenitor cells of the OC expressed properties expected of cells at a potentially earlier stage of development than those cells that are isolated from ON of the same physiological age. Such properties would be expected to include the capacity to undergo a greater extent of self-renewal, much as has been seen when the properties of O-2A/OPCs from ONs of embryonic rats and postnatal rats have been compared.[45] In respect to the properties of cortical progenitor cells, physiological considerations also appear to be consistent with our observations. The CX is one of the last regions of the CNS in which myelination is initiated, and the process of myelination also can continue for extended periods in this region.[23-25] If the biology of a precursor cell population is reflective of the developmental characteristics of the tissue in which it resides, then one might expect that O-2A/OPCs isolated from this tissue would not initiate oligodendrocyte generation until a later time than occurs with O-2A/OPCs isolated from structures in which myelination occurs earlier. In addition, cortical O-2A/OPCs might be physiologically required to make oligodendrocytes for a longer time due to the long period of continued development in this tissue, at least as this has been defined in the human CNS (see, e.g., Refs. 27 and 28).

Our findings extend upon our previous analyses of oligodendrocyte development by demonstrating expression of tissue-specific properties as well as age-specific properties by cells that share the common property of being able to generate oligodendrocytes. Moreover, the observation that cell-intrinsic differences might be associated with different levels of responsiveness to inducers of differentiation adds a new degree of complexity to our understanding of the means by which the balance between self-renewal and differentiation is modulated in dividing O-2A/OPCs once oligodendrocyte generation begins. We previously proposed that once this stage of oligodendrocyte creation is initiated, the regulation of differentiation is shifted from control by a cell-intrinsic biological clock to regulation by the environment.[15] Our present results suggest that the extent of environmental regulation that occurs is modulated by cell-intrinsic properties that modify responsiveness to environmental signals.

It will be important to determine whether the differences we have observed will be associated with differing patterns and extents of oligodendrocyte production following transplantation of these various populations *in vivo*. Although it is well established that transplanted O-2A/OPCs can readily repair demyelinating damage (see, e.g., Refs. 8, 51, and 52), it might be that cells with the characteristics of O-2A/OPCs (CX) can generate a larger number of oligodendrocytes from each injected cell than would be the case for O-2A/OPCs (ON), an outcome that would indicate a greater potential utility of O-2A/OPC (CX)-like cells in such applications.

Our results raise the intriguing possibility that at least one of the cell-intrinsic properties that regulate self-renewal and responsiveness to environmental factors is intracellular redox state. It seems particularly striking that the differences between

O-2A/OPC (CX), O-2A/OPC (OC), and O-2A/OPC (ON) populations are very much like differences we found being modulated by intracellular redox state in studies on purified ON-derived O-2A/OPCs.[5,22] In this regard, we were particularly intrigued to find that the comparative redox states of these three populations were precisely as would be predicted from our other analyses. Such results make it seem an attractive hypothesis that cell-intrinsic mechanisms contributing to redox state modulation play an important role in regulating fundamental aspects of precursor cell function. If this is correct, then deciphering what these cell-intrinsic mechanisms might be should prove of considerable interest.

Available data from the study of several biological systems provides strong reason to believe that redox modulation functions as a central integrator of multiple processes related to self-renewal and differentiation, rather than as a controller of a single unique downstream effector pathway. Many different signaling pathways appear to converge on regulation of redox state, and redox alterations can in turn modulate several different pathways of possible relevance in modulation of self-renewal and differentiation. Several components of the redox regulatory network can be altered by exposure of cell to such cell-extrinsic signaling molecules as neurotrophins,[53,54] type 1 interferon,[55] stem cell factor,[56] transforming growth factor-β,[57] inflammatory cytokines (see, e.g., Ref. 58), and thyroid hormone,[59] and also by ras activation.[60] Increased levels of oxidative stress can in turn induce elevations in proteins (such as the cyclin-dependent kinase inhibitor p21[waf1/cip1]; see Ref. 61) and could potentially modify function of transcription complexes (such as AP-1; see Ref. 62), thus affecting cell division and/or differentiation. In addition, intracellular redox state can itself impinge on many aspects of cell signaling (see, e.g., Ref. 63 for review). In this context, one of the more intriguing aspects of our studies is the observation that what appear to be relatively small changes in intracellular redox state are associated with profound differences in cellular behavior. Such observations are consistent with findings that as little as a 10% decrease in average glutathione levels significantly decreases calcium influx in peripheral blood lymphocytes stimulated with anti-CD3 antibody.[64] An ability of relatively small changes in redox state to modulate cell function would enable this fundamental component of cellular physiology to function as a highly sensitive central rheostat that integrates cell-intrinsic states with cell-extrinsic signals.

REFERENCES

1. BERTONCELLO, I., G. HODGSON & T. BRADLEY. 1985. Multiparameter analysis of transplantable hemopoietic stem cells: I. The separation and enrichment of stem cells homing to marrow and spleen on the basis of rhodamine-123 fluorescence. Exp. Hematol. **13:** 999–1006.
2. MULDER, A. & J. VISSER. 1987. Separation and functional analysis of bone marrow cells separated by rhodamine-123 fluorescence. Exp. Hematol. **15:** 99–104.
3. REID, L. 1996. Stem cell/lineage biology and lineage-dependent extracellular matrix chemistry. *In* Textbook of Tissue Engineering. R. Lanza, R. Langer & W. Chick, Eds. R.G. Landes. Austin, TX.
4. KIM, M., D. COOPER, S. HAYES & G. SPANGRUDE. 1998. Rhodamine-123 staining in hematopoietic stem cells of young mice indicates mitochondrial activation rather than dye efflux. Blood **91:** 4106–4117.
5. SMITH, J., E. LADI, M. MAYER-PRÖSCHEL & M. NOBLE. 2000. Redox state is a central modulator of the balance between self-renewal and differentiation in a dividing glial precursor cell. Proc. Natl. Acad. Sci. USA **97:** 10032–10037.

6. MILLER, R.H., C. FRENCH CONSTANT & M.C. RAFF. 1989. The macroglial cells of the rat optic nerve. Annu. Rev. Neurosci. **12:** 517–534.
7. RAFF, M.C., R.H. MILLER & M. NOBLE. 1983. Glial cell lineages in the rat optic nerve. Cold Spring Harbor Symp. Quant. Biol. **48:** 569–572.
8. GROVES, A.K. *et al.* 1993. Repair of demyelinated lesions by transplantation of purified O-2A progenitor cells. Nature **362:** 453–455.
9. NOBLE, M., K. MURRAY, P. STROOBANT, *et al.* 1988. Platelet-derived growth factor promotes division and motility and inhibits premature differentiation of the oligodendrocyte/type-2 astrocyte progenitor cell. Nature **333:** 560–562.
10. RICHARDSON, W.D., N. PRINGLE, M.J. MOSLEY, *et al.* 1988. A role for platelet-derived growth factor in normal gliogenesis in the central nervous system. Cell **53:** 309–319.
11. RICHARDSON, W.D., N. PRINGLE, M. MOSLEY, *et al.* 1988. A role for platelet-derived growth factor in normal gliogenesis in the central nervous system. Cell **53:** 309–319.
12. YAKOVLEV, A.Y., K. BOUCHER, M. MAYER-PRÖSCHEL & M. NOBLE. 1998. Quantitative insight into proliferation and differentiation of O-2A progenitor cells in vitro: the clock model revisited. Proc. Natl. Acad. Sci. USA **95:** 14164–14167.
13. BARRES, B.A., M.A. LAZAR & M.C. RAFF. 1994. A novel role for thyroid hormone, glucocorticoids and retinoic acid in timing oligodendrocyte development. Development **120:** 1097–1108.
14. MAYER, M., K. BHAKOO & M. NOBLE. 1994. Ciliary neurotrophic factor and leukemia inhibitory factor promote the generation, maturation and survival of oligodendrocytes in vitro. Development **120:** 142–153.
15. IBARROLA, N., M. MAYER-PROSCHEL, A. RODRIGUEZ-PENA & M. NOBLE. 1996. Evidence for the existence of at least two timing mechanisms that contribute to oligodendrocyte generation in vitro. Dev. Biol. **180:** 1–21.
16. MABIE, P. *et al.* 1997. Bone morphogenetic proteins induce astroglial differentiation of oligodendroglial-astroglial progenitor cells. Neuroscience **17:** 4112–4120.
17. BÖGLER, O., D. WREN, S.C. BARNETT, *et al.* 1990. Cooperation between two growth factors promotes extended self-renewal and inhibits differentiation of oligodendrocyte-type-2 astrocytes (O-2A) progenitor cells. Proc. Natl. Acad. Sci. USA **87:** 6368–6372.
18. BARRES, B.A., *et al.* 1994. A crucial role for neurotrophin-3 in oligodendrocyte development. Nature **367:** 371–375.
19. TEMPLE, S. & M.C. RAFF. 1986. Clonal analysis of oligodendrocyte development in culture: evidence for a developmental clock that counts cell division. Cell **44:** 773–779.
20. RAFF, M.C., L.E. LILLIEN, W.D. RICHARDSON, *et al.* 1988. Platelet-derived growth factor from astrocytes drives the clock that times oligodendrocyte development in culture. Nature **333:** 562–565.
21. AHLGREN, S., H. WALLACE, J. BISHOP, *et al.* 1997. Effects of thyroid hormone on embryonic oligodendrocyte precursor cell development in vivo and in vitro. Mol. Cell. Neurosci. **9:** 420–432.
22. POWER, J., M. MAYER-PROSCHEL, J. SMITH & M. NOBLE. 2002. Oligodendrocyte precursor cells from different brain regions express divergent properties consistent with the differing time courses of myelination in these regions. Dev. Biol. **245:** 362–375.
23. MACKLIN, W.B. & C.L. WEILL. 1985. Appearance of myelin proteins during development in the chick central nervous system. Dev. Neurosci. **7:** 170–178.
24. KINNEY, H.C., B.A. BRODY, A.S. KLOMAN & F.H. GILLES. 1988. Sequence of central nervous sytem myelination in human infancy. II. Patterns of myelination in autopsied infants. J. Neuropath. Exp. Neurol. **47:** 217–234.
25. FORAN, D.R. & A.C. PETERSON. 1992. Myelin acquisition in the central nervous system of the mouse revealed by an MBP-LacZ transgene. J. Neurosci. **12:** 4890–4897.
26. SKOFF, R.P., D. TOLAND & E. NAST. 1980. Pattern of myelination and distribution of neuroglial cells along the developing optic system of the rat and rabbit. J. Comp. Neurol. **191:** 237–253.
27. YAKOVLEV, P.L. & A.R. LECOURS. 1967. The myelogenetic cycles of regional maturation of the brain. *In* Regional Development of the Brain in Early Life. A. Minkowski *et al.*, Eds.: 3–70. Blackwell, Oxford.

28. BENES, F.M., M. TURTLE, Y. KHAN & P. FAROL. 1994. Myelination of a key relay zone in the hippocampal formation occurs in the human brain during childhood, adolescence and adulthood. Arch. Gen. Psychiatry **51:** 477–484.
29. WHITAKER, J.E., P.L. MOORE, R.P. HAUGLAND & R.P. HAUGLAND. 1991. Dihydrotetramethylrosamine: a long wave-length fluorogenic peroxidase substrate evaluated in vitro and in a model phagocyte. Biochem. Biophys. Res. Commun. **175:** 387–393.
30. MEISTER, A., M.E. ANDERSON & O. HWANG. 1986. Intracellular cysteine and glutathione delivery systems. J. Am. Coll. Nutr. **5:** 137–151.
31. MEISTER, A. & M.E. ANDERSON. 1983. Glutathione. Annu. Rev. Biochem. **52:** 711–760.
32. OCHI, T. 1993. Mechanism for the changes in the levels of glutathione upon exposure of cultured mammalian cells to tertiary-butylhydroperoxide and diamide. Arch. Toxicol. **67:** 401–410.
33. MARTENSSON, J. *et al.* 1991. Inhibition of glutathione synthesis in the newborn rat: a model for endogenously produced oxidative stress. Proc. Natl. Acad. Sci. USA **88:** 9360–9364.
34. ROBERTS, J., H. NAGASAWA, R. ZERA, *et al.* 1987. Prodrugs of L-cysteine as protective agents against acetaminophen-induced hepatotoxicity. 2-(Polyhydroxyalkyl)- and 2-(polyacetoxyalkyl)thiazolidine-4(R)-carboxylic acids. J. Med. Chem. **30:** 1891–1896.
35. SMILEY, S.T. *et al.* 1991. Intracellular heterogeneity in mitochondrial membrane potentials revealed by a J aggregate forming lipophilic cation JC-1. Proc. Natl. Acad. Sci. USA **88:** 3671–3675.
36. RAFF, M.C., R.H. MILLER & M. NOBLE. 1983. A glial progenitor cell that develops in vitro into an astrocyte or an oligodendrocyte depending on the culture medium. Nature **303:** 390–396.
37. RAO, M., M. NOBLE & M. MAYER-PRÖSCHEL. 1998. A tripotential glial precursor cell is present in the developing spinal cord. Proc. Natl. Acad. Sci. USA **95:** 3996–4001.
38. DURAND, B., F. GAO & M. RAFF. 1997. Accumulation of the cyclin-dependent kinase inhibitor p27/Kip1 and the timing of oligodendrocyte differentiation. EMBO J. **16:** 306–317.
39. CASACCIA-BONNEFIL, P. *et al.* 1997. Oligodendrocyte precursor differentiation is perturbed in the absence of the cyclin-dependent kinase inhibitor p27[Kip1]. Genes Dev. **11:** 2335–2346.
40. DURAND, B., M. FERO, J. ROBERTS & M. RAFF. 1998. p27[Kip1] alters the response of cells to mitogen and is part of a cell-intrinsic timer that arrests the cell cycle and initiates differentiation. Curr. Biol. **6:** 431–440.
41. TIKOO, R. *et al.* 1998. Ectopic expression of p27[Kip1] in oligodendrocyte progenitor cells results in cell cycle growth arrest. J. Neurobiol. **36:** 431–440.
42. WOLSWIJK, G. & M. NOBLE. 1989. Identification of an adult-specific glial progenitor cell. Development **105:** 387–400.
43. WOLSWIJK, G., P.N. RIDDLE & M. NOBLE. 1990. Coexistence of perinatal and adult forms of a glial progenitor cell during development of the rat optic nerve. Development **109:** 691–698.
44. WOLSWIJK, G., P.N. RIDDLE & M. NOBLE. 1991. Platelet-derived growth factor is mitogenic for O-2A[adult] progenitor cells. Glia **4:** 495–503.
45. GAO, F. & M. RAFF. 1997. Cell size control and a cell-intrinsic maturation program in proliferating oligodendrocyte precursor cells. J. Cell. Biol. **138:** 1367–1377.
46. SMALL, R.K., P. RIDDLE & M. NOBLE. 1987. Evidence for migration of oligodendrocyte-type-2 astrocyte progenitor cells into the developing rat optic nerve. Nature **328:** 155–157.
47. ONO, K., Y. YASUI, U. RUTISHAUSER & R.H. MILLER. 1997. Focal ventricular origin and migration of oligodendrocyte precursors into the chick optic nerve. Neuron **19:** 283–292.
48. WOLSWIJK, G. & M. NOBLE. 1992. Cooperation between PDGF and FGF converts slowly dividing O-2Aadult progenitor cells to rapidly dividing cells with characteristics of O-2Aperinatal progenitor cells. J. Cell. Biol. **118:** 889–900.
49. WREN, D., G. WOLSWIJK & M. NOBLE. 1992. In vitro analysis of the origin and maintenance of O-2A[adult] progenitor cells. J. Cell. Biol. **116:** 167–176.

50. ONO, K., R. BANSAL, J. PAYNE, *et al.* 1995. Early development and dispersal of oligodendrocyte precursors in the embryonic chick spinal cord. Development **121:** 1743–1754.
51. WARRINGTON, A.E., E. BARBARESE & S.E. PFEIFFER. 1993. Differential myelinogenic capacity of specific developmental stages of the oligodendrocyte lineage upon transplantation into hypomyelinating hosts. J. Neurosci. Res. **34:** 1–13.
52. UTZSCHNEIDER, D.A., D.R. ARCHER, J.D. KOCSIS, *et al.* 1994. Transplantation of glial cells enhances action potential conduction of amyelinated spinal cord axons in the myelin-deficient rat. Proc. Natl. Acad. Sci USA 53–57.
53. SAMPATH, D. & R. PEREZ-POLO. 1997. Regulation of antioxidant enzyme expression by NGF. Neurochem. Res. **22:** 351–362.
54. GABAIZADEH, R., H. STAECKER, W. LIU & T. VAN DE WATER. 1997. BDNF protection of auditory neurons from cisplatin involves changes in intracellular levels of both reactive oxygen species and glutathione. Brain Res. Mol. Brain Res. **50:** 71–78.
55. LEWIS, J., A. HUQ & P. NAJARRO. 1996. Inhibition of mitochondrial function by interferon. J. Biol. Chem. **271:** 184–190.
56. LEE, J. 1998. Inhibition of p53-dependent apoptosis by the KIT tyrosine kinase: regulation of mitochondrial permeability transition and reactive oxygen species generation. Oncogene **17:** 1653–1662.
57. ISLAM, K. *et al.* 1997. TGF-beta1 triggers oxidative modifications and enhances apoptosis in HIT cells through accumulation of reactive oxygen species by suppression of catalase and glutathione peroxidase. Free Radic. Biol. Med. **22:** 1007–1017.
58. HAMPTON, M., B. FADEEL & S. ORRENIUS. 1998. Redox regulation of the caspases during apoptosis. Ann. N.Y. Acad. Sci. **854:** 328–335.
59. PILLAR, T. & H. SEITZ. 1997. Thyroid hormone and gene expression in the regulation of mitochondrial respiratory function. Eur. J. Endocrinol. **136:** 231–239.
60. LEE, A. *et al.* 1999. Ras proteins induce senescence by altering the intracellular levels of reactive oxygen species. J. Biol. Chem. **274:** 7936–7940.
61. ESPOSITO, F. *et al.* 1997. Redox-mediated regulation of p21(waf1/cip1) expression involves a post-transcriptional mechanism and activation of the mitogen-activated protein kinase pathway. Eur. J. Biochem. **245:** 730–737.
62. XANTHOUDAKIS, S. & T. CURRAN. 1992. Identification and characterization of Ref-1, a nuclear protein that facilitates AP-1 DNA-binding activity. EMBO J. **11:** 653–665.
63. KAMATA, H. & H. HIRATA. 1999. Redox regulation of cellular signaling. Cell Signal **11:** 1–14.
64. STAAL, F. *et al.* 1994. Redox regulation of signal transduction: tyrosine phosphorylation and calcium influx. Proc. Natl. Acad. Sci. USA **91:** 3619–3622.

COX-2 and Neurodegeneration in Parkinson's Disease

P. TEISMANN,[a] M. VILA,[a] D.-K. CHOI,[a] K. TIEU,[a] D. C. WU,[a]
V. JACKSON-LEWIS,[a] AND S. PRZEDBORSKI[a,b,c]

*Neuroscience Research Laboratories of the Movement Disorder Division,
Departments of [a]Neurology and [b]Pathology and the [c]Center for Neurobiology and
Behavior, Columbia University, New York, New York 10032, USA*

ABSTRACT: Parkinson's disease (PD) is a common neurodegenerative disorder
characterized by a progressive loss of dopaminergic neurons in the substantia
nigra pars compacta. Recent observations link cyclooxygenase type-2 (COX-2)
to the progression of the disease. Consistent with this notion, studies with the
dopaminergic neurotoxin 1-methyl-4-phenyl-1,2,3,6-tetrahydropyridine
(MPTP) show that inhibition and ablation of COX-2 markedly reduce the deleterious effects of this toxin on the nigrostriatal pathway. The similarity between this experimental model and PD strongly supports the possibility that
COX-2 expression is also pathogenic in PD.

KEYWORDS: inflammation; neurotoxicity; neurodegeneration; MPTP; Parkinson's disease; reactive oxygen species; superoxide dismutase

INTRODUCTION

Inflammatory processes associated with an increased expression of cyclooxygenase (COX) and elevated prostaglandin E_2 (PGE_2) levels have been linked to a variety of neurodegenerative disorders, including Parkinson's disease (PD),
amyotrophic lateral sclerosis, and Alzheimer's disease.[1] COX, which converts
arachidonic acid to PGH_2, the prostaglandin precursor of PGE_2 and several others,
comes in eukaryotic cells in two main isoforms: COX-1, which is constitutively expressed, and COX-2, which is inducible.[2] COX-2 is rapidly upregulated at inflammatory sites and appears to be responsible for the formation of proinflammatory
PGs.[2] Thus, COX-2 may contribute to the neurodegenerative process that is seen in
Parkinson's disease[3] and that are the focus of this manuscript.

COX-2 BRAIN LOCALIZATION: EMPHASIS ON THE
NIGROSTRIATAL PATHWAY

COX-2 mRNA or protein is usually not detectable outside of a handful of discrete
areas of the brain, where it is found primarily in neurons.[4,5] COX-2 immunoreactiv-

Address for correspondence: Dr. Serge Przedborski, BB-307, Columbia University, 650 West
168th Street, New York, NY 10032. Voice: 212-305-1540; fax: 212-305-5450.
SP30@columbia.edu

Ann. N.Y. Acad. Sci. 991: 272–277 (2003). © 2003 New York Academy of Sciences.

ity is observed mainly in distal dendrites and dendritic spines and, apparently, exclusively in excitatory neurons such as glutamatergic neurons.[4] Consistent with this description, we found no evidence of definite COX-2 immunoreactivity either in normal mice or in human postmortem dopaminergic structures at the level of both the substantia nigra and the striatum, which correspond to the site of origin and of projection of the nigrostriatal neurons.

Conversely, COX-2 becomes expressed in most neurons following a variety of insults.[5] To a much lesser extent, COX-2 can also be upregulated by injury and disease in astrocytes and, more rarely, in microglial and endothelial cells.[5] These considerations are perfectly in agreement with our COX-2 immunostaining data in PD postmortem samples and in the 1-methyl-4-phenyl-1,2,3,6-trerahydropyridine (MPTP) mouse model of PD.[6] Indeed, although we did not see clear COX-2 immunoreactivity in any of the controls, except over the neurophil, strong COX-2 immunostaining was seen in cells in PD and MPTP midbrain samples. Almost all positive cells exhibited a neuronal morphology, and only a few resembled astrocytes. None appeared as microglial cells. By double immunostaining, we were able to show that the majority of COX-2–positive neurons in the MPTP mice were dopaminergic. Although Knott *et al.*[7] have found more abundant astrocytic COX-2 immunoreactivity in PD samples than we have (which could be related to technical differences), the two studies appear to agree that the majority of COX-2–positive cells in PD brains are neuronal.

COX-2 INDUCTION IN PD AND MPTP BRAINS

Among the many factors capable of inducing COX-2 expression are found many inflammatory cytokines, such as tumor necrosis factor (TNF)–α and interleukin (IL)-1β, as well as glutamate through the activation of the NMDA receptor and, presumably, inducible nitric oxide synthase (iNOS).[2] Relevant to PD and its experimental model MPTP are the demonstrations that many of the aforementioned factors are significantly increased in the cerebrospinal fluid and the substantia nigra in these two pathological situations.[3] It is worth noting, however, that while COX-2 upregulation occurs mainly in neurons, the factors potentially responsible for this induction, as suggested above, may emanate from glial cells. This raises the possibility of an interesting deleterious interplay between neuron and glia in which the first neuron to die in PD would trigger a glial response that would, by releasing proinflammatory factors, induce the expression of COX-2 in neurons, enhancing the susceptibility of dopaminergic neurons to the degenerative process. According to this scenario, COX-2 would not initiate the demise of dopaminergic neurons, but rather facilitate it. If one were to accept this scenario, one might wonder how COX-2 participates in the neurodegenerative process. In the most obvious scenario, upon COX-2 induction in dopaminergic neurons, these cells start to produce significant amounts of PGE$_2$ that would amplify the glial response and the production of glia-derived deleterious mediators such as reactive oxygen species and proinflammatory cytokines. Relevant to this hypothesis is our demonstration that following MPTP administration a robust glial response develops[8] and that mitigating this reaction attenuates dopaminergic neuronal loss.[9] At this point, however, we are not aware of any demonstration that

COX-2–derived PGE_2 plays a signaling role in linking injured neurons to the activation of glial cells.

Another route by which COX-2 could contribute to the progression of nigrostriatal neurodegeneration is via the oxidation of dopamine by COX-2 and the consequent production of dopamine quinones. In this case, glia-derived inflammatory events would lead to COX-2 induction in neurons that would employ dopamine to generate reactive quinones.[10] These reactive dopamine quinones, which are widely known to react with nucleophiles,[11] can bind covalently with cystein residues in proteins to form protein-bound 5-S-cysteinyl dopamine, a type of posttranslational modification that can seriously affect protein functions.

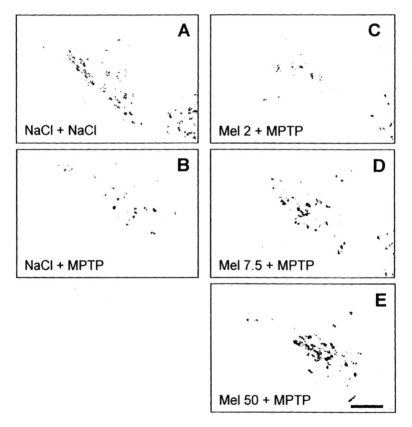

FIGURE 1. Effect of meloxicam on MPTP-induced SNpc dopaminergic neuronal death. (**A**) In saline-injected control mice, there are numerous SNpc tyrosine hydroxylase (TH)-positive neurons. (**B**) In mice treated with MPTP (30 mg/kg subcutaneous injection), the number of SNpc TH-positive neurons is reduced. (**C–E**) In mice treated with both MPTP and meloxicam, there is a noticeable attenuation of SNpc TH-positive neuronal loss. *Scale bar*: 200 μm. (Reproduced from Teismann & Ferger[13] with permission.)

TABLE 1. Effect of meloxicam on MPTP toxicity

	Saline	MPTP + saline	MPTP + meloxicam (2 mg/kg)	MPTP + meloxicam (7.5 mg/kg)	MPTP + meloxicam (50 mg/kg)
Tyrosine hydroxylase (cells/section)	76 ± 2	36 ± 4*	34 ± 6*	67 ± 4#	69 ± 3#
Nissl (cells/section)	94 ± 2	54 ± 6*	56 ± 9*	99 ± 3#	96 ± 56 ± 3#
Dopamine	13.91 ± 0.73	2.21 ± 0.40*	2.22 ± 0.53*	5.01 ± 0.47#	5.61 ± 0.35#
DOPAC	0.99 ± 0.06	0.23 ± 0.03*	0.31 ± 0.04*	0.43 ± 0.03#	0.39 ± 0.03#
HVA	1.30 ± 0.07	0.53 ± 0.06*	0.63 ± 0.08*	0.84 ± 0.05#	0.86 ± 0.04#

NOTE: Counts of tyrosine-hydroxylase positive neurons and Nissl in three sections at the third cranial nerve and dopamine, DOPAC, HVA content after saline or MPTP (30 mg/kg s.c.) in meloxicam (0, 2, 7.5, 50 mg/kg i.p.)-pretreated mice. *$P < 0.05$, fewer than saline-control mice. #$P < 0.05$, more than MPTP-injected mice and not different from control mice. Values are means ± SEM ($n = 8$–12 per group). (From Teismann & Ferger;[13] used with permission.)

ROLE OF COX-2 IN THE MPTP MOUSE MODEL OF PD

To demonstrate whether COX-2 actually plays a deleterious role in PD, we and other investigators have examined the effects of COX-2 inhibition on MPTP-induced dopaminergic neurotoxicity. In an earlier report, acetylsalicylic acid and salicylic acid provided protection against MPTP neurotoxicity in mice, whereas diclofenac failed to do so.[12] Because the failure to observe neuroprotection by diclofenac could be due to poor brain entry, we have revisited the issue using meloxicam, a specific COX-2 inhibitor with better brain penetration.[13] In this subsequent study, the authors found that MPTP caused a significant reduction in striatal dopamine levels as well as in dopaminergic neuron numbers in the substantia nigra, which was markedly attenuated by meloxicam (FIG. 1 and TABLE 1). In another MPTP study, mutant mice deficient in COX-2 were used instead of pharmacological inhibitors. This study generated essentially the same outcomes.[14] These latter data confirm the significant role of COX-2 in MPTP-induced neurodegeneration.

CONCLUSION

COX-2 has emerged as a potential pathogenic factor in several neurodegenerative disorders, including PD. Several studies have shown that COX-2 protein is upregulated in dopaminergic neurons in PD and in its experimental model, MPTP. Although the actual mechanism by which COX-2 is involved in the nigrostriatal neurodegeneration remains to be elucidated, the fact that both the inhibition and abrogation of COX-2 in MPTP-treated mice attenuates significantly the loss of dopaminergic neurons provides compelling evidence of its role in the pathogenesis of PD.

ACKNOWLEDGMENTS

The authors wish to thank Mr. Brian Jones for his help in the preparation of this manuscript. The authors wish also to acknowledge the support of the NIH/NIHNDS (Grants R29 NS37345, RO1 NS38586 and NS42269, and P50 NS38370); the NIH/ NIA (Grant AG13966); the U.S. Department of Defense (Grants DAMD 17-99-1- 9471 and DAMD 17-03-1); the Lowenstein Foundation; the Lillian Goldman Charitable Trust; the Parkinson's Disease Foundation; the Muscular Dystrophy Association; the ALS Association; and Project ALS. P.T. is a recipient of a scholarship from the German Research Foundation (DFG TE 343/1-1).

NOTE ADDED IN PROOF

Since the submission of this manuscript, we have published an article [Teismann, P., *et al.* 2003. Cyclooxygenase-2 is instrumental in Parkinson's disease neurodegeneration. Proc. Natl. Acad. Sci. USA **100**(9): 5473–5478] further supporting a critical role for COX-2 in both the pathogenesis and selectivity of the PD neurodegenerative process. In this paper, we show that COX-2 is upregulated in brain dopaminergic neurons of both PD and MPTP mice and that COX-2 induction occurs through a JNKc-Jun–dependent mechanism after MPTP administration. We demonstrate that targeting COX-2 does not protect against MPTP-induced dopaminergic neurodegeneration by mitigating inflammation. Instead, we provide evidence that COX-2 inhibition/ablation prevents the formation of the oxidant species dopamine-quinone, which has been implicated in the pathogenesis of PD.

REFERENCES

1. WYSS-CORAY, T. & L. MUCKE. 2002. Inflammation in neurodegenerative disease: a double-edged sword. Neuron **35:** 419–432.
2. O'BANION, M.K. 1999. Cyclooxygenase-2: molecular biology, pharmacology, and neurobiology. Crit. Rev. Neurobiol. **13:** 45–82.
3. VILA, M. *et al.* 2001. The role of glial cells in Parkinson's disease. Curr. Opin. Neurol. **14:** 483–489.
4. KAUFMANN, W.E. *et al.* 1997. Cyclooxygenases and the central nervous system. Prostaglandins **54:** 601–624.
5. HURLEY, S.D. *et al.* 2002. Cyclooxygenase inhibition as a strategy to ameliorate brain injury. J. Neurotrauma **19:** 1–15.
6. PRZEDBORSKI, S. & M. VILA. 2001. MPTP: a review of its mechanisms of neurotoxicity. Clin. Neurosci. Res. **1:** 407–418.
7. KNOTT, C. *et al.* 2000. Inflammatory regulators in Parkinson's disease: iNOS, lipocortin-1, and cyclooxygenases-1 and -2. Mol. Cell. Neurosci. **16:** 724–739.
8. LIBERATORE, G.T. *et al.* 1999. Inducible nitric oxide synthase stimulates dopaminergic neurodegeneration in the MPTP model of Parkinson disease. Nat. Med. **5:** 1403–1409.
9. WU, D.C. *et al.* 2002. Blockade of microglial activation is neuroprotective in the 1-methyl-4-phenyl-1,2,3,6-tetrahydropyridine mouse model of Parkinson disease. J. Neurosci. **22:** 1763–1771.
10. HASTINGS, T.G. 1995. Enzymatic oxidation of dopamine: the role of prostaglandin H synthase. J. Neurochem. **64:** 919–924.
11. GRAHAM, D.G. 1978. Oxidative pathways for catecholamines in the genesis of neuromelanin and cytotoxic quinones. Mol. Pharmacol. **14:** 633–643.

12. AUBIN, N. *et al.* 1998. Aspirin and salicylate protect against MPTP-induced dopamine depletion in mice. J. Neurochem. **71:** 1635–1642.
13. TEISMANN, P. & B. FERGER. 2001. Inhibition of the cyclooxygenase isoenzymes COX-1 and COX-2 provide neuroprotection in the MPTP-mouse model of Parkinson's disease. Synapse **39:** 167–174.
14. FENG, Z. *et al.* 2002. Cyclooxygenase-2-deficient mice are resistant to 1-methyl-4-phenyl-1,2,3,6-tetrahydropyridine-induced damage of dopaminergic neurons in the substantia nigra. Neurosci. Lett. **329:** 354.

Striatopallidal Changes in a Preclinical Rat Model of Parkinson's Disease

A. E. GRISSELL, T. M. BUCHANAN, AND M. A. ARIANO

Department of Neuroscience, The Chicago Medical School, North Chicago, Illinois 60064, USA

KEYWORDS: Parkinson's disease; dopamine; striatum

INTRODUCTION

Parkinson's disease (PD) is characterized by motor symptoms due to substantial nigrostriatal dopamine (DA) loss (~80%). To investigate the neurochemical alterations that occur prior to motor symptoms, an early preclinical model of PD has been produced. Malonate was infused into one substantia nigra causing a partial, unilateral striatal DA depletion. HPLC analysis detected striatal DA loss (~50%) at 4 weeks. Subtle behavioral changes, indicated by asymmetry of limb use, confirmed a DA imbalance.[1] Morphological analysis of the DA-depleted striatum showed enhanced D2 DA receptor staining, signifying receptor upregulation due to partial DA loss;[2] activated (cleaved) caspase-3, an indication of cellular homeostatic imbalances; and 8-oxoguanine, a marker of oxidative nucleic acid damage. Further, alterations occurred specifically in the striatopallidal projection system, based upon coincident expression of enkephalin as a phenotypic marker of the efferents with the neurochemical markers.

ANIMAL PREPARATION

Twenty-eight male Sprague-Dawley rats (~225 g) were lesioned unilaterally using malonate infusion (3 µmoles in 1 µl) into the right substantia nigra. Rats were killed 4 weeks after malonate infusions.

HPLC ANALYSIS

Striata were dissected, frozen on dry ice, and stored at −86°C until HPLC analysis.[3] Striatal DA content was averaged (±SEM): intact 14.09 ± 2.22 ng/mg protein versus DA-depleted 8.01 ± 3.38 ng/mg protein ($P < 0.001$, $N = 14$). DOPAC:DA ratios: intact $0.26 \pm .03$; DA-depleted $0.32 \pm .07$ ($P = .008$).

Address for correspondence: Dr. Marjorie A. Ariano, Department of Neuroscience, The Chicago Medical School, 3333 Green Bay Road, North Chicago, Illinois 60064. Voice: 847-578-3412; fax: 847-578-8515.

arianom@finchcms.edu

Ann. N.Y. Acad. Sci. 991: 278–280 (2003). © 2003 New York Academy of Sciences.

BEHAVIORAL ASSESSMENT

Rat forelimb use was evaluated as described in Tillerson *et al.*[1] Comparisons between ipsilateral (right side, DA-depleted) or contralateral (left side, intact) forelimb use as a percentage of total movements made were calculated, then averaged.

MORPHOLOGICAL EXAMINATION

Frozen brains ($N = 14$) were cut at 10 µm in the coronal plane, mounted on slides, and fixed by immersion in freshly prepared 4% paraformaldehyde (in PBS) for 5 min. The sections were processed for routine, double-labeled immunofluorescence to determine changes in striatopallidal (enkephalin-positive) striatal neurons on the intact versus the DA-depleted side. Image acquisition and analysis used methods described previously.[4]

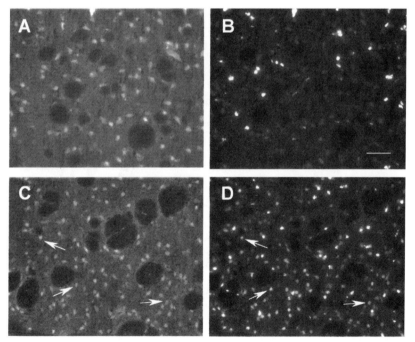

FIGURE 1. Striatopallidal cleaved caspase-3 staining is found in the preclinical PD rat. Enkephalin can identify the projection system and shows the density and shape of medium spiny projection neurons in the intact **(A)** and DA-depleted **(C)** sides. Caspase-3 is cleaved in response to cellular stress and changes in homeostasis produced by DA loss. Cleaved caspase-3 levels were enhanced in DA-depleted **(D)** compared to backgrounds detected in glial cells in intact striatum **(B)**. Many striatopallidal neurons express cleaved caspase-3 in the DA-depleted striatum (*arrows* in **C, D**). *Calibration bar* is 100 µm for all images.

RESULTS

The preclinical PD rat provides a credible model of preclinical stages of PD. Rats have subtle behavior imbalances correlated to the partial striatal DA loss, which showed preferential use of the forepaw ipsilateral to the DA depletion (27.78%, 29.44%, 31.67%) versus the intact side (11.67%, 8.89%, 5.56%) at 2 weeks, 3 weeks, and 4 weeks postinfusion ($N = 9$). Morphological correlates include slight elevation in D2 DA receptor staining and significant ($P < .001$) elevation in expression of cleaved caspase-3 and 8-oxoguanine within the striatopallidal projection pathway ipsilateral to the nigrostriatal DA loss (FIGURE 1), evaluated using cellular luminosity histogram analyses.[4]

CONCLUSIONS

These neurochemical enhancements were unexpected in light of the level (~50%) and duration (4 weeks) of the striatal DA loss. These findings suggest substantial postsynaptic (striatal) changes occur in the early stages of PD and provide a mechanism to evaluate initial neurochemical alterations that may be modified to retard or stop the insidious progression of PD. These results demonstrate the complexity of PD and caution our thinking of the disorder as principally dopaminergic in scope.

ACKNOWLEDGMENT

This work was supported by Department of Defense Grant DAMD17-99-1-9542.

REFERENCES

1. TILLERSON, J.L., A.D. COHEN, J. PHILHOWER, et al. 2001. Forced limb-use effects on the behavioral and neurochemical effects of 6-hydroxydopamine. J. Neurosci. 21: 4427–4435.
2. GERFEN, C.R. & W.S. YOUNG 3RD. 1988. Distribution of striatonigral and striatopallidal peptidergic neurons in both patch and matrix compartments: an in situ hybridization histochemistry and fluorescent retrograde tracing study. Brain Res. 460: 161–167.
3. MORROW, B.A., A.J. REDMOND, R.H. ROTH & J.D. ELSWORTH. 2000. The predator odor, TMT, displays a unique, stress-like pattern of dopaminergic and endocrinological activation in the rat. Brain Res. 864: 146–151.
4. ARIANO, M.A., N. ARONIN, M. DIFIGLIA, et al. 2002. Striatal neurochemical changes in transgenic models of Huntington's disease. J. Neurosci. Res. 68: 716–729.

Neurotoxicity-Induced Changes in Striatal Dopamine Receptor Function

ANNA-LIISA BROWNELL, IRIS Y. CHEN, XUKUI WANG, MEIXIANG YU,
AND BRUCE G. JENKINS

*Department of Radiology, Massachusetts General Hospital,
Boston, Massachusetts 02114, USA*

KEYWORDS: dopamine receptor; dopamine transporter; striatum

Impairment of dopaminergic neurotransmission can be primary, as in Parkinson's disease or secondary, as in Huntington's disease (HD). The secondary dopamine dysfunction is related to the progressive loss of the striatal neurons bearing the postsynaptic dopamine D1 and D2 receptors. PET studies have shown a significant decrease, at an annual rate of 2–6.5%[2], in striatal glucose metabolism[1] and in dopamine D1 and D2 receptor binding in both asymptomatic and symptomatic HD patients.

Huntington's disease can be modeled by 3-nitropropionic acid (3-NP), which is an inhibitor of succinate dehydrogenase.[3] It causes mitochondrial inhibition and striatal degeneration. We used *in vivo* PET studies to investigate 3-NP–induced acute and prolonged neurotoxic effects on striatal dopamine receptors and transporters in a rat model. 3-NP was administered twice a day at a dose of 10 mg/kg i.p. to eight rats (male Spraque-Dawley rats from Charles River Laboratories, average weight 300 g) until symptomatic gait was observed or for a maximum of 5 days. Imaging studies of dopamine D1 and D2 receptors and transporters were conducted before 3-NP administration and 2 and 7 days and 4 and 16 weeks after 3-NP administration. To validate the striatal deficit, an additional PET study of glucose metabolism was done two days after the cessation of 3-NP using ^{18}F-2-fluorodeoxy-D-glucose (^{18}F-FDG). Studies of dopamine D1 receptors were done using ^{11}C-SCH (Schoering 23660) as a tracer. Dopamine D2 receptors were imaged by ^{11}C-raclopride, and dopamine transporters using 2β-carbomethoxy-3β-4-fluorophenyl tropane (^{11}C-CFT). All the PET imaging studies were conducted using an in-house built tomographic instrument.[4]

FIGURE 1 shows PET studies conducted 2 days after 3-NP administration. The glucose study revealed large striatal lesions. At that time a moderate decrease of dopamine D1 and D2 receptor binding and an increase in dopamine transporter binding were observed. After that, progressive decrease was observed in pre and postsynaptic dopamine receptor function (TABLE 1, FIG. 1).

Address for correspondence: Anna-Liisa Brownell, Department of Radiology, Massachusetts General Hospital, 55 Fruit St., Boston, MA 02114.
abrownell@partners.org

Ann. N.Y. Acad. Sci. 991: 281–283 (2003). © 2003 New York Academy of Sciences.

TABLE 1. 3-NP–induced degeneration of the binding of striatal dopamine D1 and D2 receptors and transporters

	Percent change in the binding of dopamine		
Time after 3-NP	D1 receptors	D2 receptors	Transporters
2 days	-4 ± 2	-5 ± 2	$+6 \pm 3$
4 weeks	-24 ± 8	-23 ± 7	-10 ± 3
4 months	-36 ± 9	-33 ± 8	-12 ± 4

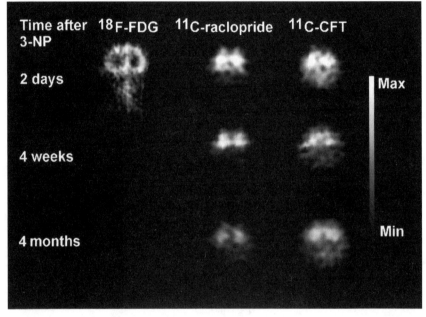

FIGURE 1. Longitudinal follow-up studies of dopamine D2 receptors (^{11}C-raclopride) and dopamine transporters (^{11}C-CFT) after 3-NP toxicity. Coronal slices show the binding distribution at the midstriatal level. Study of glucose utilization with ^{18}F-FDG shows large striatal lesions 2 days after 3-NP.

Even though HD is associated mainly with the impairment of postsynaptic dopamine receptors as a result of neural loss,[1,2] dopamine transporter binding might have a significant role in predicting the time course of dopaminergic degeneration. We found temporal variation in dopamine transporter binding in the 3-NP rat model. A similar observation has been published in a quinolinic acid rat model.[5] The reports of dopamine transporter function in HD patients include increased, unchanged, or decreased dopamine transporter binding.[6,7] Altogether, these observations might present degeneration at different time points and might well support our observation of the transient mechanism.

ACKNOWLEDGMENT

This work was supported by the DOD Grant DAMD17-99-1-9555.

REFERENCES

1. ANDREWS, T.C., *et al.* 1998. Advances in the understanding of early Huntington's disease using the functional imaging techniques of PET and SPECT. Mol. Med. Today **4**(12): 532–539.
2. ANDREWS, T.C., *et al.* 1999. Huntington's disease progression, PET and clinical observations. Brain **122**(Pt. 12): 2353–2363.
3. ALSTON, T.A., *et al.* 1977. 3-Nitropropionate, the toxic substance of Indigofera, is a suicide inactivator of succinate dehydrogenase. Proc. Natl. Acad. Sci. USA **74**: 3767–3771.
4. BROWNELL, G.L., *et al.* 1985. High resolution tomograph using analog coding. *In* The Metabolism of the Human Brain. Studies with Positron Emssion Tomography. T. Greitz *et al.,* Eds.: 13–19. Raven Press. New York.
5. ARAUJO, M.D. *et al.* 2000. Deficits in striatal dopamine D2 receptors and energy metabolism detected by in vivo mirco PET imaging in a rat model of Huntington's disease. Exp. Neurol. **166**: 287–297.
6. SUZUKI, M. *et al.* 2001. Vesicular neurotransmitter transporters in Huntington's disease: initial observations and comparison with traditional synaptic markers. Synapse **41**(4): 329–336.
7. GINOVART, N. *et al.* 1997. PET study of pre- and post-synaptic dopaminergic markers for neurodegenerative process in Huntington's disease. Brain **120**: 503–514.

The Developmental Time Course of Glial Cell Line–Derived Neurotrophic Factor (GDNF) and GDNF Receptor α-1 mRNA Expression in the Striatum and Substantia Nigra

JINWHAN CHO,[a] NIKOLAI G.KHOLODILOV,[a] AND ROBERT E. BURKE[a,b]

Departments of [a]Neurology and [b]Pathology, The College of Physicians and Surgeons, Columbia University, New York, New York 10032, USA

KEYWORDS: glial cell line–derived neurotrophic factor (GDNF); GDNF receptor α-1 (GFR α-1); natural cell death; Northern analysis; phosphoimager

INTRODUCTION

In most developing neural systems, a natural cell death (NCD) event occurs that eliminates 50% or more of the neuronal population. One central neuronal population of particular interest consists of the dopamine (DA) neurons of the substantia nigra (SN), the population that degenerates to the greatest extent in Parkinson's disease. Of central interest to the neurobiology of this disease are the neurotrophic factors that support the viability of these neurons during development and that ultimately determine their number in the mature brain. There is evidence that NCD in dopamine neurons of the SN is regulated during development by interaction with their target, the striatum, but the neurotrophic factors that mediate this regulation are unknown. One candidate is glial cell line–derived neurotrophic factor (GDNF), which was originally identified on the basis of its ability to support the development of embryonic mesencephalic DA neurons in culture.[1] However, little is known about the time course of developmental expression of GDNF and its receptor GFR α-1 in the developing rat brain in relation to the time course of the postnatal NCD event. We therefore examined GDNF and GFR α-1 expression to understand better the possible role of GDNF as a physiologic striatal target-derived neurotrophic factor in relation to the NCD event in SN DA neurons.

RESULTS

The expression levels of GDNF and GFR α-1 in the striatum and SN were studied by Northern analysis for rats at postnatal days 2, 6, 10, 14, and 28, as well as for

Address for correspondence: Robert E. Burke, Department of Neurology, Room 308, Black Building, Columbia University, 650 West 168th Street, New York, New York 10032. Voice: 212-305-7374; fax: 212-305-5450.

rb43@columbia.edu

Ann. N.Y. Acad. Sci. 991: 284–287 (2003). © 2003 New York Academy of Sciences.

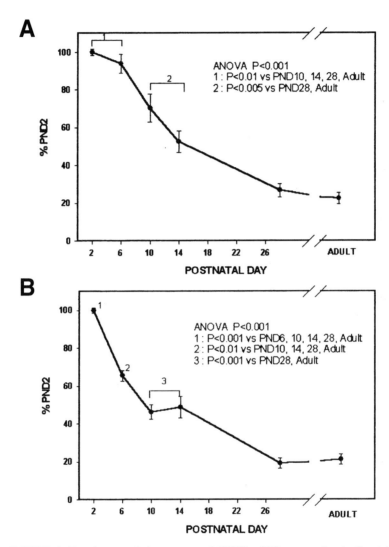

FIGURE 1. Developmental time course of GDNF mRNA expression in the striatum **(A)** and in the SN **(B)**. Expression of GDNF is highest in the striatum at postnatal day 2 and progressively decreases after postnatal day 6. In the SN, GDNF mRNA also decreases after postnatal day 2 and shows a small plateau between postnatal days 10 and 14.

adult rats. Northern blot analysis showed a single major band at 900 bp for GDNF, and two major bands were identified for GFR α-1, at about 4.0 and 8.0 kb. We analyzed radioactive bands using a phosphoimager and expressed them as a relative percentage of the radioactivity at postnatal day 2. Expression of GDNF is highest in the striatum at postnatal day 2 and progressively decreases after postnatal day 6 (FIG. 1A). In the SN, GDNF mRNA also decreases after postnatal day 2 and shows a small

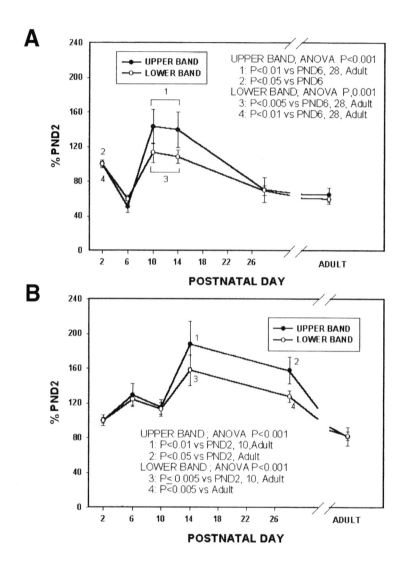

FIGURE 2. Developmental time course of GFR α-1 mRNA expression in the striatum (A) and in the SN (B). Expression of GFR α-1 does not parallel that of GDNF. In the SN, expression of GFR α-1 is highest between postnatal days 14 and 28 and then decreases in adulthood. Expression of GFR α-1 in the striatum is biphasic, with peaks at postnatal day 2 and postnatal days 10–14.

plateau between postnatal days 10 and 14 (FIG. 1B). However, expression of GFR α-1 does not parallel that of GDNF. In the SN, expression of GFR α-1 is highest between postnatal days 14 and 28 and then decreases in adulthood. Expression of GFR α-1 in the striatum is biphasic, with peaks at postnatal day 2 and postnatal days 10–14 (FIG. 2).

CONCLUSIONS

In both striatum and SN, GDNF mRNA expression is highest during the first postnatal week, suggesting that this is the time period when it is most likely to play a role in regulating dopamine neuron development. In the nigrostriatal axis, its expression is highest in the striatum, most consistent with a role as a target-derived factor. Nevertheless, abundant expression is also observed in the SN, suggesting that it may also have a local role in regulating development.

The expression of GFR α-1 mRNA is also developmentally regulated, but its temporal pattern of expression is more complex and does not parallel that of GDNF. In the nigrostriatal axis, its expression is higher in SN than striatum, as would be expected were SN DA neurons responsive to GDNF derived from the striatal target. However, in SN expression peaks at postnatal day 14, when GDNF striatal mRNA begins to wane. The reasons for this discrepancy are unknown. It is possible that GFR α-1 mRNA rises at postnatal day 14 as a compensatory response when competition for striatum-derived GDNF becomes most intense. Alternatively, it is possible that SNpc neurons produce GFR α-1 for presentation to other neurons in *trans*.[2]

ACKNOWLEDGMENTS

This work was supported by NIH/NINDS Grants NS26836 and NS38370 and by the Parkinson's Disease Foundation and the Lowenstein Foundation.

REFERENCES

1. LIN, L.H. *et al.* 1993. GDNF: a glial cell line-derived neurotrophic factor for midbrain dopaminergic neurons. Science **260:** 1130–1132.
2. SAARMA, M. 2001. GDNF recruits the signaling crew into lipid rafts. Trends Neurosci. **24:** 427–429.

Subcellular Compartmentalization of P-ERKs in the Lewy Body Disease Substantia Nigra

CHARLEEN T. CHU AND JIAN-HUI ZHU

Department of Pathology, Division of Neuropathology, University of Pittsburgh School of Medicine, Pittsburgh, Pennsylvania 15213, USA

KEYWORDS: extracellular signal–regulated kinase (ERK); Lewy body disease; substantia nigra; mitochondria; mitogen-activated protein kinase

Extracellular signal–regulated kinases (ERKs) are involved in regulating neuronal survival, differentiation, and plasticity. Recent studies also indicate that ERKs can play a detrimental role in models of oxidative neuronal injury.[1,2] Our previous studies showed discrete cytoplasmic accumulations of phophorylated ERKs (P-ERKs) in Parkinson's disease and other Lewy body diseases, and in 6-hydroxydopamine–treated neuronal cell cultures.[3] As the effects of ERK phosphorylation are critically dependent upon subcellular localization and access to downstream targets, we investigated the subcellular distribution of P-ERKs in Lewy body disease using double-label confocal microscopy. The association of P-ERK granules with a subset of (sometimes enlarged) mitochondria suggests a potential interaction between mitochondrial function and the ERK signaling pathway in degenerating dopaminergic neurons.

METHODS

Substantia nigra sections from a diffuse Lewy body disease patient were stained for P-ERKs as described previously[3] and then incubated with organelle-specific antibodies and appropriate Cy3-conjugated secondary antibodies. Negative controls included double labeling of sections substituting nonimmune mouse or rabbit IgG for the primary antibodies. The slides were observed using a Zeiss laser scanning confocal imaging system.

RESULTS AND DISCUSSION

Immunofluorescence staining showed coarse, granular, or vesicular-appearing accumulations of P-ERKs in substantia nigra neurons. The immunoreactivity of the P-ERKs was confined to the cytoplasm and did not colocalize with nuclear stains.[3]

Address for correspondence: Charleen T. Chu, M.D., Ph.D., Division of Neuropathology, Room A-516, UPMC Presbyterian, 200 Lothrop Street, Pittsburgh, Pennsylvania 15213. Voice: 412-647-3744; fax: 412-647-5602.

chu@np.awing.upmc.edu

Ann. N.Y. Acad. Sci. 991: 288–290 (2003). © 2003 New York Academy of Sciences.

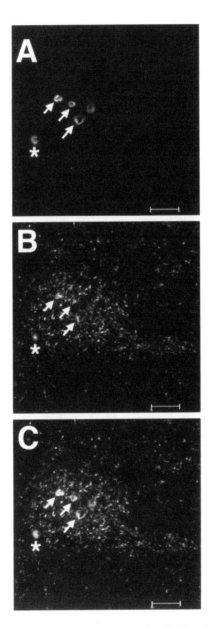

FIGURE 1. Double labeling of P-ERK (**A**) with the 60-kDa mitochondrial protein (**B**). In the overlap image (**C**), note that regions of colocalization (*arrows*) often appear as smaller punctate areas within the P-ERK profile. Enlarged mitochondria occasionally appear to be associated centrally within vesicular-appearing P-ERK profiles (*star*).

P-ERK granules were occasionally colocalized with the early endosome marker Rab5, but not with markers of the lysosome (cathepsin D), 20S proteasome (β subunit), or endoplasmic reticulum (cytochrome P450 reductase). P-ERK immunoreactivity was more commonly co-localized with 60-kDa (FIG. 1) and 110-kDa mitochondrial proteins, and with manganese superoxide dismutase. The areas of colocalization, verified by orthogonal analysis, usually appeared as smaller punctate areas within the P-ERK profile. A second type of association was also observed in which vesicular-appearing P-ERK accumulations appeared to envelop, rather than colocalize with, enlarged mitochondria (FIG. 1, star).

Sustained activation of ERKs is associated with 6-OHDA toxicity in B65 (see Ref. 2) and SH-SY5Y cell lines (C.T. Chu, unpublished data), and MEK inhibitors confer significant protection. P-ERK staining is cytoplasmic, attaining a discrete punctate appearance following commitment to cell death.[3] Moreover, substantia nigra neurons in patients with the full spectrum of Lewy body diseases display unusual, discrete cytoplasmic, but not nuclear, accumulations of P-ERK immunoreactivity.[3] In this study, we found that the P-ERK granules can be associated with an early endosomal marker, but were more commonly associated with mitochondrial markers.

Partial colocalization of a subset of P-ERK granules with an early endosome marker, Rab5, may reflect physiologic recruitment and assembly of Ras-ERK signaling cascades on endosomal surfaces.[4] Recent evidence that ERK1 can phosphorylate Rab5 further suggests the possibility for cross-talk between the Ras-ERK signaling pathway and the endocytic machinery.

Mitochondria are vulnerable to various insults and can undergo enlargement and structural disorganization, associated with decreased membrane potential and reduced ATP production. The association of P-ERK granules with a subset of (sometimes enlarged) mitochondria suggests a potential interaction between mitochondrial function and the ERK signaling pathway in dopaminergic neurons. P-ERKs have been reported to form signaling modules with other MAP kinases in cardiac mitochondria.[5] Alternatively, it is possible that these structures reflect sequestration of damaged mitochondria.

REFERENCES

1. STANCIU, M., Y. WANG, R. KENTOR, *et al.* 2000. Persistent activation of ERK contributes to glutamate-induced oxidative toxicity in a neuronal cell line and primary cortical neuron cultures. J. Biol. Chem. **275:** 12200–12206.
2. KULICH, S.M. & C.T. CHU. 2001. Sustained extracellular signal-regulated kinase activation by 6-hydroxydopamine: implications for Parkinson's disease. J. Neurochem. **77:** 1058–1066.
3. ZHU, J.-H., S.M. KULICH, T.D. OURY & C.T. CHU. 2002. Cytoplasmic aggregates of phosphorylated extracellular signal-regulated kinase in Lewy body diseases. Am. J. Pathol. **161:** 2087–2098.
4. RIZZO, M.A., K. SHOME, S.C. WATKINS & G. ROMERO. 2000. The recruitment of Raf-1 to membranes is mediated by direct interaction with phosphatidic acid and is independent of association with Ras. J. Biol. Chem. **275:** 23911–23918.
5. BAINES, C.P., J. ZHANG, G.W. WANG, *et al.* 2002. Mitochondrial PKCepsilon and MAPK form signaling modules in the murine heart: enhanced mitochondrial PKCepsilon-MAPK interactions and differential MAPK activation in PKCepsilon-induced cardioprotection. Circ. Res. **90:** 390-397.

Altered Striatal Neuronal Morphology Is Associated with Astrogliosis in a Chronic Mouse Model of Parkinson's Disease

A. G. DERVAN,[a] S. TOTTERDELL,[b] Y.-S. LAU,[c] AND G. E. MEREDITH[a]

[a]*Department of Cellular and Molecular Pharmacology, Chicago Medical School, North Chicago, Illinois 60064, USA*

[b]*Department of Pharmacology, University of Oxford, Oxford OX1 3QT, United Kingdom*

[c]*Department of Pharmacology, University of Missouri–Kansas City, Kansas City, Missouri 64108, USA*

KEYWORDS: astrocyte; dendrite; spine; MPTP; dopamine; gliosis; medium spiny neuron; glutamate

INTRODUCTION

Neostriatal medium spiny neurons (MSNs) lose their dopaminergic (DA) innervation in Parkinson's disease (PD). This loss is followed by a cascade of events that ultimately changes the structure of MSNs and the activity of basal ganglia circuits, resulting in the development of PD symptomatology. The specific mechanisms leading to MSN morphological change are not well understood but may involve glutamate hyperactivity.[1] Astrocytes provide trophic support for neurons and their associated synapses. They also possess receptor systems for recycling glutamate.[2] With central nervous system insults, astrocytes react, presumably to restore homeostasis. However, once reactive, their ability to carry out normal supportive functions is impaired.[3] In the present study, we examined the association between resident astrocytes and MSN morphology after DA loss in a chronic mouse model of PD.[4,5]

METHODS

Adult C57/bl mice were treated with 1-methyl-4-phenyl-1,2,3,6-tetrahydropyridine (MPTP) hydrochloride (25 mg/kg, sc in saline) and probenecid (250 mg/kg, ip in DMSO) or probenecid alone (controls) for 5 weeks (10 doses). All animals were assessed with an acceleration test on a rotarod; 3–5 weeks after treatment, the animals were anesthetized (pentobarbital, 130 mg/kg) and perfused transcardially with

Address for correspondence: Dr. G.E. Meredith, Department of Cellular and Molecular Pharmacology, Chicago Medical School, Finch University of Health Sciences, 3333 Green Bay Road, North Chicago, Illinois 60064. Voice: 847-578-8680; fax: 847-578-3268.
gloria.meredith@finchcms.edu

Ann. N.Y. Acad. Sci. 991: 291–294 (2003). © 2003 New York Academy of Sciences.

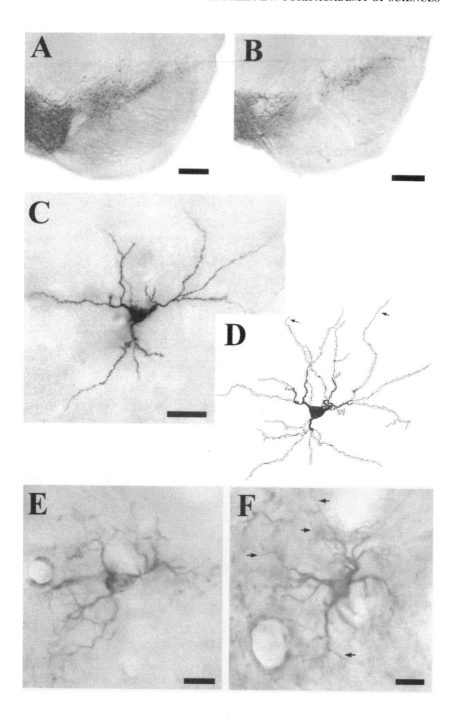

FIGURE 1. *See following page for legend.*

fixative; 300-μm slices through the striatum were cut alternately with 50-μm sections. In slices, neurons counterstained with DAPI (0.001%) were iontophoretically injected with biotinylated Lucifer yellow. Slices were then resectioned (40 μm) and reacted with nickel-enhanced DAB. Adjacent sections were immunoreacted for tyrosine hydroxylase (TH) or glial fibrillary acidic protein (GFAP). Reconstructed intracellularly filled neurons were morphometrically analyzed, and the density of GFAP-immunopositive (+) cells and fibers was studied. Control and treated groups were compared with standard statistics.

RESULTS AND DISCUSSION

When compared to controls, MPTP/probenecid (MPTP/p)-treated mice were significantly impaired on the rotarod ($P < 0.01$), and showed reduced striatal TH innervation and few TH+ neurons in the substantia nigra (FIGS. 1A,B). MSNs (FIGS. 1C,D) did not differ between groups in dendritic length, surface area, or spine density. However, distal dendrites were significantly more tortuous ($P < 0.05$), had fewer spines ($P < 0.05$), and tended ($P = 0.1$) to be longer in MPTP/p mice than in controls. As for astrocytes, GFAP+ cells typically had short, fine processes in controls (FIG. 1E), but numerous long, thick extensions (FIG. 1F), typical of reactive astrocytes, after MPTP/p treatment. GFAP+ cell and fiber densities were significantly increased ($P < 0.01$) by 40% and 36%, respectively, compared to controls.

Morphological change seen in experimental models of PD appears to depend upon the severity of DA depletion and, as data here suggest, changes in resident astrocytes. Complete 6-OHDA lesions produce atrophy and major spine loss.[6,7] However, more partial lesions remodel distal dendrites with little spine loss (present results and Meredith *et al.*[7]). Astrocytes, which are vital for brain homeostasis because they clear glutamate and influence calcium dynamics,[8] proliferate after injury and release growth factors. Such factors may help maintain the integrity of dendrites, especially small distal processes vulnerable to calcium overload.[1] Nevertheless, striatal glutamate levels rise following DA loss,[1,9] and astrocytes, once reactive, essentially lose their ability to recycle it.[3] They also activate microglia that produce proinflammatory cytokines.[3,8] In PD, astrogliosis is rarely observed in the striatum, yet postmortem studies show that striatal neurons are severely altered structurally.[10] This may mean that inflammation occurs early in the disease process, a hypothesis that is strongly supported by the present results.

FIGURE 1. TH immunoreactivity in the midbrain of (**A**) probenecid control and (**B**) 4 weeks post-MPTP/probenecid-treated mouse. (**C**) Intracellularly injected MSN of an MPTP/probenecid-treated mouse and (**D**) its digitized reconstruction. Note the sparse spines on dendrites (*arrows*). Typical astrocytes in (**E**) control and (**F**) MPTP/probenecid-treated striata. Note numerous fine processes (*arrows*) in (**F**). *Scale bars*: A,B = 200 μm, C = 20 μm, E,F = 10 μm.

ACKNOWLEDGMENTS

This study was funded by USPHS Grant R01 NS41799 from NIH/NINDS and a Wellcome Trust Biomedical Collaboration Grant.

REFERENCES

1. INGHAM, C.A. *et al.* 1998. Plasticity of synapses in the rat neostriatum after unilateral lesion of the nigrostriatal dopaminergic pathway. J. Neurosci. **18:** 4732–4743.
2. AMUNDSON, R.H. *et al.* 1992. Uptake of [^{3}H]serotonin and [^{3}H]glutamate by primary astrocyte cultures. II. Differences in cultures prepared from different brain regions. Glia **6:** 9–18.
3. RIDET, J.L. *et al.* 1997. Reactive astrocytes: cellular and molecular cues to biological function. Trends Neurosci. **20:** 570–577.
4. PETROSKE E. *et al.* 2001. Mouse model of parkinsonism: a comparison between sub-acute MPTP and chronic MPTP/p treatment. Neuroscience **106:** 589–601.
5. MEREDITH, G.E. *et al.* 2002. Lysosomal malfunction accompanies alpha-synuclein aggregation in a progressive mouse model of Parkinson's disease. Brain Res. **956:** 156–165.
6. INGHAM, C.A. *et al.* 1989. Spine density on neostriatal neurons changes with 6-hydroxydopamine lesions and with age. Brain Res. **503:** 334–338.
7. MEREDITH G.E. *et al.*1995. The effects of dopamine depletion on the morphology of medium spiny neurons in the shell and core of the rat nucleus accumbens. J. Neurosci. **15:** 3808–3820.
8. EDDELSTON, M. & L. MUCKE. 1993. Molecular profile of reactive astrocytes—implications for their role in neurologic disease. Neuroscience **54:** 15–36.
9. ROBINSON, S. *et al.* 2001. Blockade of NMDA receptors by MK-801 reverses the changes in striatal glutamate immunolabeling in 6-OHDA-lesioned rats. Synapse **42:** 54–61.
10. McNEILL, T.H. *et al.* 1988. Atrophy of medium spiny I striatal dendrites in advanced Parkinson's disease. Brain Res. **455:** 148–152.

Is the Initial Insult in Parkinson's Disease and Dementia with Lewy Bodies a Neuritic Dystrophy?

JOHN E. DUDA,[a,b] BENOIT I. GIASSON,[a] VIRGINIA M-Y. LEE,[a] AND JOHN Q. TROJANOWSKI[a]

[a]Center for Neurodegenerative Disease Research, University of Pennsylvania, Philadelphia, Pennsylvania 19104, USA

[b]Parkinson's Disease Research, Education and Clinical Center, Philadelphia VA Medical Center, Philadelphia, Pennsylvania 19104, USA

KEYWORDS: Parkinson's disease; dementia with Lewy bodies; neuritic dystrophy; alpha-synuclein

The role that intracytoplasmic α-synuclein (α-syn) inclusions including Lewy bodies (LBs) and Lewy neurites (LNs) play in the neurodegenerative process in Parkinson's disease (PD) and dementia with Lewy bodies (DLB) remains controversial. Whether they are a primary insult that begins a cascade towards eventual neuronal death or a secondary adaptive response is still debated. Recently, we have published three lines of evidence suggesting that LNs, and the interruption of axonal transport that they may engender, is an integral component in this neurodegenerative process. First, with novel antibodies to α-syn, we have demonstrated a burden of neuritic pathology in PD, DLB, and concomitant DLB and AD (AD/DLB) that is far greater than previously recognized.[1] In this report, we documented a large, previously unrecognized burden of neuritic pathology in the striatum of the Lewy body disorders. Moreover, with immunofluorescent double labeling we were able to confirm that at least some of the neuritic aggregates were located within axons of nigrostriatal pathway neurons. In addition, we have also examined the burden of this pathology in the cerebral cortex of the Lewy body disorders. When we performed a similar semiquantitative analysis of neuritic burden in the cingulate cortex from patients representing the complete range of synucleinopathies as well as several control groups, we observed a similar density pattern to what we observed in the striatum. Specifically, the highest density was seen in cases of AD/DLB, followed by DLB, and then PD; little or no pathology was seen in multiple system atrophy, AD, progressive su-

Address for correspondence: John Q. Trojanowski, Center for Neurodegenerative Disease Research, University of Pennsylvania, 3600 Spruce St., 3 Maloney, Philadelphia, PA 19104. Voice: 215-662-6399; fax: 215-349-5909.
trojanow@mail.med.upenn.edu

Ann. N.Y. Acad. Sci. 991: 295–297 (2003). © 2003 New York Academy of Sciences.

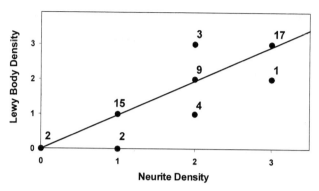

FIGURE 1. Independent semiquantitative analysis of Lewy neurite (LN) density and Lewy body (LB) density was performed on the anterior cingulate gyrus from 53 patients with DLB/AD, DLB, or PD. Sections were immunostained with an anti-synuclein monoclonal antibody, Syn 514.[1] The following assessment strategy was used to estimate the density of α-syn inclusions: 3 = frequent; 2 = moderate; 1= sparse; and 0 = few to none. When the density of LN (*x axis*) in the cingulate cortex is correlated with LB density (*y axis*) in the same cortex, a correlation of $R^2 = 0.906$, $P < 0.0001$ is achieved. *Numbers* represent the numbers of cases at each data point.

pranuclear palsy, corticobasal degeneration, idiopathic striatonigral degeneration, and normal controls. In addition, we performed a semiquantitative analysis of the abundance of neuritic pathology and an independent assessment of LB density in the cingulate cortex of 53 cases of AD/DLB, DLB, and PD and found a strong correlation ($R^2 = 0.906$, $P < 0.0001$) (FIG. 1) between the two. Taken together with many recent studies correlating cortical LB density and the dementia of LB disorders,[2–4] it is reasonable to hypothesize a similar correlation between cortical neurite density and dementia.

The second line of evidence supporting the role of neuritic dystrophy in LB disorders is the observation that neuritic aggregates are the predominant pathology in a case of familial PD from the Contursi kindred with a pathogenic A53T mutation in the α-syn gene.[5] We reexamined the initial autopsy from the kindred[6] using α-syn and tau immunochemistry and found an overwhelming burden of neuritic pathology and virtual absence of LBs in this patient. This patient is particularly interesting in that he died an accidental death prior to the end stage of the disease and therefore gives us a pathological "snapshot" earlier in the disease process. When compared to the pathology at the end stage of this kindred in other cases (unpublished results and personal communication with Dr. D.W. Dickson) that have more typical PD pathology, it is tempting to postulate widespread neuritic pathology as an early pathological aberration.

Finally, we have developed an A53T transgenic mouse model that displays an age-dependent neurodegenerative process that includes development of primarily neuritic α-syn aggregates and a concomitant motor phenotype with rapid progression to paralysis and death.[7] The close temporal association between the development of α-syn aggregates and the onset of the motor phenotype in these mice support a pathogenic role for these inclusions and allow us to examine the consequences of neuritic inclusions. With α-syn immunoelectron microscopy of the ventral roots of affected mice, we are able to confirm the deposition of fibrillar α-syn aggregates within the axonal compartment; the intraaxonal accumulation of vesicles, mitochondria, vacuoles, and neurofilaments, suggesting an interruption of axonal transport; and axonal degeneration. Therefore, it is possible to hypothesize that intraaxonal aggregates are an early component of the disease process and lead to an interruption of axonal transport with resultant axonal degeneration that is the ultimate pathological cause of the motor phenotype observed in these animals.

Collectively, these observations engender a "neuritic dystrophy hypothesis" of pathophysiology for the Lewy body disorders wherein various environmental, genetic, or intrinsic factors cause a conformational change in the structure of α-syn to β-pleated sheet and a propensity to aggregate into pathological inclusions. These inclusions can occur in the cell soma as LBs or in the axonal compartment and grow in size by accumulating additional α-syn and trapping other proteins and/or organelles. In the axonal compartment, these inclusions expand until they congest the axonal compartment, resulting in an interruption of axonal transport. This cessation of axonal transport disallows distal axonal viability and eventually leads to axonal degeneration with the possibility of resultant neuronal degeneration. Further examination of the human diseases as well as many of our current models of the Lewy body disorders may improve our understanding of the role of neuritic dystrophy and eventually lead to novel therapeutic interventions to prevent disease progression in these disorders.

REFERENCES

1. DUDA, J.E., B.I. GIASSON, M.E. MABON, *et al.* 2002. Novel antibodies to synuclein show abundant striatal pathology in Lewy body diseases. Ann. Neurol. **52:** 205–210.
2. HARDING, A.J. & G.M. HALLIDAY. 2001. Cortical Lewy body pathology in the diagnosis of dementia. Acta Neuropathol. **102:** 355–363.
3. HURTIG, H.I., J.Q. TROJANOWSKI, J. GALVIN, *et al.* 2000. Alpha-synuclein cortical Lewy bodies correlate with dementia in Parkinson's disease. Neurology **54:** 1916–1921.
4. MATTILA, P.M., J.O. RINNE, H. HELENIUS, D.W. DICKSON & M. ROYTTA. 2000. Alpha-synuclein-immunoreactive cortical Lewy bodies are associated with cognitive impairment in Parkinson's disease. Acta Neuropathol. **100:** 285–290.
5. DUDA, J.E., B.I. GIASSON, M.E. MABON, D.C. MILLER, *et al.* 2002. Concurrence of alpha-synuclein and tau brain pathology in the Contursi kindred. Acta Neuropathol. **104:** 7–11.
6. GOLBE, L.I., G. DI IORIO, V. BONAVITA, *et al.* 1990. A large kindred with autosomal dominant Parkinson's disease. Ann. Neurol. **27:** 276–282.
7. GIASSON, B.I., J.E. DUDA, S.M. QUINN, *et al.* 2002. Neuronal alpha-synucleinopathy with severe movement disorder in mice expressing A53T human alpha-synuclein. Neuron **34:** 521–533.

Neuroplasticity in the MPTP-Lesioned Mouse and Nonhuman Primate

MICHAEL W. JAKOWEC,[a] BETH FISHER,[a] KERRY NIXON,[a]
ELIZABETH HOGG,[a] CHARLES MESHUL,[b] SAMUEL BREMMER,[b]
TOM McNEILL,[a] AND GISELLE M. PETZINGER[a]

[a]Department of Neurology, University of Southern California,
Los Angeles, California 90033, USA

[b]Department of Behavioral Neuroscience, VA Medical Center/Oregon Health and Science
University, Portland, Oregon 97201, USA

KEYWORDS: neuroplasticity; MPTP-lesioned mouse; nigrostriatal dopaminergic neurons

INTRODUCTION

Systemic administration of the neurotoxicant MPTP (1-methyl-4-phenyl-1,2,3,6-tetrahydropyridine) to C57 BL/6J mice and squirrel monkey (*Saimiri sciureus*) leads to the destruction of nigrostriatal dopaminergic neurons, the depletion of striatal dopamine, and the onset of parkinsonian features including bradykinesia. Interestingly, both mice and nonhuman primates demonstrate neurochemical and behavioral recovery from this neurotoxic-induced injury to the basal ganglia. The molecular mechanisms underlying neuroplasticity in these models are not fully understood. The focus of our studies is to elucidate the molecular, morphological, and neurochemical basis for recovery including interventions, such as exercise, that may enhance recovery.

METHODS

Male 8-week-old mice were administered MPTP in a series of four injections (20 mg/kg, ip, free-base, every 2 h). Brain tissue was collected at postlesion days 7, 14, 30, 60, and 90. Another group of mice were subjected to treadmill exercise starting 4 days after MPTP lesioning, recording velocity and duration (maximum 1 h). Brain tissue was collected after 30 days of treadmill training. Squirrel monkeys were administered MPTP in a series of six injections (2 mg/kg, sc, free-base, 2 weeks between each injection). Motor behavior was assessed using a modified Parkinson's

Address for correspondence: Michael W. Jakowec, Ph.D., Department of Neurology, MCH-142, 1333 San Pablo Street, University of Southern California, Los Angeles, California 90033. Voice: 323-442-1057; fax: 323-442-1055.
mjakowec@surgery.usc.edu

Ann. N.Y. Acad. Sci. 991: 298–301 (2003). © 2003 New York Academy of Sciences.

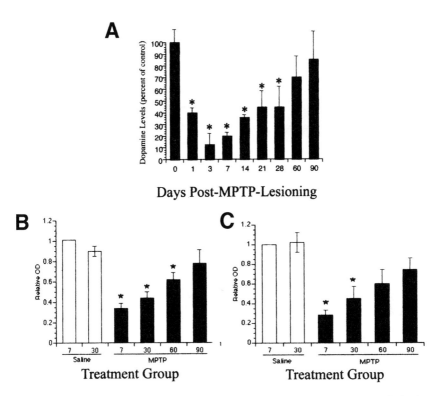

FIGURE 1. Time course analysis of striatal dopamine function after MPTP lesioning in the C57 BL/6J mouse. **(A)** HPLC analysis of striatal dopamine levels ($N = 6$ per time point). Western immunoblot analysis of **(B)** striatal TH protein and **(C)** striatal DAT protein. *Asterisks* indicate significant difference ($P < 0.05$) based on one-way ANOVA compared to saline control ($N = 6$ per time point).

rating scale for the squirrel monkey. Brain tissue was harvested at either 6 weeks or 9 months after the last injection of MPTP.

RESULTS

At 7 days postlesioning, mice had a 90% depletion of striatal dopamine (by HPLC analysis) and a 70% loss of nigrostriatal neurons (by unbiased stereological counting techniques). Analysis of the time course of striatal dopamine showed return to near prelesioned levels 90 days after injury (FIG. 1A). Expression of striatal tyrosine hydroxylase (TH) and dopamine transporter (DAT) protein (by Western immunoblotting) showed return to within 75% of prelesioned levels by 90 days postlesioning (FIGS. 1B,C).

Analysis of the time course of motor behavior in squirrel monkeys showed a reversal of motor deficits to prelesioned levels 12 weeks after the last injection of

(A)

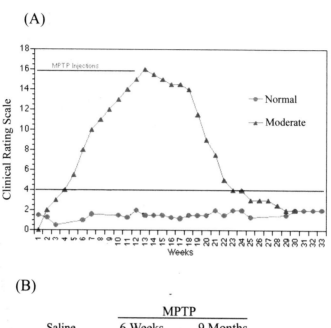

(B)

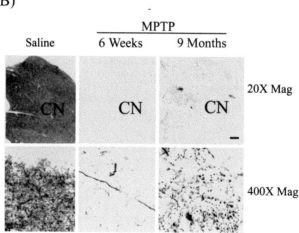

FIGURE 2. The time course of motor behavior in the MPTP-lesioned squirrel monkey. (A) Analysis using a clinical rating scale indicates the recovery of motor deficit 12 weeks after the last injection of MPTP ($N = 4$ animals per group). (B) Immunocytochemical analysis of TH protein in the caudate nucleus (CN) indicates severe depletion at 6 weeks after the last injection of MPTP but only partial return 9 months after the last injection of MPTP. The **upper three panels** in **B** are derived from the dorsal caudate nucleus, while the **lower three panels** are derived from theuppermost dorsal-lateral quadrant of the caudate nucleus/ white matter junction. The *scale bar* in **upper right panel** represents 1 mm.

MPTP (FIG. 2). The expression of TH and DAT proteins in the caudate and putamen showed a 90% depletion at 6 weeks but returned to only 35% of prelesioned levels at 9 months. Despite the partial recovery of TH, monkeys demonstrated normal motor behavior. Unbiased stereological analysis of SNpc neurons based on TH immunoreactivity with Nissl substance staining in both parkinsonian (harvested at 6 weeks postlesioning) and recovered (harvested at 9 months postlesioning) monkeys is being used to determine if there is a significantly different number of midbrain dopaminergic neurons between these groups (Petzinger *et al.*, in preparation).

In the treadmill exercise paradigm, MPTP-lesioned mice showed enhanced behavioral recovery. After 30 days of exercise, both velocity and endurance reached levels similar to the normal exercise animals. Molecular analysis of the exercised MPTP-lesioned animals showed suppression of striatal DAT protein compared to the nonexercised MPTP-lesioned control group. Immunoelectron microscopy analysis showed that MPTP alone increased the density of nerve terminal glutamate and that exercise reversed this increase (Fisher *et al.*, in preparation).

DISCUSSION

Results from these studies show that both TH and DAT protein return participate in behavioral recovery after MPTP lesioning. The partial return of TH and DAT protein in the squirrel monkey in conjunction with the complete behavioral recovery suggests that nondopaminergic systems may be involved in neuroplasticity after injury to the basal ganglia. One important system may involve glutamate.

The treadmill exercise paradigm shows that exercise alters both the glutamatergic and dopaminergic systems as part of neuroplasticity in the injured basal ganglia. These alterations that accompany behavioral recovery can take place at either the molecular level (DAT protein expression) or morphological level (changes in glutamate density of nerve terminal glutamate immunolabeling). Ongoing studies indicate that expression of TH and dopamine receptors (D1 and D2 subtypes) are also altered in our exercise paradigm (Fisher *et al.*, in preparation).

The elucidation of the molecular mechanisms underlying neuroplasticity in the MPTP-lesioned mouse and nonhuman primate will identify novel therapeutic targets and will provide insight into the application of current strategies including transplantation.

ACKNOWLEDGMENTS

These studies are supported by the National Institutes of Health, the U.S. Army, the Parkinson's Disease Foundation, the Lisette and Norman Ackerberg Foundation, the Baxter Foundation, the Zumberge Foundation, and the VA Merit Review Program (to C.M.).

An Experimental Infection by Filterable Forms of *Nocardia asteroides* and Late-Onset Movement Disorder in Mice

S. KOHBATA[a] AND C. KADOYA[b]

[a]*Department of Microbiology, Gifu University School of Medicine, Gifu City, Gifu 500-8076, Japan*

[b]*Department of Neurosurgery, University of Occupational and Environmental Health, Kitakyushu, Fukuoka 807-8555, Japan*

KEYWORDS: *Nocardia asteroides*; filterable nocardiae; Parkinson's disease

Filterable nocardiae, morphologically identical to lipochrome bodies in Parkinson's disease,[1] are not gram-positive bacteria isolated from broth cultures of *Nocardia asteroides* by filtration.[2,3] They fluoresced brilliantly green-yellow under ultraviolet light when stained with acridine orange and were strongly periodic acid–Schiff stain (PAS) positive on day 1 of incubation in broth cultures. They became acid fast after day 2 of incubation. The 5-h cultures were used as inoculum for the experimental infection. The 14-h cultures were used as antigen for the preparation of anti-filterable nocardiae antiserum according to the modified method.[4]

After the mice were inoculated via the tail vein, they appeared to be healthy and to move as quickly as control mice. By early in month 5, the mice were moving slowly. When the tail was picked up, they failed to respond abruptly, and when they did move, they moved slowly. They appeared to have difficulty with a particular motion, the twisting of the body trunk, at month 5. At month 6, they hung limply when suspended. Soon after, they bent their backs and held their forepaws, assuming a peculiar posture, resembling sleeping bats, which they maintained.

Their brains were collected, fixed, and embedded in paraffin. Serial coronal sections were prepared. The sections were stained for Nissl substance with cresyl violet for dopamine neurons with anti-tyrosine hydroxylase antibody,[5] or for filterable nocardiae with carbolfuchsin, PAS, and anti-filterable nocardiae antiserum. The midbrain section revealed that the pars compacta dopamine neurons were severely damaged at month 5 and lost bilaterally at month 6. Filterable nocardiae were demonstrated as acid-fast particles within many macroglia in nearby sinusoidal vessels

Address for correspondence: S. Kohbata, Department of Microbiology, Gifu University School of Medicine, Tsukasa-machi 40, Gifu City, Gifu 500-8076, Japan. Voice: 81-582-65-1241; fax: 81-562-67-0156.

skohbata@cc.gifu-u.ac.jp

Ann. N.Y. Acad. Sci. 991: 302–303 (2003). © 2003 New York Academy of Sciences.

of the midbrain. These were apparent early in month 5 and continued to be evident during the month. At month 6, they were seen as immunoreactive deposits within many macroglia distributed through the substantia nigra. The acid-fast filterable nocardiae, observed early in month 5, are reminiscent of acid-fast lipochrome bodies in the early phases of Parkinson's disease.[1] The immunological detection of filterable nocardiae in Parkinson's disease is now under study.[6] Filterable nocardiae were also detected as immunopositive deposits within many macroglia distributed through the substantia nigra at week 5, but they were not detected later.

Filterable nocardiae, which may be able to invade the midbrain substantia nigra, were probably eliminated by host immune responses. Reinvasion of the midbrain by filterable nocardiae, early in month 5 through month 6, indicates their extraneural focus of infection rather than their neural persistence in host tissues.

The results suggest that an infection of the midbrain with filterable nocardiae may occur and cause the severe damage of the pars compacta dopamine neurons related to the movement disorder.

REFERENCES

1. KOHBATA. S., *et al*. 1998. Accumulation of acid-fast lipochrome bodies in glial cells of the midbrain nigral lesion in Parkinson's disease. Clin. Diag. Lab. Immunol. **5:** 888–893.
2. KOHBATA, S. 1996. Acid-fastness of *Nocardia asteroides* GUH-2 cultured in brain heart infusion broth supplemented with paraffin. Microbiol. Immunol. **40:** 711–716.
3. KOHBATA, S. 1998. Tinctorial properties of spherical bodies in broth cultures of *Nocardia asteroides* GUH-2. Microbiol. Immunol. **42:** 151–157.
4. KOHBATA, S., *et al*. 1986. Cytopathogenic effect of *Salmonella typhi* GIFU 10007 on M cells of murine ileal Peyer's patches in ligated ileal loops: An ultra-structural study. Microbiol. Immunol. **30:** 1225–1237.
5. KOHBATA, S. & B.L. BEAMAN. 1991. L-Dopa-responsive movement disorder caused by *Nocardia asteroides* localized in the brains of mice. Infect. Immunity **59:** 181–191.
6. KOHBATA, S., *et al*. 2002. An infection with filterable forms of *Nocardia asteroides* in the midbrain nigral lesion in Parkinson's disease. Paper presented at the Seventh International Congress of Parkinson's Disease and Movement Disorders, Miami, FL, November 11, 2002.

A Characterization of Dopaminergic Neurodegeneration in Organotypic Cultures

GERALDINE J. KRESS AND IAN J. REYNOLDS

Department of Pharmacology, University of Pittsburgh,
Pittsburgh, Pennsylvania 15261, USA

KEYWORDS: Parkinson's disease; 6-hydroxydopamine; substantia nigra; cell death

Parkinson's disease is a neurodegenerative disorder involving the progressive dopaminergic degeneration of the nigrostriatal pathway. A major obstacle in the prevention and treatment of this disease is determining the cause of degeneration. Many studies have linked oxidative stresses, such as those arising from dysfunctional mitochondria, as playing a role.[1] Additionally, compounds such as 6-hydroxydopamine (6-OHDA) also cause oxidative stresses by accumulating in dopaminergic neurons, oxidizing, and producing free radicals and hydrogen peroxide. Interestingly, 6-OHDA selectively harms dopamine cells of the substantia nigra but not those of the ventral tegmental area.

Several studies of dopaminergic neurotoxins have been performed in whole animal models and in dissociated cell culture, but none in organotypic cultures. Therefore, we propose to study dopaminergic cell death in cortex-striatum-substantia nigra organotypic cultures prepared from P1-3 rats. Organotypic cultures provide a useful intermediate between dissociated cell cultures and *in vivo* models because (1) they possess mature dopaminergic neurons and supporting glial cells; (2) they form synaptic connections; (3) they are relatively long-lived; and (4) they retain the simplicity of *in vitro* systems. In our organotypic culture, adapted from Plenz and Kitai,[2] the slices were grown for 18–23 days before experimentation.

Prior to 6-OHDA application, slices were stained with 5,7-dihydroxytryptamine (DHT). DHT is a fluorophore selectively taken up by dopaminergic cells via the dopamine transporter without displaying any visible toxic effects. DHT was used to locate and quantify the number of dopaminergic cells in live slices. Moreover, prior to 6-OHDA application, the viability of the slice was examined with propidium iodide (PI), a fluorophore that stains dead cells. Slices were excluded from the study if the initial amount of PI staining was high. After PI and DHT staining, 6-OHDA was applied, then washed extensively, and returned to the incubator. After 6-OHDA

Address for correspondence: Ian J. Reynolds, Ph.D., Department of Pharmacology, School of Medicine, University of Pittsburgh, Pittsburgh, PA 15261. Voice: 412-648-2134; fax: 412-624-0794.

iannmda+@pitt.edu

Ann. N.Y. Acad. Sci. 991: 304–306 (2003). © 2003 New York Academy of Sciences.

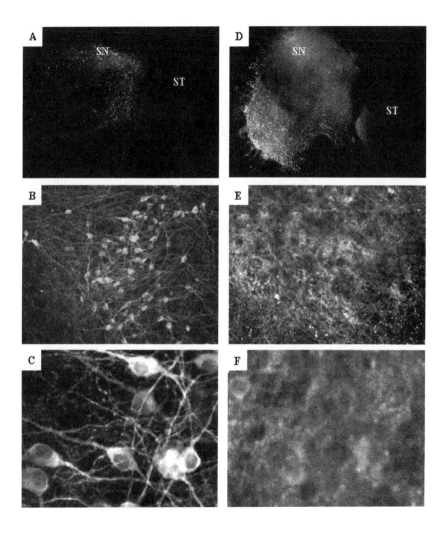

FIGURE 1. Cortex-striatum-substantia nigra organotypic cultures were treated with media or 200 µM 6-hydroxydopamine for 1 hour, washed, and evaluated 7 days after treatment. Cultures were fixed and immunostained for tyrosine hydroxylase (TH) and then visualized with Alexa Fluor 488 conjugate. Control treatment cultures in **A**, **B**, and **C** illustrate TH cell bodies in the substantia nigra and innervating processes into the striatum. Cells bodies and processes are bright and intact. **D**, **E**, and **F** illustrate altered TH staining 7 days after 6-OHDA treatment. The TH staining is diffuse and less associated with cell bodies and processes.

treatment, the slices were examined with PI staining to assess nonspecific death and then fixed for immunohistochemical determinations.

Control slices illustrated in FIGURE 1A, B, and C show bright, intact tyrosine hydroxylase (TH)–positive cell bodies in the substantia nigra with processes innervating the striatum. The PI staining of control slices is nearly undetectable (data not shown). With high 6-OHDA concentrations (5 mM) for short exposure times (15 minutes), gross injury was evident by the detachment of the slice from the substrate. The determined amount of 6-OHDA applied to the slice to produce low nonspecific death was 200 μM for 1 hour; the slice was then visualized 7 days post stimulus with PI staining (data not shown). FIGURE 1D, E, and F show a type of TH staining very different from that of the control. There is an overall loss of TH staining in the substantia nigra and striatum, which is diffuse and less associated with cell bodies and processes. This altered pattern of staining may be indicative of a selective injury process. Also, this altered pattern of TH staining after 6-OHDA is not what we expected on the basis of studies *in vivo* and in dissociated cell cultures where TH staining is lost using this kind of injury paradigm. Moreover, it is difficult to do an objective quantitative assessment of this kind of rearrangement of staining using simple measures of fluorescence intensity.

In conclusion, we have demonstrated that a change occurs in TH staining with low nonspecific cell death that may reflect selective dopaminergic injury after 6-OHDA. However, additional studies, perhaps with other markers of cell injury, will be necessary to establish whether alterations in TH staining following 6-OHDA actually reflect cell injury.

REFERENCES

1. BETARBET, R., *et al.* 2002. Animal models of Parkinson's disease. Bioessays **24:** 308–318.
2. PLENZ, D. & S.T. KITAI. 1996. Organotypic cortex-striatum-mesencephalon cultures: nigrostriatal pathway. Neurosci. Lett. **209:** 177–180.

Developmental Cell Death and Oxidative Stress

Lessons from Nigral Dopamine Neurons

LAURENT GROC,[a–c] TANGELLA JACKSON HUNTER,[a] HAO JIANG,[a,b]
LAURENT BEZIN,[d] AND ROBERT A. LEVINE[a–c]

[a]William T. Gossett Neurology Laboratories, Henry Ford Health System,
Detroit, Michigan 48202, USA

[b]John D. Dingell Veterans Administration Medical Center,
Detroit, Michigan 48201, USA

[c]Department of Pharmaceutical Sciences, Wayne State University,
Detroit, Michigan 48201, USA

[d]CNRS-UMR5578, Lyon, France

KEYWORDS: developmental cell death; dopamine; oxidative stress; substantia
nigra

Neuronal death during development appears to be a key event for the maturation of the nervous system. The mechanisms underlying developmental death are poorly understood, although several *in vitro* studies have suggested the involvement of oxidative stress.[1] As shown in FIGURE 1, oxidative stress in neurons (e.g., dopaminergic) can be mediated by reactive oxygen species (ROS) that induce cellular damage such as lipid peroxidation (lipid byproducts derived from the breakdown of polyunsaturated fatty acids). Oxidative stress may also involve nitric oxide metabolism. ROS can be scavenged by the antioxidant enzymes superoxide dismutase, catalase, and glutathione peroxidase (GPx),[2] which are usually activated during periods of oxidative stress. High oxidative stress exceeds the capacity of antioxidant enzymes and leads to ROS-induced cellular damage, particularly lipid peroxidation. On the contrary, when the activity of these enzymes is upregulated sufficiently, the amount of lipid peroxidation is kept at a low level (FIG. 1).

Developmental apoptotic death of dopamine neurons in the rat substantia nigra occurs mainly around birth, with a major peak at postnatal day (P) 3.[3] Understanding intrinsic mechanisms causing developmental apoptotic death that is not induced by external insults (e.g., neurotoxins) may shed light on the causes of apoptotic death of nigral dopamine neurons in Parkinson's disease, because the same mechanisms may mediate the premature loss of nigral dopamine neurons in Parkinson's disease.

Address for correspondence: Robert A. Levine, Ph.D., W.T. Gossett Neurology Laboratories, Henry Ford Health System, 1 Ford Place, Detroit, MI 48202. Voice: 313-874-3771; fax: 208-545-3455.

bob-levine@earthlink.net or laurent.groc@physiol.gu.se

Ann. N.Y. Acad. Sci. 991: 307–310 (2003). © 2003 New York Academy of Sciences.

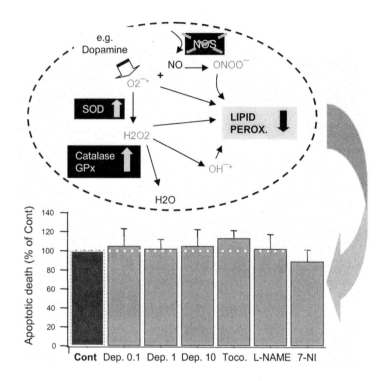

FIGURE 1. (Upper panel) Antioxidant treatments during the perinatal period increased antioxidant enzyme activities (*black boxes*) and decreased the level of lipid peroxidation likely due to a decrease in reactive oxygen species (ROS). **(Lower panel)** Lowering oxidative stress as well as nitric oxide formation did not change the level of developmental cell death of nigral dopamine neurons (deprenyl, 0.1, 1, and 10 mg/kg; α-tocopherol 1 g/kg; L-NAME, 60 mg/kg; 7-NI, 30 mg/kg; $n = 5$–10 per group, $P > 0.05$).

Although adult nigral dopaminergic neurons are destroyed by neurotoxins that induce oxidative stress,[2] the involvement of oxidative stress in developmental apoptosis of these neurons has remained an open question. To address this question, we used two complementary approaches: (1) to compare the level of oxidative stress markers in the substantia nigra during developmental apoptotic and nonapoptotic periods,[4] and (2) to attempt to block developmental dopamine neuronal death using antioxidants[4,5] and inhibitors of nitric oxide synthesis.[6]

Approach 1. Two major byproducts derived from the breakdown of polyunsaturated fatty acids (e.g., malonaldehyde) were measured to estimate the level of lipid peroxidation.[4] During the main apoptotic period (P3), lipid peroxidation was lower than that during a nonapoptotic period (P8). The low level of lipid peroxidation was not due to overactivation of antioxidant enzymes, because the activities of superoxide dismutase, catalase, and GPx were constant during apoptotic and nonapoptotic periods.[4] These results suggest that the level of oxidative stress during the peak of apoptosis at P3 is low.

Approach 2. To test further if oxidative stress triggers apoptotic death of nigral dopamine neurons at crucial stages during perinatal development, we examined whether antioxidant drug treatments during pre- and postnatal periods could prevent this death process.[4–6] Antioxidant treatments with deprenyl and α-tocopherol increased the activity of antioxidative enzymes and reduced lipid peroxidation,[4,5,7] and nitric oxide synthase inhibitors (L-NAME, 7-NI) significantly reduced the formation of nitric oxide (FIG. 1, upper panel). However, none of those treatments reduced the developmental death of nigral dopamine neurons (FIG. 1, lower panel). Moreover, no change in the structure of the substantia nigra, as monitored by tyrosine hydroxylase immunocytochemistry, was observed after antioxidant treatments.[5,6] These treatments also had no effect on the locomotor activity of adult rats.[7]

Our findings suggest that neither ROS nor nitric oxide is a major inducer or mediator of *in vivo* developmental death of nigral dopamine neurons.[4–7] In related studies, we have also shown that oxidative stress is unlikely to be involved in the apoptotic death of PC12 cells after withdrawal of trophic support.[8] It therefore seems unlikely that ROS, which are highly reactive and rather nonspecific molecules, mediate the highly controlled process of developmental cell death.[9] The increased levels of ROS previously observed in different *in vitro* or *in vivo* neurodegenerative models of developmental cell death[1] may be a passive result rather than a causal factor in apoptosis. Which cellular pathways, then, may be responsible for the death of the dopamine neurons during development? There is evidence for the involvement of caspase 3,[10] Bcl-2 family members,[11,12] as well as the proteasome complex.[13] Moreover, the involvement of transcription factors, such as Nurr1, in the late postnatal cell death process has been hypothesized.[14] However, more investigations are needed to fully clarify the relevant pathways. Once the underlying mechanisms causing apoptosis of nigral dopamine neurons during development are elucidated, it will be possible to investigate whether these same mechanisms are inappropriately activated in Parkinson's disease.

REFERENCES

1. CASTAGNE, V., M. GAUTSCHI, K. LEFEVRE, *et al.* 1999. Relationships between neuronal death and the cellular redox status. Focus on the developing nervous system. Prog. Neurobiol. **59:** 397–423.
2. CADET, J.L. & C. BRANNOCK. 1998. Free radicals and the pathobiology of brain dopamine systems. Neurochem. Int. **32:** 117–131.
3. OO, T.F. & R.E. BURKE. 1997. The time course of developmental cell death in phenotypically defined dopaminergic neurons of the substantia nigra. Dev. Brain Res. **98:** 191–196.
4. GROC, L., L. BEZIN, J.A. FOSTER, *et al.* 2001. Lipid peroxidation-mediated oxidative stress and dopamine neuronal apoptosis in the substantia nigra during development. Neurochem. Int. **39:** 127–133.
5. GROC, L., R.A. LEVINE, J.A. FOSTER, *et al.* 2000. Evidence of deprenyl-insensitive apoptosis of nigral dopamine neurons during development. Brain Res. Dev. Brain Res. **120:** 95–98.
6. GROC, L., T. JACKSON HUNTER, H. JIANG, *et al.* 2002. Nitric oxide synthase inhibition during development: effect on apoptotic death of dopamine neurons. Brain Res. Dev. Brain Res. **138:** 147–153.
7. GROC, L., L. BEZIN, H. JIANG, *et al.* 2002. Inhibition of oxidative stress during developmental cell death: cellular and behavioral effects. Chem. Biol. Pteridines Folates 399–404. Kluwer Academic Publishers. The Netherlands.

8. ANASTASIADIS, P.Z., H. JIANG, L. BEZIN, et al. 2001. Tetrahydrobiopterin enhances apoptotic PC12 cell death following withdrawal of trophic support. J. Biol. Chem. **276:** 9050–9058.

9. JACOBSON, M.D. 1996. Reactive oxygen species and programmed cell death. Trends Biochem. Sci. **21:** 83–86.

10. JEON, B.S., N.G. KHOLODILOV, T.F. OO, et al. 1999. Activation of caspase-3 in developmental models of programmed cell death in neurons of the substantia nigra. J. Neurochem. **73:** 322–333.

11. GROC, L., L. BEZIN, H. JIANG, et al. 2001. Bcl-2 and cyclin expression and apoptosis in rat substantia nigra during development. Neurosci. Lett. **306:** 198–202.

12. JACKSON-LEWIS, V., M. VILA, R. DJALDETTI, et al. 2000. Developmental cell death in dopaminergic neurons of the substantia nigra of mice. J. Comp. Neurol. **424:** 476–488.

13. EL-KHODOR, B.F., N.G. KHOLODILOV, O. YARYGINA & R.E. BURKE. 2001. The expression of mRNAs for the proteasome complex is developmentally regulated in the rat mesencephalon. Brain Res. Dev. Brain Res. **129:** 47–56.

14. SAUCEDO-CARDENAS, O., J.D. QUINTANA-HAU, W.-D. LE, et al. 1998. Nurr1 is essential for the induction of the dopaminergic phenotype and the survival of ventral mesencephalic late dopaminergic precursor neurons. Proc. Natl. Acad. Sci. USA **95:** 4013–4018.

Identification of a Novel Gene Linked to Parkin via a Bidirectional Promoter

PAUL J. LOCKHART,[a] ANDREW B. WEST,[b] CASEY A. O'FARRELL,[a] AND MATTHEW J. FARRER[a]

[a]Laboratories of Neuroscience and [b]Program for Molecular Neuroscience, Mayo Clinic Jacksonville, Jacksonville, Florida 32224, USA

KEYWORDS: Parkinson's disease; Parkin; transcription regulation; bidirectional promoters

Mutations of the Parkin gene (*Parkin*) on chromosome 6q25-27 are the predominant cause of familial early-onset, autosomal-recessive parkinsonism (AR-JP). Parkin is a multidomain protein, with ubiquitin-protein (E3) ligase activity, that has a role in the proteasome-mediated degradation of target substrates. Previously, we identified and characterized the promoter structure and regulatory regions of *Parkin*.[1] In the process, we identified a novel gene that initiates 204 bp upstream of *Parkin* and spans over 0.6 Mb of genomic DNA, antisense to *Parkin*. We have named this novel gene *Parkin coregulated gene* or *PACRG*.[2] Northern blot analysis demonstrated that *PACRG* was expressed in many tissues and was co-expressed with *Parkin* in several, including brain, heart, and muscle (FIG. 1). Database analysis identified homologous proteins encoded in the mouse and the fly databases (FIG. 2); however, no functional domains were detected across the complete protein sequence. Currently, the function of *PACRG* is unknown.

Electronic prediction analysis suggested that *Parkin* and *PACRG* shared a bidirectional promoter with common transcription factor binding sites (data not shown). To test this hypothesis, we designed a series of overlapping promoter fragments and inserted them (in both orientations) upstream of a promoterless luciferase reporter construct (pGL3-Basic, Promega). Dopaminergic BE(2)-M17 neuroblastoma cells were transfected with the constructs, and promoter activity was assessed by a dual-luciferase assay (Promega). Transcriptional activation of the reporter was observed 72 bp upstream/sense of the *Parkin* transcriptional start site (TSS) and 173

Address for correspondence: Dr. Paul J. Lockhart, Laboratories of Neuroscience, Mayo Clinic Jacksonville, 4500 San Pablo Road, Jacksonville, FL 32224. Voice: 904-953-2483; fax: 904-953-7370.

lockhart.paul@mayo.edu

Ann. N.Y. Acad. Sci. 991: 311–314 (2003). © 2003 New York Academy of Sciences.

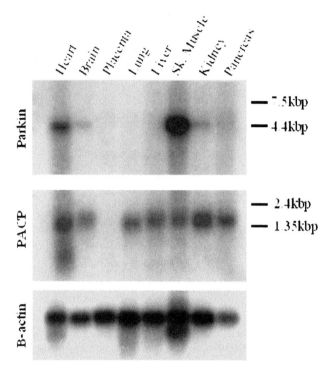

FIGURE 1. Expression analysis of *PACRG*. Probes for *Parkin*, *PACRG*, and *beta-actin* were hybridized to a multiple human tissue blot (Clontech).

bp upstream/sense of the *PACRG* TSS (FIG. 3). These results suggest that a common bidirectional region of transcription activation for *Parkin* and *PACRG* is located in the region −72 to −38 bp upstream/sense of the *Parkin* TSS. This sequence contains a noncanonical myc site (CGCGTG), recently demonstrated to bind N and C-myc/ Max transcription factors and mediate expression of Pax3.[3] We are currently testing the possibility that *Parkin/PACRG* transcription might be regulated by a similar mechanism.

To confirm that *PACRG* was expressed and translated *in vivo*, we generated peptide antibodies specific for *PACRG* and performed Western analysis of mouse and human brain extracts. Two independent antibodies gave similar results. A protein of the predicted size (approximately 30 kDa) was detected in human and mouse brain extracts and in HEK293 cells transfected with *PACRG* expression constructs (data not shown). This protein was not observed when the antibody was incubated

```
Human        ----MVAEKETLSLNKCPDKMPKRTK-LLAQQPLPVHQPH-SLVSEG------FTVKAMM  48
Mouse        -------------------MPKRTK-LLPQQTFQVHQPR-SLVSEG------FTVKAMM  32
Drosophila   MAMAQTARTATARRPTHDYHRPTRSKSANPAQLRPLSGIHGAAVSSRPRYVPPFSIQSQQ  60
                 :  :       .     *.*:*   . *   :   : : **.      *:::::

Human        KNSVVRG------PPAAGAFKERPTKP--------------------------------  69
Mouse        KNSVVRG------PPVAGAFKERPAKP--------------------------------  53
Drosophila   KNTVVIDGPIHETAPKTASARSRVPNPKILRRQQKSMSTFNLGMGLNGCSTGGANDPGRG  120
             **:**  .        .* :.: :.* .:*

Human        TAFRKFYERGDFPIALEHDSKGNKIAWKVEIEKLDYHHYLPLFFDGLCEMTFPYEFFARQ  129
Mouse        TTFRKCYERGDFPIALEHDSKGNKIAWKVEIEKLDYHHYLPLFFDGLSEMTFPYEFFARR  113
Drosophila   TLFRMYFDRGDLPIKMEYLCGGDKIGWTVDIEKLDYSLYLPLFFDGLAETKHPYKTYARQ  180
             * **  ::***:** :*: . *:**.*.*:****** ********.* ..**: :**:

Human        GIHDMLEHGGNKILPVLPQLIIPIKNALNLRNRQVICVTLKVLQHLVVSAEMVGKALVPY  189
Mouse        GIHDMLEHGGNKILPVIPQLIIPIKNALNLRNRQIICVTLKVLQHLVVSSEMVGEALLPY  173
Drosophila   GVTDLLLAGGEKIHPVIPQLILPLKNALSTRNLEVMCTTLKIIQQLVMSSDLVGPALVPF  240

             *: *:* **:** **:****:*:**** ** :::*.***::*:**:*:::** **:*:

Human        YRQILPVLNIFKNMNVNSGDGIDYSQQKRENIGDLIQETLEAFERYGGENAFINIKYVVP  249
Mouse        YRQILPILNIFKNMNVNSGDGIDYSQQKRENIGDLIQETLEAFERYGGEDAFINIKYMVP  233
Drosophila   YRQLLPMFNAFKVKNLNCGDEIDYAQKNNLNLGDLIDETLQVLELHGGEDAFINIKYMVP  300
             ***:**::* ** *:*.** ***:*:: *:****:***::* :***:*******:**

Human        TYESCLLN 257            ▨▨▨▨ =Predicted alpha-helix domain
Mouse        TYESCLLN 241            ▬▬▬▬ =Predicted beta sheet domain
Drosophila   TYESCYLN 308
             ***** **
```

FIGURE 2. *PACRG* protein homology. Alignment of human (AF546872), mouse (BAB24230), and *Drosophila* (AAF57542) *PACRG* is given. Predicted secondary structure is indicated, as determined by Nnpredict (http://www.cmpharm.ucsf.edu).

with an excess of the immunizing peptide or when the filter was probed with preimmune serum samples.

In summary, we have identified a novel gene that shares a 35-bp region of bidirectional transcription activation with the *Parkin* gene. Bidirectional promoters have been described to drive genes that function in a common biological pathway, such as subunits of the trifunctional protein complex.[4] Although the function of

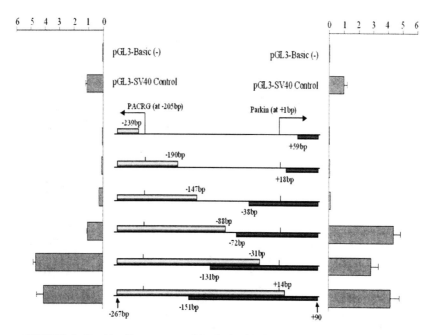

FIGURE 3. Dual luciferase assay of the *Parkin/PACRG* promoter region. Deletion constructs were inserted into the pGL3-Basic vector in the sense (*dark bar*) or antisense (*light bar*) orientation relative to *Parkin*. Resulting luciferase activity in transiently transfected BE(2)-M17 neuroblastoma cells is given adjacent to each construct. Units are relative to the SV-40 control promoter, defined as one. Data are representative of six independent experiments, and *error bars* are 2 × SEM. Positions of deletion constructs are given relative to the *Parkin* transcriptional start site.

PACRG is currently unknown, we are currently investigating the possibility that *PACRG* may function in the same biological pathway as *Parkin*.

REFERENCES

1. WEST, A., *et al.* 2001. Identification and characterization of the human parkin gene promoter. J. Neurochem. **78:** 1146–1152.
2. WEST, A., *et al.* 2003. Identification of a novel gene linked to parkin via a bi-directional promoter. J. Mol. Biol. **326:** 11–19.
3. BLACKWELL, T.K., *et al.* 1993. Binding of myc proteins to canonical and noncanonical DNA sequences. Mol. Cell Biol. **13:** 5216–5224.
4. ORII, K.E., *et al.* 1999. Genes for the human mitochondrial trifunctional protein alpha- and beta-subunits are divergently transcribed from a common promoter region. J. Biol. Chem. **274:** 8077–8084.

Gene Expression Analysis of the MPTP-Lesioned Substantia Nigra in Mice

R. M. MILLER, C. CASACELI, L. CHEN, AND H. J. FEDEROFF

Department of Neurology, Center for Aging and Developmental Biology, University of Rochester School of Medicine, Rochester, New York 14642, USA

KEYWORDS: genes; Parkinson's disease; MPTP; substantia nigra

INTRODUCTION

Parkinson's disease (PD) is a clinical syndrome triggered by disparate mechanisms. That the clinical and neuropathological features are indistinguishable among the different forms suggests a convergent, shared pathway. The earliest shared steps of this cascade, including compensatory responses, represent ideal targets for therapeutic development.

One approach is the use of robust exploratory methodologies to identify candidate molecules or pathways that can be implicated in one or more models of PD. An assortment of new technologies is available to assist in this discovery. To increase the reliability of target identification and then confirm involvement of a particular molecule in any biologic process, additional strategies are needed. To this end, we have undertaken an integrative bionomic approach whereby multiple methodologies are used to establish the involvement of candidate molecules in dopamine neuron cell injury, compensation, and cell death. We applied the integrated bionomics approach to the discovery of new molecular targets for PD in the 1-methyl-4-phenyl-1,2,3,6-tetrahydropyridine (MPTP)-treated mouse model (30 mg/kg MPTP-HCl; 4 doses ip over 8 days). Two time points following MPTP intoxication were examined. Using four data mining methods (MAS 5.0 and DMT, dChip,[1] and SAM[2]), we found that the expression of many genes decreased in MPTP-treated mice relative to saline-treated controls at the 24-hour time point. At 7 days, there were both increased and decreased genes.

RESULTS

Gene expression analysis using Affymetrix U74A oligonucleotide arrays of MPTP- and saline-treated mice was employed to discover novel and potentially important molecular changes in the substantia nigra (SN) following dopaminergic cell injury. Raw intensity data (.cel files) were analyzed using two independent methods

Address for correspondence: H.J. Federoff, M.D., Ph.D., University of Rochester School of Medicine, 601 Elmwood Ave., Rochester, NY 14642. Voice: 585-273-2190; fax: 585-506-1957.
    howard_federoff@urmc.rochester.edu

Ann. N.Y. Acad. Sci. 991: 315–318 (2003). © 2003 New York Academy of Sciences.

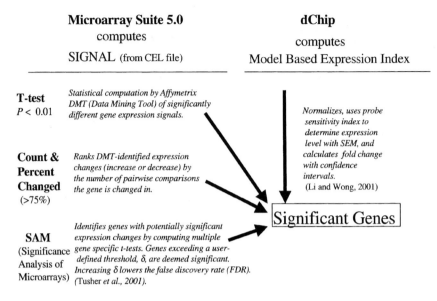

FIGURE 1. Affymetrix .cel files were analyzed with MAS 5.0 or dChip to generate gene expression levels for each sample. Gene expression levels in saline- and MPTP-treated samples were then compared to identify significant changes. Each method (*t*-test, pair-wise comparisons, SAM, and dChip) was used to create a list of genes whose difference exceeded a predefined significance threshold.

to generate expression levels for each gene, which were then used to compare levels between MPTP and saline arrays (FIG. 1). As expected, we found that the expression of several genes related to the dopaminergic phenotype, including tyrosine hydroxylase (TH) and dopamine transporter (DAT), was decreased in MPTP-treated mice. Other functional classes were affected as well, notably transcription factors, kinases, and phosphatases, and messages coding for proteins involved with protein transport and degradation (TABLE 1). We found that the expression of 126 genes was

TABLE 1. Functional classification of mRNAs

Functional class	MML genes: 126 total in 4/4 methods	MME & MML genes: 23 total in 4/4 methods
Transcription/translation	15	4
Kinase/phosphatase	9	3
Signaling	11	2
Developmental	3	0
Bioenergetics	5	2
Protein turnover/transport	8	2
Other	11	3
Unknown	63	8

A.   Analysis of MPTP 24 hr (MME) vs. Saline-Treated Mice

	T-test	Inc./Dec.	SAM	dChip
# significant genes:	3258	1073	218	1161

MERGE:

#genes in 4/4 methods: 126

B.   Analysis of MPTP 7 day (MML) vs. Saline-Treated Mice

	T-test	Inc./Dec.	SAM	dChip
# significant genes:	558	328	221	638

MERGE:

#genes in 4/4 methods: 44

FIGURE 2. Summary of significantly different gene totals for each method separately and merged. MPTP-treated mice sacrificed at 24 hours following the last dose were compared to saline-treated littermates **(A)**. MPTP-treated mice sacrificed 7 days after the last dose were compared to saline-treated littermates **(B)**.

decreased, as determined by all four methods employed, 24 hours after the final MPTP injection (FIG. 2). Seven days after the final MPTP dose, 23 of these genes were still decreased, whereas an additional 21 genes were significantly different (up or down, by all four methods) in the MPTP-treated mouse SN (FIG. 2B). In addition to the use of multiple data analysis techniques, we also verified our gene expression findings using quantitative real-time polymerase chain reaction (PCR) (TABLE 2). As predicted by the microarray results (genes called significant in four of four analysis

TABLE 2. Validation of MML and MME by quantitative RT-PCR

	Primer and probe set	Confirmed	Direction of change
Merged significant genes: 4/5 or 5/5	DAT	yes	D
	TH	yes	D
	E1kL motif kinase	yes	D
	AchE	yes	D
	PTP, D type	not detected	D
Single-method significant genes	Kinesin 3a	no	NC
	VAMP 2	no	NC
	MAP-6	no	NC

methods), expression of TH, DAT, emk, and AchE was significantly decreased by re-al- time PCR. Further validation of these candidates is in progress. We have been un-able to validate genes called significant in three or fewer methods (i.e., kinesin 3A, VAMP-2, and MAP-6).

REFERENCES

1. LI, C & W.H. WONG. 2001. Model-based analysis of oligonucleotide arrays: model val-idation, design issues and standard error application. Genome Biol. **2:** 32.1–32.11.
2. TUSHER, V.G., R. TIBSHIRANI & G. CHU. 2001. Significance analysis of microarrays applied to the ionizing radiation response. Proc. Natl. Acad. Sci. USA **98:** 5116–5121.

Neuroimaging and Proteomic Tracking of Neurodegeneration in MPTP-Treated Mice

HOWARD E. GENDELMAN,[a,b] CHRISTOPHER J. DESTACHE, [a,c]
MARINA L. ZELIVYANSKAYA,[a,b] JAY A. NELSON,[a,d] MICHAEL D. BOSKA,[a,d]
TONI M. BISKUP,[a,b] MICHAEL K. McCARTHY,[a,b] KIMBERLY A. CARLSON,[a,b]
CRAIG NEMECHEK,[a,b] ERIC J. BENNER,[a,b] AND R. LEE MOSLEY[a,b]

[a]Center for Neurovirology and Neurodegenerative Disorders, University of Nebraska
Medical Center, Omaha, Nebraska 68198-5215, USA

[b]Department of Pathology and Microbiology, University of Nebraska Medical Center,
Omaha, Nebraska 68198-5215, USA

[c]Department of Pharmacy Practice, Creighton University, Omaha, Nebraska 68178, USA

[d]Department of Radiology, University of Nebraska Medical Center, Omaha, Nebraska
68198-5215, USA

KEYWORDS: mouse; dopamine; neurodegeneration; 1-methyl-4-phenyl-1,2,3,6-tetrahydropyridine (MPTP); single-photon emission computed tomography (SPECT); magnetic resonance imaging (MRI); magnetic resonance spectroscopic imaging (MRSI); proteomics; tyrosine hydroxylase; dopamine transporter (DAT); 2β-carboxymethoxy-3β-(4-iodophenyl)tropane (β-CIT); D2 receptors; iodobenzamide (IBZM)

Our laboratory is developing an integrated testing paradigm for human Parkinson's disease aimed at early diagnosis and therapeutic monitoring of disease utilizing 1-methyl-4-phenyl-1,2,3,6-tetrahydropyridine (MPTP)-treated mice. Such MPTP-treated animals mirror the biochemical and histopathological aspects of human Parkinson's disease.[1] In our studies, male 8–11-week-old C57BL/6NCrlBR mice from Charles River Laboratories were administered four intraperitoneal (ip) injections (1 every 2 hours) of 21.8 mg MPTP·HCl (18 mg free base)/10 mL phosphate-buffered saline (PBS)/kg body weight. Excipient control mice received 10 mL PBS/kg body weight intraperitoneally over the same time period. MPTP induced typical dopaminergic neurodegeneration in the substantia nigra pars compacta (SNpc) and the striata, as determined by immunohistochemistry with antibody to tyrosine hydroxylase (TH).[2] A 63% loss of TH immunoreactive neurons was observed in the SNpc by 7 days after MPTP treatment as compared to controls ($P = 0.001$). Reverse

Address for correspondence: R. Lee Mosley, Ph.D., University of Nebraska Medical Center, 985215 Nebraska Medical Center, Omaha, NE 68198-5215. Voice: 402-559-2510; fax: 402-559-8922.
rlmosley@unmc.edu

Ann. N.Y. Acad. Sci. 991: 319–321 (2003). © 2003 New York Academy of Sciences.

phase–high performance liquid chromatography (HPLC) with electrochemical detection[3] of striatal lysates showed a 70% reduction in dopamine levels of MPTP mice ($P < 0.03$) with no significant differences in dopamine metabolites. Additionally, the loss of striatal termini and nigral neurons was evaluated by coregistration of single-photon emission computed tomography (SPECT)[4,5] and magnetic resonance (MR)/MR spectroscopic imaging (MRI/MRSI). SPECT analysis of striatal D2 receptors with [^{123}I]-iodobenzamide ([^{123}I]-IBZM)[5] and dopamine transporter (DAT) with [^{123}I]-2β-carboxymethoxy-3β-(4-iodophenyl)tropane ([^{123}I]-β-CIT)[4] demonstrated 30% and 32% reductions, respectively, in MPTP-treated mice compared to controls. Coregistration of SPECT and MRI confirmed the striatal location of [^{123}I]-IBZM and [^{123}I]-β-CIT ligand-receptor specificity. MRSI evaluation of 36-mm^3 midbrain volumes circumscribing the SN from day 5 MPTP-treated mice showed significantly reduced levels of N-acetylaspartate (42%), choline (25%), and glutamate (26%) and increased myoinositol (34%) compared to those in control animals. These meta-bolic changes are consistent with neuronal degradation and prominent gliosis.

To detect alterations in protein profiles induced by MPTP treatment, lysates from the midbrain of mice at 1, 2, 3, 4, and 7 days after intoxication were evaluated by proteomic tests using surface-enhanced laser desorption/ionization (SELDI) from adsorbed NP20 protein chips (Ciphergen Biosystems, Fremont, CA). Duplicate determinations from three mice per time point were compared to samples obtained from excipient controls treated on day 0, and phenomic profiles were generated by the evaluation of relative protein concentrations as a function of mass/charge. Protein concentrations of each molecular weight species at each time point that differed significantly were identified by Student's t test as candidates for further evaluation as a function of time. ANOVA indicated the existence of 45 different proteins for which the variance in protein expression was significantly affected over time post-MPTP treatment. Kinetic analysis of protein expression and histopathology obtained from the substantia nigra revealed that 35 of these midbrain protein species presented kinetic profiles that correlated with the frequency of silver-stained degenerating neurons, which peak by day 2 and, similar to TH immunoreactive neurons, reach a nadir by day 4 post-MPTP treatment.[2] Four protein profiles correlated with CD3$^+$ T cell infiltration into the substantia nigra; however, because of the small population of T cells found in the brain of MPTP-treated mice and consequent low contribution of proteins in midbrain lysates, the possibility could not be ruled out that these profiles may reflect mechanistic responses from other cell types. The remaining proteins exhibited expression kinetics for which no correlations could be made with the kinetic profile of any one cell type and appear to reflect a combination of kinetic profiles, suggesting that these protein species may be commonly expressed by a variety of MPTP-responsive cell types. We have recently initiated studies integrating SELDI proteomic and microsequence (ProteomiX, Thermo Finnigan) analyses to determine the identities of neural proteins whose expression is altered by MPTP treatment.

Overall, the utility of SPECT, MRI, and MRSI and the coregistration of these neuroimages with histopathological techniques in the MPTP model will provide additional information concerning disease processes during dopaminergic neurodegeneration. Moreover, the elucidation of noninvasive definitive neuroimages and unique protein profiles in the brain during the degenerative process could provide novel insights into the neuropathogenesis of disease as well as uncovering proteins that could be used for diagnosis and/or therapeutic monitoring of human Parkinson's disease.

REFERENCES

1. HEIKKILA, R.E., A. HESS & R.C. DUVOISIN. 1984. Dopaminergic neurotoxicity of 1-methyl-4-phenyl-1,2,5,6- tetrahydropyridine in mice. Science **224:** 1451–1453.
2. JACKSON-LEWIS, V., M. JAKOWEC, R.E. BURKE & S. PRZEDBORSKI. 1995. Time course and morphology of dopaminergic neuronal death caused by the neurotoxin 1-methyl-4-phenyl-1,2,3,6-tetrahydropyridine. Neurodegeneration **4:** 257–269.
3. JACKSON-LEWIS, V. & G. LIBERATORE. 2000. Effects of a unilateral stereotaxic injection of Tinuvin 123 into the substantia nigra on the nigrostriatal dopaminergic pathway in the rat. Brain Res. **866:** 197–210.
4. GOODMAN, M.M., M.P. KUNG, G.W. KABALKA, *et al.* 1994. Synthesis and characterization of radioiodinated N-(3-iodopropen-1-yl)-2 beta-carbomethoxy-3 beta-(4-chlorophenyl)tropanes: potential dopamine reuptake site imaging agents. J. Med. Chem. **37:** 1535–1542.
5. KUNG, H.F., R. KASLIWAL, S.G. PAN, *et al.* 1988. Dopamine D-2 receptor imaging radiopharmaceuticals: synthesis, radiolabeling, and *in vitro* binding of (R)-(+)- and (S)-(−)-3-iodo-2-hydroxy-6-methoxy-*N*-[(1-ethyl-2-pyrrolidinyl)methyl]benzamide. J. Med. Chem. **31:** 1039–1043.

PCBs and Dopamine Function

Neurological Effects of Polychlorinated Biphenyls: Does Occupational Exposure Alter Dopamine-Mediated Function?

RICHARD F. SEEGAL

Wadsworth Center, New York State Department of Health and School of Public Health, University at Albany, Albany, New York 12201, USA

KEYWORDS: polychlorinated biphenyls; occupational exposure; dopamine; neurological function

Polychlorinated biphenyls (PCBs), once heavily used in industry, are now widespread environmental contaminants that are suggested to be associated with developmental and cognitive deficits in infants and children born to mothers who consumed food products contaminated with PCBs and other toxicants.[1] These data, supported by studies of laboratory animals exposed during development to PCBs, as reviewed by Seegal,[2] suggest that the developing central nervous system (CNS) is sensitive to this toxicant. However, both *in vitro* and *in vivo* data (to be described) suggest that: (1) susceptibility extends beyond the perinatal period, and (2) PCBs induce long-term alterations in dopamine (DA) function, including reductions in *de novo* synthesis and inhibition of monoamine transporter function. These findings, in turn, provide a biologically based rationale for examining neurological function in a cohort of aging former capacitor workers who had been exposed to extraordinarily high levels of PCBs.

PCBs ALTER DOPAMINE FUNCTION *IN VITRO*

PCBs reduce DA content in tissues derived from laboratory rodents, including pheochromocytoma (PC12) cells, adult striatal tissue, and synaptosomes exposed *ex vivo* to PCBs, and they elevate media DA concentrations.[3] These changes in DA function may, in part, involve PCB-induced inhibition of monoamine transporters, including the membrane dopamine transporter (DAT) and the intracellular vesicular

Address for correspondence: Dr. Richard F. Seegal, Wadsworth Center, New York State Department of Health and School of Public Health, University at Albany, Albany, NY 12201. Voice: 518-473-4378; fax: 518-486-1505.

seegal@wadsworth.org

Ann. N.Y. Acad. Sci. 991: 322–325 (2003). © 2003 New York Academy of Sciences.

monoamine transporter (VMAT).[4,5] The consequences of such transporter inhibition include increased free cytosolic DA, elevations in both tissue and media concentrations of 3,4-dihydroxyphenylacetic acid (DOPAC), and enhanced formation of DA quinones and semiquinones, leading to generation of hydrogen peroxide and other reactive oxygen species.[6]

PCBs ALTER DOPAMINE FUNCTION *IN VIVO*

The alterations in DA function just described may explain the neurochemical and neuropathological consequences of long-term exposure of the adult nonhuman primate to PCBs. Thus, in adult nonhuman primates exposed to PCBs for 20 weeks, an exposure that results in serum concentrations similar to those seen in former workers, basal ganglia DA concentrations were significantly reduced.[7] Furthermore, when additional nonhuman primates were exposed to similar levels of PCBs but were then removed from exposure for 24 or 44 weeks prior to sacrifice, brain DA concentrations remained depressed and were not significantly different from DA levels in nonhuman primates sacrificed during exposure,[8] despite dramatic reductions in serum PCB levels (FIG. 1). This pattern suggests long-term, if not permanent, changes in DA function. A likely explanation for these persistent reductions in basal ganglia DA concentrations is based on our findings that the number of tyrosine hydroxylase–positive neurons in the nonhuman primate substantia nigra pars compacta was reduced by approximately 50% (FIG. 2).

These laboratory findings, incorporating both *in vitro* and *in vivo* techniques, provide compelling evidence that PCBs alter central DA function, including inhibition of monoamine transporter function, leading to premature death of central DA neurons. When combined with the aforedescribed studies in nonhuman primates, the

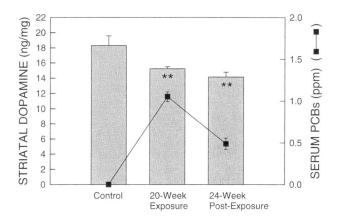

FIGURE 1. Striatal dopamine and serum PCB concentrations in nonhuman primates (macaques, *Macaca nemestrina*) exposed as adults to PCBs (Aroclor 1016, 20 weeks, 3.2 mg/kg/day) and sacrificed either immediately or 24 weeks following exposure. **$P \leq$ 0.01 compared to controls; $n = 3$–5 animals per exposure condition.

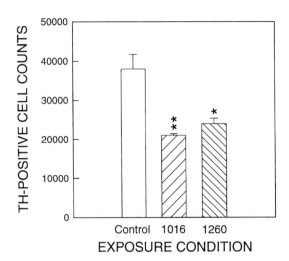

FIGURE 2. Tyrosine hydroxylase (TH)–positive cell counts in the substantia nigra of nonhuman primates exposed to 3.2 mg/kg/day of PCBs for 66 weeks before sacrifice. *$P \leq$ 0.05, **$P \leq 0.01$ compared to controls; $n = 3$ animals per exposure condition.

primarily *in vitro* studies suggest that high-level (e.g., occupational) exposure of adults to PCBs may have long-term consequences on DA-mediated function, including possible deficits in cognition and motor control. We have an opportunity to test that hypothesis in an aging cohort of former workers, who have been exposed to PCBs at concentrations so high that serum levels, measured 3 years after exposure ceased,[9] were at least 100-fold higher than those in nonoccupationally exposed individuals. Neurological and neuropsychological examinations of these workers will allow us to determine: (1) the relationships between PCB body burdens and observable dysfunctions and (2) whether pathology similar to that seen in adult nonhuman primates exposed to PCBs also occurs in aging former capacitor workers as determined by β-CIT SPECT imaging of basal ganglia DAT.

REFERENCES

1. JACOBSON, J.L. & S.W. JACOBSON. 1996. Intellectual impairment in children exposed to polychlorinated biphenyls in utero. N. Engl. J. Med. **335:** 783–789.
2. SEEGAL, R.F. 2001. Neurochemical effects of polychlorinated biphenyls: a selective review of the current state of knowledge. *In* PCBs: Recent Advances in Environmental Toxicology and Health Effects. L.W. Robertson & L.G. Hansen, Eds.: 241–255. University Press of Kentucky. Lexington, KY.
3. SEEGAL, R.F. 2003. Effects of polychlorinated biphenyls on neuronal signaling. *In* Dioxins and Health, 2nd edit. A. Schecter & T. Gasiewicz, Eds.: 433–455. Wiley. Hoboken, NJ.
4. MARIUSSEN, E. & F. FONNUM. 2001. The effect of polychlorinated biphenyls on the high affinity uptake of the neurotransmitters, dopamine, serotonin, glutamate and GABA, into rat brain synaptosomes. Toxicology **159:** 11–21.

5. MARIUSSEN, E., P.L. ANDERSSON, M. TYSKLIND & F. FONNUM. 2001. Effect of poly-chlorinated biphenyls on the uptake of dopamine into rat brain synaptic vesicles: a structure-activity study. Toxicol. Appl. Pharmacol. **175:** 176–183.

6. LAVOIE, M.J. & T.G. HASTINGS. 1999. Dopamine quinone formation and protein modi-fication associated with the striatal neurotoxicity of methamphetamine: evidence against a role for extracellular dopamine. J. Neurosci. **19:** 1484–1491.

7. SEEGAL, R.F., B. BUSH & K.O. BROSCH. 1991. Comparison of effects of Aroclors 1016 and 1260 on nonhuman primate catecholamine function. Toxicology **66:** 145–163.

8. SEEGAL, R., B. BUSH & K.O. BROSCH. 1994. Decreases in dopamine concentrations in adult non-human primate brain persist following removal from polychlorinated biphenyls. Toxicology **86:** 71–87.

9. LAWTON, R.W., M.R. ROSS, J. FEINGOLD & J.F. BROWN, JR. 1985. Effects of PCB expo-sure on biochemical and hematological findings in capacitor workers. Environ. Health Perspect. **60:** 165–184.

A Murine Model of ALS-PDC with Behavioral and Neuropathological Features of Parkinsonism

J. D. SCHULZ,[a] J. M. B. WILSON,[a] AND C. A. SHAW[a,b,c,d]

[a]Neuroscience Graduate Program and Departments of [b]Ophthalmology,
[c]Physiology, and [d]Experimental Medicine, University of British Columbia,
Vancouver, British Columbia 6T 1Z4, Canada

KEYWORDS: parkinsonism; amyotrophic lateral sclerosis (ALS); dementia

Amyotrophic lateral sclerosis–parkinsonism dementia complex (ALS-PDC) is an unusual neurological disease that occurs among the Chamorro people of Guam. It can express as ALS, an Alzheimer's disease-like disorder with parkinsonism features, or as a combined form with both motor and cognitive deficits. Kurland[1] and others recognized the importance of understanding the Guamanian disorders in the hopes of unlocking crucial clues to related neurodegenerative disorders worldwide. The strongest epidemiologic link to ALS-PDC is the correlation to consumption of flour made from the seed of *C. circinalis*, a species of cycad.[2] Cycad is known to contain potent toxins, some of which can be removed by the extensive washing procedures used by the Chamorros.[1] Early work using unwashed cycad and isolated components of cycad seeds in animal models failed to support a role for cycad as a causal agent in ALS-PDC.[3] However, to our knowledge, the critical *in vivo* animal experiments using washed cycad had never been performed.

To test the hypothesis that cycad neurotoxicity could be causal to ALS-PDC, we fed washed cycad flour to mice as part of their diet and used a battery of behavioral tests and histological assays to assess developing and end-state neural degeneration. (See Wilson *et al.*[4] for a complete description of the experimental methods.)

Cycad-fed mice showed significant decreases in motor, olfactory, and cognitive functions that correlated with neuron degeneration in substantia nigra, spinal cord, olfactory bulb, neocortex, and the hippocampus, as well as a decrease of dopaminergic terminals in the striatum. In regard to motor function, deficits were demonstrated by a significant loss of the leg extension reflex, which is indicative of motor neuron dysfunction (FIG. 1A). In addition, measurements of gait length, a marker of basal ganglia function that correlates significantly with cell loss in the substantia

Address for correspondence: Dr. C.A. Shaw, Neuroscience Graduate Program, Departments of Ophthalmology, Physiology, and Experimental Medicine, University of British Columbia, Vancouver, BC 6T 1Z4, Canada. Voice: 604-875-4111, ext. 68375; fax: 604-874-4376.
cshaw@interchange.ubc.ca

Ann. N.Y. Acad. Sci. 991: 326–329 (2003). © 2003 New York Academy of Sciences.

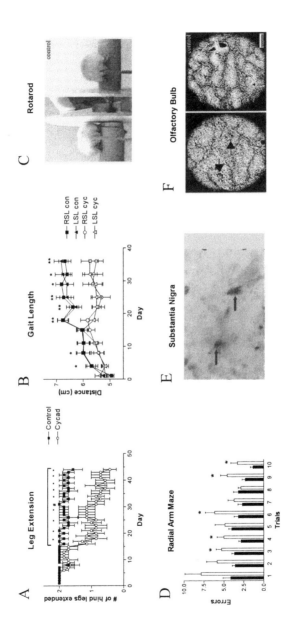

FIGURE 1. Motor and cognitive effects of cycad feeding. (**A**) Leg extension deficits in cycad-fed vs. control mice. (**B**) Gait length in the same animals. (**C**) On the rotarod, cycad-fed animals consistently leaned against either side of the barriers and adopted a hunched, "legs in" position. (**D**) Radial arm data showed significant learning and memory deficits in cycad-fed mice on reference memory tasks. (**E**) Histological assessment of cell death showing caspase-3 positive cells in the substantia nigra (*arrows*). (**F**) Caspase-3–positive cells were also observed in the olfactory bulb (*arrows*) along with a highly altered glomerular morphology. Significance: *$P < 0.05$, **$P < 0.001$, #$P < 0.0001$, ANOVA.

A

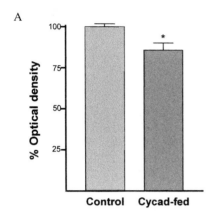

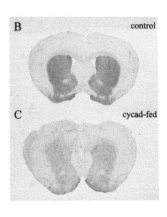

FIGURE 2. Effect of cycad feeding on tyrosine hydroxylase (TH) immunoreactivity. **(A)** Quantification of striatal TH staining shows a decrease of 16% in cycad-fed mice ($n = 3$ mice/group, $P < 0.05$, two-tailed t-test). Sections of the striatum **(B,C)** showed decreased expression of TH in cycad-fed mice.

nigra and striatum, showed a significant alteration in cycad-fed mice (FIG. 1B). Cycad-fed and control animals tested on a variable speed rotarod failed to show different latencies to "fall." However, cycad-fed mice displayed an unusual hunched, "legs in" position that was never observed in control animals (FIG. 1C) and a significant decrease in time to fall at high rotarod speeds.

Cognitive function was assessed with a radial arm maze, an indicator of working and reference memory with which cycad-fed mice demonstrated significant deficits (FIG. 1D). In addition, the olfactory system showed significant impairment (data not shown).

Apoptotic cell death was assessed with immunohistochemical assays for TUNEL or caspase-3. Apoptotic cells were observed in the olfactory bulb and the substantia nigra (FIG. 1E,F) as well as in the neocortex and the hippocampus of cycad-fed mice (data not shown). Assays for tyrosine hydroxylase (TH) immunoreactivity revealed a significant 16% decrease in striatal dopaminergic terminals of cycad-fed mice (FIG. 2A-C). In some animals, we also observed a decrease in nigral TH immunoreactivity that had not yet reached significance (data not shown). These results are significant as a basal ganglia dopaminergic deficit is the hallmark of Parkinson's disease and thus links the murine ALS-PDC model to parkinsonism pathology.

Our data suggest that we are observing the early stages of a disorder that, given time, would develop into a more classic end-stage form of ALS-PDC with greater behavioral and neuropathological outcomes. If true, we believe the murine model of ALS-PDC will be invaluable in the elucidation of preclinical pathology that leads to neurodegenerative disorders.

ACKNOWLEDGMENTS

This work was supported by the ALS Association, Parkinson's Disease Foundation, Scottish Rite Charitable Foundation of Canada, Natural Science and Engineering Research Council of Canada, and the U.S. Army Medical Research and Materiel Command (#DAMD17-02-1-0678) (to C.A.S.).

REFERENCES

1. KURLAND, L.T. 1988. Amyotrophic lateral sclerosis and Parkinson's disease complex on Guam linked to an environmental toxin. Trends Neurosci. **11:** 51–53.
2. KURLAND, L.T. *et al.* 1994. Amyotrophic lateral sclerosis–parkinsonism dementia complex on Guam: epidemiological and etiological perspectives. *In* Motor Neuron Disease. A. Willams, Ed.: 109–130. Chapman & Hall. London.
3. LILENFELD, D.E. *et al.* 1994. Guam neurodegeneration. *In* Neurodegenerative Diseases. D.B. Calne, Ed.: 895–908. W.B. Saunders. Philadelphia.
4. WILSON, J.M.B. *et al.* 2002. Behavioural and neurological correlates of ALS-parkinsonism dementia complex in adult mice fed washed cycad flour. Neuromolecular Med. **1:** 207–221.

Neuroprotective Ganglioside Derivatives

K. CONN,[a,b] S. DOHERTY,[c] P. EISENHAUER,[a,b,c] R. FINE,[a,b]
J. WELLS,[a,b] AND M. D. ULLMAN[a,c]

[a]VA Hospital, Bedford, Massachusetts 01730, USA

[b]Boston University School of Medicine, Boston, Massachusetts 02118, USA

[c]University of Massachusetts Medical School Shriver Center, Waltham, Massachusetts 02452, USA

KEYWORDS: gangliosides; neuroprotective agents

Natural and semisynthetic gangliosides protect neurons from injury. The hydrophilic property of gangliosides, however, restricts their blood-brain barrier (BBB) permeability when given peripherally. This hinders their use as neuroprotective agents. Gangliosides are amenable to chemical derivatization, so that semisynthetic derivatives with both cytoprotective properties and improved ability to cross the BBB can be produced. Therefore, ganglioside functional group derivatives that provide cytoprotection and effectively cross the BBB are being sought. This will provide a basis to understand neuroprotective mechanisms. Insight into neuroprotective mechanisms also requires an understanding of cell death processes. Thus, studies into 1-methyl-4-phenylpyridinium (MPP$^+$)-induced changes in gene expression are also ongoing.

Semisynthetic GM1 derivatives were synthesized and tested for their ability to protect SH-SY5Y human neuroblastoma cells from MPP$^+$ toxicity. SH-SY5Y cells were cultured at 37°C in a 95% air, 5% CO$_2$ humidified incubator and maintained in DMEM-high glucose supplemented with 10% fetal bovine serum. For cytoprotection experiments, 10×10^3 cells per well were plated in a 48-well cell culture plate and differentiated in the presence of 10 μM retinoic acid. After 4 days, medium was replaced with that containing 0.5% fetal calf serum and the test ganglioside (690 nM) 1 hour before exposure to MPP$^+$. Ganglioside was again added on the day after MPP$^+$ treatment.

For experiments on gene expression, 5×10^5 cells were plated in 100 mm^2 culture dishes in 10 mL of DMEM medium containing 10% fetal bovine serum, 100 units/mL penicillin, and 100 mg/mL streptomycin and cultured for 4 days. Freshly prepared toxin was added to the cultures and incubated for the requisite times. RNA iso-

Address for correspondence: M. David Ullman, VA Hospital (182B), 200 Springs Road, Bedford, MA 01730. Voice: 781-687-2636; fax: 781-687-3515.
david.ullman@umassmed.edu

Ann. N.Y. Acad. Sci. 991: 330–332 (2003). © 2003 New York Academy of Sciences.

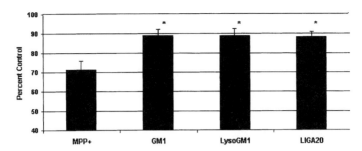

FIGURE 1. GM1, LysoGM1, and LIGA20 cytoprotection. Under the conditions described in the text, GM1, lysoGM1, and LIGA20 showed comparable cytoprotection. Values are percent control ± SEM. $n = 4$. *Differs from MPP$^+$ only, one-way ANOVA, Tukey-Kramer post-hoc test, $P < 0.05$.

lation and RT-PCR microarray and Western blot analyses have previously been described.[1,2]

For cytoprotection experiments, dose response and preincubation experiments performed with GM1 indicated that a 1-hour preincubation of 690 nM GM1 provided maximal cytoprotection against 1 mM MPP$^+$. This same preincubation period and concentration was used for lysoGM1 (GM1 amine, no ceramide fatty acid) and LIGA20 (GM1 with a dichloroacetate ceramide fatty acid). GM1, lysoGM1, and LIGA 20 were tested for their ability to protect SH-SY5Y cells from MPP$^+$ toxicity, and they showed comparable cytoprotection (FIG. 1). Further testing, however, is required to examine the effects of preincubation time and concentration on ganglioside-derivative cytoprotection. Nonetheless, these results imply that the ceramide fatty acid does not significantly influence cytoprotection in this model system or that the derivatives have different mechanisms of action. The ceramide fatty acid, however, most likely contributes significantly to blood-brain barrier permeability.

To better understand possible ganglioside-derivative cytoprotective mechanisms in cell death processes, the toxic effects of MPP$^+$ on mitochondrial gene expression were initially investigated in undifferentiated SH-SY5Y cells. It was found that MPP$^+$ decreased expression of NADH:ubiquinone oxidoreductase (complex I) subunit 4 (ND4), a mitochondrial gene important for electron transport chain complex I function.[1] MPP$^+$ did not affect expression of other mitochondrial (16S and COX1) or nuclear (B14) genes, indicating a degree of specificity for MPP$^+$-induced decreased ND4 expression.

Gene microarray analysis (Clontech) also indicated that MPP$^+$ exposure increased the endoplasmic reticulum (ER) stress-related gene GADD153. RT-PCR analysis demonstrated that GADD153 mRNA levels increased linearly up to 72 hours. Western blot analysis indicated that GADD153 protein levels increased to 24 hours, and caspase 3 activation increased linearly from 24–72 hours.[2] This suggests that increased GADD153 expression and ER stress may also contribute to the initiation of an active cell death mechanism in the SH-SY5Y cells. In parallel cultures treated with toxins whose primary mode of action is either via mitochondrial impairment (rotenone) or via oxidative stress (6-hydroxy dopamine or H$_2$O$_2$),

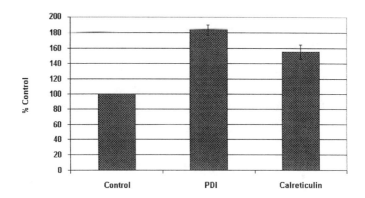

FIGURE 2. Expression of select ER stress genes in SH-SY5Y cells after exposure to MPP^+ (1 mM). RT-PCR analyses were performed using RNA isolated 72 hours after exposure to 1 mM MPP^+. Gene expression was normalized to G3PDH. Values are percent control ± SEM.

GADD153 expression was not increased.[2] This supports the possibility that a cellular mechanism different from mitochondrial impairment or oxidative stress—for example, ER stress—contributes to MPP^+ toxicity. In further support of an ER-stress–related mechanism, MPP^+ increases the expression of at least two other ER stress genes, protein disulfide isomerase (PDI) and calreticulin (FIG. 2). Thus, MPP^+-induced cell death may entail multiple pathways, and perhaps successful neuroprotection will require multiple therapeutic agents and/or therapeutic agents with multiple mechanisms of action such as gangliosides.[3] Knowledge of functional group requirements for ganglioside cytoprotection and a better understanding of cell death mechanisms will provide a basis for delineating their cytoprotective mechanisms and for targeting molecular structures to specific components of cell death processes.

ACKNOWLEDGMENTS

This work was supported by DoD Grant DAMD 170110779 and by Veterans Affairs Merit (K.C.) and REAP grants.

REFERENCES

1. CONN, K.J., M.D. ULLMAN, P.B. EISENHAUER, *et al.* 2001. Decreased expression of the NADH-ubiquinone oxidoreductase (complex I) subunits 4 and 6 in 1-methyl-4-phenyl-pyridinium (MPP^+)-treated SH-SY5Y neuroblastoma cells. Neurosci. Letts. **306:** 145-148.
2. CONN, K.J., G. WEN-WU, M.D. ULLMAN, *et al.* 2002. Upregulation of GADD153/CHOP in MPP^+-treated SH-SY5Y cells. J. Neurosci. Res. **68:** 755-760.
3. LEDEEN, R.W., S.-I. HAKAMORI, A.J. YATES, *et al.* 1998. Sphingolipids as signaling modulators in the nervous system. Ann. N.Y. Acad. Sci. **845:** 1–431.

Redox- and Metalloregulated RNA Bioaptamer Targets of Proteins Associated with Parkinson's and Other Neurodegenerative Diseases

Factors of Relevance in the Life Cycle of Cells

JOSEF H. WISSLER

ARCONS Applied Research Institute, D-61231 Bad Nauheim, Germany

KEYWORDS: Parkinson's parkin; Alzheimer's amyloid precursor; Huntington's huntingtin; prion PrP; S100 EF-hand; calgranulin; psoriasin proteins; RNA bioaptamer; angiotropin CuRNP ribokine; copper-ribonucleoprotein; angiogenesis; morphogenesis; Cu, zinc transition metalloregulation; nucleic acid-binding R3H domain; Fenton redox reaction; receptor for advanced glycosylation end products (RAGE); amyotrophic lateral sclerosis; fragile X syndrome; ubiquitinylation; proteosome; RNA-chaperone; 3D-rapid prototyping molecular model

INTRODUCTION

Some proteins of neuronal tissue and their genes involved in Parkinson's and other neurodegenerative diseases with complex clinical features (synucleopathies) have been considered unrelated, such as Parkinson's parkin, Alzheimer's amyloid precursor, prion (PrP), Huntington's huntingtin, S100 EF-hand, and other amyloidogenic proteins. Their physiological functions are still under debate. Parkin was shown to have conserved Cu,Zn-metalloregulator and also nucleic acid binding sites[1,2] in terms of short basic residue, SR/K/RS peptide segments, and conserved compact R3H (RxxxH) motifs besides known ring- and in-between-ring (IBR) finger domains (FIG. 1). R3H is a domain that binds single-stranded nucleic acids; it is related to regulatory canonical metal binding domains.[3–5] Secondary structure predictions and patterns of residue conservation suggest nucleation of helix-β-hairpin and adoption of helix structures upon binding of transition metal (Cu,Zn) ions and RNA.[3–5] Findings for S100 EF-hand, Alzheimer's precursor, huntingtin, and prion proteins were similar.[1,2,6–14] This suggests relationships in functions on a common structural basis in proteins by binding metalloregulated RNA or oligonucleotides. As shown,[9–14] some sequence-defined RNA bioaptamers (natural RNA targets selected by evolution) impart novel biofunctions to certain proteins that these do not have on their own.

Address for correspondence: Professor Josef H. Wissler, Ph.D., ARCONS Institute for Applied Research, Education and Didactics, Postfach 1327, D-61231 Bad Nauheim, Germany. Voice: +49-6032-31716; fax: +49-6032-31725.

jhw@arcons-research.de

Ann. N.Y. Acad. Sci. 991: 333–338 (2003). © 2003 New York Academy of Sciences.

```
Parkin      R3H     AA   265   HLYCVTRLNDRQFVHDPQLGYSLPCVAGCPNSLI.KE...LHHFRILGEEQ
Parkin      H3R     AA   114   GDSVGLAVILHTDSRKDSPPAGSPAGRSIYNSFYVYC..KGPCQRVQPGKL
Parkin      H3R     AA    87   DPRNAAGGCEREPQSLTR...VDLSSSVLPGDSVGLAVILHTDSRKDSPPA

APP         R3H     AA    29   AEPQIAMFCGRLNMHMNVQNGK...WDSD..PSGTK...TCIDTKEGILQY

Huntingtin  R3H     AA   774   CGTLICSILSRSRFHVGDWMGTIRTLTGNTFSLADCIPLLRKTLKDESSVT
Huntingtin  R3H     AA   884   FLEAKAENLHRGAHHYTGLLKLQERVLNNVVIHLLG..DEDPRVRHVAAAS
Huntingtin  R3H     AA  2898   AESLVKLSVDRVNVHSPHRAMAALGLMLTCMYTGKE...KVSPGRTSDPNP

PrP         R3H     AA   126   GGYMLGSAMSRPIIHFGSDYED.RYYRE..NMHRYP...NQVYYRPMDEYS
PrP         R3H     AA   141   FGSDYEDRYYRENMHRYPNQVYYRPMDEYSNQNNFVHDCVNITIKQHTVTT
```

FIGURE 1. Homology of (Cu,Zn)-metalloregulated nucleic acid-binding sites in Parkinson's parkin, Alzheimer's amyloid precursor (APP), Huntington's huntingtin and prion (PrP) proteins in terms of compact helix-nucleating and stabilizing R3H (RxxxH) domain.[1,2] Additional RNA-binding domains in terms of short basic residue and SR/K/RS peptide segments and canonical metalloregulator sites (e.g., HxxxH, octarepeats, ring fingers, etc.) are not indicated in this figure. Sequences arbitrarily cut off at amino terminal. R3H domain in parkin is separate from following in-between-ring finger (IBR) and second ring finger domain. It is noteworthy that parkin contains an additional antisense R3H (H3R), which extends almost symmetrical to the amino and carboxy terminal of the protein. APP contains further nucleic acid binding sites not noted in this compilation. The two R3H domains in PrP were shown to be surface located and therefore accessible to RNA bioaptamers.[23] The first R3H is highly conserved in mammalian PrP, whereas the second in some species is subject to mutation to R3H/N/Y.[1,2,6–8] It is noteworthy that R3H in the different proteins does not have the same detailed structure, indicating that proteins have functions, imparted by RNA bioaptamers, that are not identical, but related. Sequence source: NCBI protein data bank.

MATERIALS AND METHODS

Materials, methods, and definition of terms in use are described elsewhere.[9–14]

RESULTS AND DISCUSSION

In search of the endogenous RNA bioaptamers that fit to binding properties of proteins, methods were established to isolate and characterize sequence-defined intracellular and extracellular modified and edited, redox-sensitive, metal (Cu,Zn,Ca,Mg,Na,K) ion-regulated small RNA or oligonucleotides.[10–14] Thus, cytokine (ribokine) families of Cu ion-complexed ribonucleoproteins (CuRNP) were defined in structure and bioactivity (angiotropin). They consist of OH* radical redox reaction-sensitive, highly modified and edited, 5′-end-phosphorylated metalloregulated extracellular RNA bioaptamers (72-78 nucleotides) that impart novel biological roles to S100A12-like EF-hand proteins (calgranulin-C, hippocampal neurite differentiation factor, and angiotropin-related proteins, ARP) for cellular differentiation and morphogenetic reactions.[9–14] Structures and properties are shown elsewhere.[12–14] Biomolecular switching between functions is operated by metal ions and Fenton-type OH*-radical redox reactions with RNA modification by formation of labile adenosine-N^1-oxide in transit to isoguanosine nucleotides. Cu ions are necessary and not replaceable by Ca, Mg, and Zn ions for tightly complexing RNA to

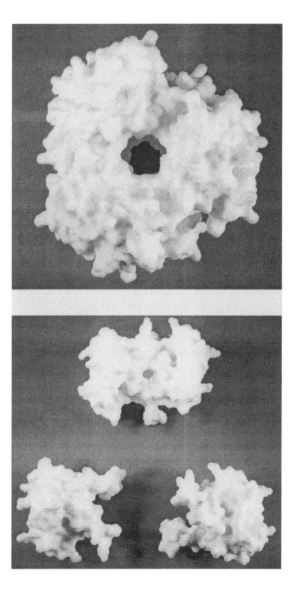

FIGURE 2. Accurate three-dimensional rapid prototyping molecular image models ($\sim 2 \times 10^7$-fold magnification) of an RNA-binding S100A12 ARP protein based on crystallographic data. [12,20–22] Sequences and properties are shown elsewhere.[9–14] **Bottom panel, lower two models:** Solvent (water)-accessible surface of two monomers in different positions (twisted by 90°) to form a dimer **(upper model).** The monomer[9–14] shows vicinally space-positioned helix-nucleating and stabilizing metal-binding domains and a 3-D groove for binding a Cu ion-prestructured small RNA. [12,20] By conformational rearrangement on dimerization, the metal binding domains are surface located in the dimer. **Upper model:** Solvent (water)-accessible surface of a slightly twisted hexamer as an RNA chaperone-shaped assembly with crater-like pits and horn-like protuberances, formed upon metallo(Ca,Cu)-

proteins and OH* radical formation by Fenton-type redox reactions. Findings were similar for intracellular oligo RNA bioaptamers as targets for proteins, such as transfer factors of delayed-type hypersensitivity reactions, psoriasin.[7,8,15–18]

To investigate functions, a novel method was applied.[19,20] Accurate three-dimensional rapid prototyping molecular image models (3-D RPM) of metalloregulated proteins can now be constructed when structural data of proteins are available in terms of X-ray crystallographic or NMR data—that is, retrievable from the Brookhaven Data Bank.[19] This allows detailed surface topography analysis of molecules in $\sim 2 \times 10^7$-fold magnified 3-D scale plastic image. Thus, for example, based on crystallographic data,[21,22] a 3-D RPM (FIG. 2) of Ca,Zn,Mg,Cu ion-regulated RNA-binding S100A12 EF-hand ARP monomer[9–14] shows vicinally space-positioned helix-nucleating and stabilizing metal-binding domains and a 3-D groove for binding a Cu ion–prestructured small RNA.[12,20] Upon metalloregulated oligomerization via dimers to hexamers, slightly twisted chaperone-shaped assemblies with crater-like pits and horn-like protuberances are formed, having an elliptically shaped internal tubular channel of ~4 nm in length. The internal diameter enlarging from ~1 nm at two entries to ~2.5 nm at the center allows transient homing and reforming of small RNA. It suggests RNA chaperone–shaped assemblies at cellular receptors in dependence of metal (Ca,Cu) ions.[20] Based on NMR-derived structure data, similar functional relationships are suggested for other (prion) proteins associated with neurodegenerative disease.[1,2,23] Because crystallography or NMR-derived structure data for parkin and other proteins are unavailable so far, such studies have to wait to be applied to them. However, in view of the known role of parkin in ubiquitinylation and possibly proteasomal processes in which involvement of RNA was shown, metallo(Cu,Zn)-regulated functions of parkin in supramolecular structure reformation/degradation comparable to chaperones likewise may be regulated or imparted by RNA bioaptamers. The considerations show the proteins also sharing properties with RNA-binding proteins in amyotrophic lateral sclerosis and fragile X syndrome.[24]

SUMMARY AND CONCLUSIONS

The results suggest proteins in neuronal tissues having common sequence homologies in helix-nucleating and stabilizing domains associated with defined functions (RNA chaperones and reformation). They may bind endogenous Cu ion-prestructured, OH* radical redox-sensitive, modified and edited oligo-RNA. Therefore, neurodegenerative disorders may be seen as related to disorders or impairment of functions imparted by binding of endogenous metalloregulated RNA bioaptamers to proteins that these do not have on their own. Thus, synucleopathies in which these

---

regulated oligomerization from monomers via dimers at cellular receptors for advanced glycosylation end products (RAGE). It has an elliptically shaped internal tubular channel of ~4 nm in length. Enlargement of the internal diameter from ~1 nm at two entries to ~2.5 nm at the center allows transient homing and reforming of small RNA.[12,20] The entries to the channel allow passage of reformed extracellular single-stranded oligoRNA (ssRNA) into the cell via RAGE to induce a cellular differentiation process.

proteins are involved may result from impaired redox- and metalloregulated RNA–protein interactions and reformation. Such disorders or impairment may deviate metal ion– and RNA-devoid protein structures to unfolding/misfolding and, thus, to disease. The propensity of some proteins to form redox- and metalloregulated RNA-chaperone–shaped assemblies for reforming RNA structures in cellular processes emphasizes the kinetics and thermodynamics of cellular topochemistry, binding, and turnover of RNA bioaptamers as factors of relevance in the life cycle of (neuronal) cells.

REFERENCES

1. WISSLER, J.H. & E. LOGEMANN. 2000. Bioinformatics applied to neurodegenerative diseases suggests physiological prion (PrP), Alzheimer's amyloid precursor (APP), Parkinson's parkin (P) and Huntington's huntingtin (H) proteins being (Cu/Zn)-metalloregulated RNA-binding protein families. Mol. Biol. Cell Suppl. **11**: 132a.
2. WISSLER, J.H. & E. LOGEMANN. 2001. Proteins of neurodegenerative diseases scrapie (cellular prion, PrP), Alzheimer (amyloid precursor, APP), Parkinson (parkin, P) and Huntington (huntingtin, H) are related in canonical (Cu/Zn)-metalloregulator and RNA-binding (R3H) domains. Biophys. J. **80**: 566a.
3. HIGAKI, J.N., R.J. FLETTERICK & C.S. CRAIK. 1992. Engineered metalloregulation in enzymes. Trends Biochem. Sci. **17**: 100–104.
4. VARANI, G. 1997. RNA-protein intermolecular recognition. Acc. Chem. Res. **30**: 189–195.
5. GRISHIN, N.V. 1998. The R3H motif: a domain that binds single-stranded nucleic acids. Trends Biochem. Sci. **23**: 329–330.
6. WISSLER, J.H. & E. LOGEMANN. 2000. Prion proteins (PrP) have conserved nucleic acid-binding (R3H) motifs: leads of ribokine structure to function and transfer of bioinformation in PrP infectivity. Biophys. J. **78**: 290A.
7. WISSLER, J.H. & E. LOGEMANN. 2000. Prion proteins (PrP) have conserved (HxxxH/N/G) metalloregulator (Cu/Zn) and nucleic acid-binding (R3H) domains: leads of nutrition factors and transfer of bioinformation in PrP infectivity. FASEB J. **14**: A794.
8. WISSLER, J.H. & E. LOGEMANN. 2000. Bioinformatics applied to prion proteins (PrP) suggest metalloregulated RNA-binding protein families with helix-nucleating and stabilizing canonical metalloregulator (HxxxH/N/G) and RNA-binding (R3H) domains. Biol. Chem. **381**: S234.
9. WISSLER, J.H., W.M. AMSELGRUBER, M. SCHWEIGER & E. LOGEMANN. 1997. Structure, function and cellular localization of angiotropin, a non-mitogenic leukocytic endothelial cell RNP-morphogen (ribokine) for organoid capillary pattern formation. Mol. Biol. Cell Suppl. **8**: 231a.
10. WISSLER, J.H. & E. LOGEMANN. 1998. RNA structure and modification of copper-RNP complex of angiotropin ribokines (non-mitogenic leukocytic endothelial cell morphogens). FASEB J. **12**: A1463.
11. WISSLER, J.H. & E. LOGEMANN. 2000. Ribokines with modified and edited extracellular eRNA: endogenous metallo-regulated copper-ribonucleoprotein cytokines (CuRNP) and their components (S100-EF-hand protein, RNA, precursors) in cellular signal transduction. Biol. Chem. **381**: S246.
12. WISSLER, J.H. 2001. Engineering of blood vessel patterns by angio-morphogens (angiotropins): non-mitogenic copper-ribonucleoprotein cytokines (CuRNP ribokines) with their metalloregulated constituents of RAGE-binding S100-EF-hand proteins and extracellular RNA bioaptamers in vascular remodeling of tissue and angiogenesis *in vitro*. Materialwiss. Werkstofftech. (Mat. Sci. Eng. Technol.) **32**: 984–1008.
13. WISSLER, J.H. 2002. Engineering of capillary patterns in muscle by a nonmitogenic copper-ribonucleoprotein angiomorphogen (angiotropin CuRNP ribokine). Ann. N.Y. Acad. Sci. **961**: 292–297.

14. WISSLER, J.H., E. LOGEMANN, H.E. MEYER, et al. 1986. Structure and function of a monocytic blood vessel morphogen (angiotropin) for angiogenesis in vivo and in vitro: a copper-containing metallo-polyribonucleo-polypeptide as a novel and unique type of monokine. In Protides of the Biological Fluids. H. Peeters, Ed. 34: 517–536. Pergamon Press. Oxford.

15. WISSLER, J.H. 1999. Prion modeling: potential of copper-mediated ribokine formation and relation of molecular mechanisms in bioinformation transfer of prion "infectivity" to virus-independent factors of transfer of (delayed-type) cell-mediated immunity. FASEB J. 13: A1510 and Biol. Chem 380: S208.

16. WISSLER, J.H. & E. LOGEMANN. 1999. Transfer factors of delayed-type hypersensitivity (TF-DTH): structure of copper-RNP cytokines (ribokines) and cellular and enzymatic biofunctions of their S100-EF-hand protein and oligonucleotide (RNA, dsDNA) units. FASEB J. 13: A1472 and Biol. Chem. 380: S208.

17. WISSLER, J.H. & E. LOGEMANN. 2001. Prion proteins (PrP) that (Cu,Zn)-metalloregulated bind RNA are related to transfer factors of delayed-type hypersensitivity: mechanisms of transfer of bioinformation and PrP infectivity. FASEB J. 15: A938.

18. WISSLER, J.H. 2001. Clonal selection of bioaptamers and diversity of oligonucleotide biolibraries in antibody-independent, antigen-specific delayed-type hypersensitivity (DTH), spongiform encephalopathy (TSE) and related transfer ("infectivity") reactions. Biol. Chem. 382: S99.

19. LAUB, M., T. SEUL, E. SCHMACHTENBERG & H.P. JENNISSEN. 2001. Molecular modelling of bone morphogenetic protein-2 (BMP-2) by 3D-rapid prototyping. Materialwiss. Werkstofftech. (Mat. Sci. Eng. Technol.) 32: 926–930.

20. WISSLER, J.H., M. LAUB & H.P. JENNISSEN. 2002. Non-mitogenic angio-morphogenesis by angiotropin: 3D-rapid-prototyping molecular modeling suggests RNA-chaperone-shaped assemblies of S100-proteins (calgranulins) at receptors for advanced glycosylation end products (RAGE) of endothelial cells. Mol. Biol. Cell Suppl. 13: 69a.

21. MOROZ, O.V., A.A. ANTSON, G.N. MURSHUDOV, et al. 2001. The three-dimensional structure of human S100A12. Acta Crystallogr. D Biol. Crystallogr. 57: 20–29.

22. MOROZ, O.V., A.A. ANTSON, E.J. DODSON, et al. 2002. The structure of S100A12 in a hexameric form and its proposed role in receptor signalling. Acta Crystallogr. D Biol. Crystallogr. 58: 407–413.

23. WISSLER, J.H., M. LAUB & H.P. JENNISSEN. 2003. 3D-Rapid prototyping molecular image models of cellular prion proteins (PrP^C) based on NMR data: metalloregulated interactions with copper-structured RNA bioaptamers and relation to RNA chaperones. FASEB J. 17: A595.

24. KAYTOR, M.D. & H.T. ORR. 2001. RNA targets of the fragile X protein. Cell 107: 555–557.

Dopaminergic Stimulatory Polypeptides from Immortalized Striatal Cells

ALFRED HELLER,[a] MARTIN GROSS,[b] SUZANNE HESSEFORT,[a]
NANCY BUBULA,[a] AND LISA WON[a]

[a]Department of Neurobiology, Pharmacology and Physiology, and [b]Department of
Pathology, The University of Chicago, Chicago, Illinois 60637, USA

KEYWORDS: dopamine; serotonin; trophic factor; cell lines; reaggregate
culture; mesencephalon; corpus striatum; nigrostriatal projection

Somatic cell fusion has been utilized as an approach to the immortalization of neurons for the purpose of obtaining monoclonal cell lines expressing neurotrophic factors.[1] Such fusions have permitted the generation of monoclonal hybrid cells derived from neurons of the nigrostriatal projection expressing specific transmitter phenotypes.[1–3] The cells include a striatal cell line (X61) that served as a source of possible trophic agents[3] and a mesencephalic cell line (MN9D) expressing a dopaminergic (DA) phenotype that was used as a test object.[2]

Cell lysates of the striatal X61 line have been shown to contain factors that have a stimulatory effect on both immortalized DA hybrid cells and primary DA neurons.[4] The DA stimulatory activity resides in a low-molecular-weight polypeptide fraction of less than 5 kDa.

The effect of this polypeptide fraction was examined on primary neurons using the three-dimensional reaggregate system that permits culture of mesencephalic DA and serotonergic (5-HT) cells in the presence or absence of appropriate target cells.[1] In the absence of target cells (mesencephalic-tectal aggregates), no axonal arbors are formed and most monoaminergic neurons disappear, presumably secondary to cell death. Some neurons survive and form fairly large processes, which appear to be dendritic in character and make autotypic connections with other DA neurons. We have already reported on the effect of the crude X61 stimulatory factor on DA neurons in such cultures in terms of increased DA content.[4] Here we describe the effect of the partially purified stimulatory factor on the morphology of both DA and 5-HT neurons by means of immunocytochemical methods.

A partially purified preparation (UF4) from X61 cell lysate was added (20 μL/mL) to the aggregate culture medium from day 1 to day 15 of culture. Aggregate sections were examined for DA neurons using an antibody against tyrosine hydroxylase, and

Address for correspondence: Alfred Heller, M.D., Ph.D., Department of Neurobiology, Pharmacology and Physiology, The University of Chicago, 947 East 58th Street, Chicago, IL 60637. Voice: 773-702-3513; fax: 773-702-3774.
effe@midway.uchicago.edu

Ann. N.Y. Acad. Sci. 991: 339–341 (2003). © 2003 New York Academy of Sciences.

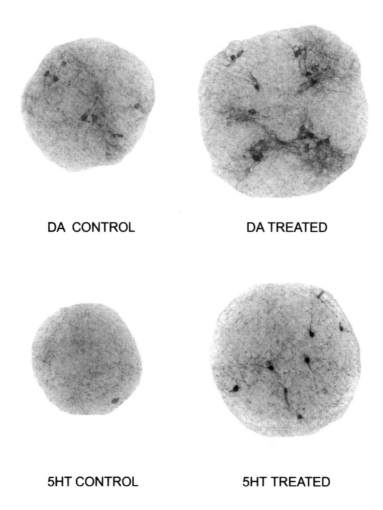

DA CONTROL   DA TREATED

5HT CONTROL   5HT TREATED

FIGURE 1. Immunocytochemical visualization of monoaminergic neurons in mesencephalic-tectal aggregates following treatment with UF4, a partially purified fraction obtained from the lysate of an immortalized clonal hybrid cell (X61) derived from embryonic murine corpus striatum.

for 5-HT neurons by an antibody against 5-HT. The results of this experiment are shown in FIGURE 1. With UF4 treatment, substantial numbers of densely stained DA neurons with extensive processes are observed. By contrast, while DA neurons are present in the untreated controls, such dense groupings of heavily stained cells with extensive processes are, at best, extremely rare. UF4-treated aggregates also contain 5-HT neurons and axons that are more densely stained than the cells observed in the untreated controls. Neurochemical analysis of the aggregates revealed a 30% increase in aggregate DA ($P < 0.001$) and a 52% increase in aggregate 5-HT following treatment with the UF4 partially purified preparation. Homovanillic acid, a major metabolite of DA, was increased by 75% ($P < 0.001$) in the media from UF4-treated aggregates.

A low-molecular-weight polypeptide fraction, obtained from lysate of immortalized monoclonal cells derived from the striatum, is, therefore, capable of increasing DA levels of both a monoclonal cell line (MN9D) and primary DA and 5-HT neurons in three-dimensional reaggregate culture. In addition, the polypeptide fraction increases the immunocytochemical staining of both cell bodies and processes of the monoaminergic neurons. Purification and sequencing of the active polypeptides will permit assessment of their efficacy in the reversal of the motor dysfunction that occurs secondary to degeneration of the DA nigrostriatal projection.

ACKNOWLEDGMENT

This research was supported by DAMD 17-01-1-0819.

REFERENCES

1. HELLER, A., *et al.* 1992. Study of dopaminergic neuronal differentiation and survival by use of three-dimensional reaggregate tissue culture and monoclonal hybrid cell lines. *In* Progress in Parkinson's Disease Research. F. Hefti & W.J. Weiner, Eds.: 403–426. Futura. New York.
2. CHOI, H.K., *et al.* 1991. Immortalization of embryonic mesencephalic dopaminergic neurons by somatic cell fusion. Brain Res. **552:** 67–76.
3. WAINWRIGHT, M.S., *et al.* 1995. Immortalized murine striatal neuronal cell lines expressing dopamine receptors and cholinergic properties. J. Neurosci. **15:** 676–688.
4. HELLER, A., *et al.* 2000. Cellular dopamine is increased following exposure to a factor derived from immortalized striatal neurons. Neurosci. Lett. **295:** 1–4.

Glutathione and Ascorbate

Their Role in Protein Glutathione Mixed Disulfide Formation during Oxidative Stress and Potential Relevance to Parkinson's Disease

GAIL D. ZEEVALK, LAURA P. BERNARD, AND JULIE EHRHART

Department of Neurology, UMDNJ-Robert Wood Johnson Medical School, Piscataway, New Jersey 08854, USA

KEYWORDS: glutathione; ascorbate; protein-glutathione-mixed disulfide; oxidative stress

Recent advances have identified several genetic mutations as causative factors in familial Parkinson's disease (PD). Yet, the sporadic form of the disease, representing 85–95% of the Parkinson population, has had no such evidence forthcoming. Instead, sporadic PD is associated with a selective loss of total glutathione in the substantia nigra, deficits in mitochondrial metabolism, and clear evidence of ongoing oxidative damage. The glutathione system and its associated enzymes are one of the cell's major defenses against oxidative damage. Given the 40–50% loss of total glutathione in sporadic PD,[1] the consequences of this deficit on the remaining nigral population and progression of the disease need to be considered. An appreciation of this, however, requires an understanding of the various functions carried out by the glutathione system. The most widely studied functions of glutathione are H_2O_2 removal, catalyzed by glutathione peroxidase, and toxin conjugation, catalyzed by a family of glutathione S-transferases. Less studied is the role of glutathione in protein glutathione mixed disulfide (PrSSG) formation, where the sulfhydryl moiety on a cysteine residue on a protein can undergo reversible sulfhydryl linkage with glutathione (see Ref. 2 for review). Both thiolation and dethiolation of proteins with glutathione are catalyzed by glutaredoxin. This enzyme was recently identified in the cytosol of brain neurons.[3] We[4] and others[5] have demonstrated a mitochondrial form of the enzyme. Glutaredoxin also contains dehydroascorbate reductase activity,[6] which is needed to maintain the reduced form of the antioxidant ascorbate in cells. Oxidative stress can increase PrSSG formation in cell cytosol and mitochondria (see Ref. 7 for discussion). The function of this increase in glutathionylation of proteins during oxidative stress remains controversial. It has been suggested to provide a beneficial role in protecting sulfhydryl groups on proteins from irreversible

Address for correspondence: Gail D. Zeevalk, Department of Neurology, UMDNJ-Robert Wood Johnson Medical School, Building UBHC, 675 Hoes Lane, Piscataway, NJ 08854. Voice: 732-235-3494; fax: 732-235-5295.

zeevalgd@umdnj.edu

Ann. N.Y. Acad. Sci. 991: 342–345 (2003). © 2003 New York Academy of Sciences.

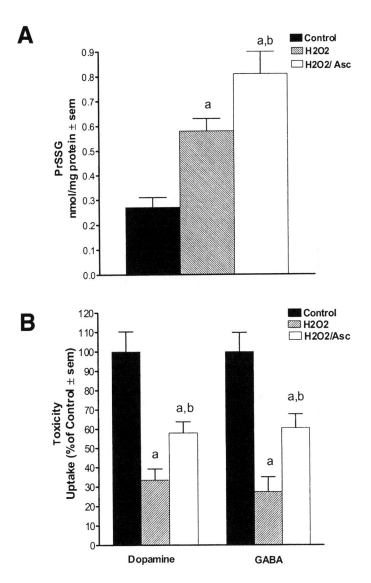

FIGURE 1. Rat mesencephalic cultures were exposed to 100 μM H_2O_2 in the presence or absence of 400 μM ascorbate for 6 h and **(A)** analyzed for protein glutathione mixed disulfides (PrSSG) or **(B)** returned to toxin-free medium and recovery for 72 h prior to assessing toxicity by measurement of the high-affinity uptake of ^{3}H-dopamine and ^{14}C-GABA. *Black bars* = control; *hatched bars* = exposed to H_2O_2 only; *white bars* = exposed to H_2O_2 in the presence of ascorbate. a = different from control; b = different from H_2O_2 alone (ANOVA, Tukey post hoc test).

oxidation as well as a detrimental role caused by alteration of protein function (see Ref. 7 for discussion). Given the dual function of glutaredoxin in thiolation/dethiolation and ascorbate reduction, the present study was carried out to examine interactions between ascorbate and glutathione protein thiolation to provide insight into the role of this enzyme and PrSSG formation during oxidative stress.

An oxidative stress was imposed in embryonic day 15 rat mesencephalic cultures by exposure to 100 μM H_2O_2 for 6 h in a bicarbonate-buffered Krebs-Ringer in the presence or absence of 400 μM ascorbate. Cultures were either immediately processed for total PrSSG levels (FIG. 1A) as described previously[7] or returned to toxin-free medium and allowed to recover for 72 h prior to assessing toxicity of dopamine and GABA neurons by a functional assay to measure dopamine and GABA transporter activity (FIG. 1B) as described in detail elsewhere.[7] H_2O_2 was equally toxic to mesencephalic dopamine and GABA neurons, and toxicity was partially attenuated by ascorbate. Mixed disulfide levels increased twofold with H_2O_2 exposure. Protection by ascorbate was accompanied by a further stimulation of PrSSG formation. No elevation in mixed disulfides was observed with ascorbate in the absence of an oxidative stress (data not shown).

To provide a more comprehensive picture of the effects of ascorbate on glutathione status during oxidative stress, cultures were exposed to 100 μM H_2O_2 plus or minus ascorbate for 6 h, and intra- and extracellular oxidized glutathione (GSSG) and reduced glutathione (GSH) and PrSSG levels were determined (TABLE 1). H_2O_2 exposure significantly decreased intracellular GSH, increased GSSG, and subsequently increased the oxidation status of the redox pair GSSG/GSH. The decrease in intracellular GSH could be accounted for by a large efflux of GSH into the extracellular space. Extracellular GSSG was also elevated. Ascorbate spared intracellular GSH and abrogated the rise in GSSG, thus maintaining the GSSG/GSH redox status. Evaluation of the effects of ascorbate suggested that maintenance of intracellular GSH and GSSG by ascorbate was due to an attenuation of efflux of GSH and stimulated incorporation of intracellular GSSG into mixed disulfides. In contrast, efflux of GSSG was not diminished by ascorbate. Glutaredoxin with its dual action as a dehydroascorbate reductase and thioltransferase could provide a link to coordinate these events as shown schematically in FIGURE 2. The reaction sequence depicted in FIGURE 2 would provide a threefold benefit to cells during oxidative stress. It would (1) recycle DHA back to ascorbate, (2) remove excess intracellular GSSG by incor-

TABLE 1. Effect of ascorbate on glutathione status during oxidative stress

	Intracellular				Extracellular	
	GSH	GSSG	GSSG/ GSH	PrSSG	GSH	GSSG
Control	24.0 ± 1.0	0.79 ± 0.06	0.033	0.27 ± 0.04	4.0 ± 0.35	0.35 ± 0.09
H_2O_2	19.4 ± 0.9^a	1.42 ± 0.12^a	0.073	0.58 ± 0.05^a	12.8 ± 1.1^a	1.25 ± 0.22^a
Asc + H_2O_2	22.7 ± 1.1^b	1.05 ± 0.17	0.046	$0.81 \pm 0.09^{a,b}$	$7.7 \pm 1.3^{a,b}$	1.09 ± 0.19^a

NOTE: Results (nmol/mg protein ± SEM) are from five experiments run in duplicate.
[a]Different from control.
[b]Different from H_2O_2 alone.

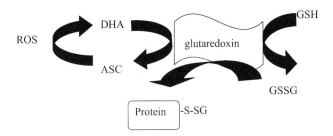

FIGURE 2. Schematic diagram of the coupled reduction of ascorbate and stimulation of glutathione protein mixed disulfides by glutaredoxin during oxidative stress. Ascorbate (ASC), by serving to remove free radicals such as superoxide and hydroxyl radicals, becomes oxidized to dehydroascorbate (DHA). Glutaredoxin, using GSH as an electron donor, reduces DHA back to ascorbate and forms GSSG in the process. GSSG can then serve as substrate for glutaredoxin in the formation of a protein mixed disulfide.

poration into protein, and (3) through mixed disulfide formation protect vulnerable sulfhydryl groups from irreversible oxidation to sulfinic or sulfonic acids, thus reducing the oxidized protein burden. Once the oxidative stress had abated, glutaredoxin, using GSH as electron donor, could further serve to reverse protein thiolation and return proteins to their reduced state. The significant loss of glutathione in the substantia nigra in PD will likely affect the ability of the glutathione system to carry out its various functions. In addition to H_2O_2 and toxin removal, the effects on protein glutathionylation and dethiolation should also be considered, as effective antioxidant therapy will need to carry out all the roles played by glutathione.

REFERENCES

1. JENNER, P, D.T. DEXTER, J. SIAN, *et al.* 1992. Oxidative stress as a cause of nigral cell death in Parkinson's disease and incidental lewy body disease. Ann. Neurol. **32:** S82–S87
2. MIEYAL, J.J., U. SRINIVASAN, D.W. STARKE, *et al.* 1995. Glutathionyl specificity of thioltransferases: mechanistic and physiological implication. *In* Biothiols in Health and Disease. L. Packer & E. Cadenas, Eds.: 305–372. Marcel Decker. New York
3. BALIJEPALLI, S, P.S. TIRUMALAI, K.V. SWAMY, *et al.* 1999. Rat brain thioltransferase: regional distribution, immunological characterization, and localization by fluorescent in situ hybridization. J. Neurochem. **72:** 1170–1178.
4. EHRHART, J., M. GLUCK, J. MIEYAL & G.D. ZEEVALK. 2002. Functional glutaredoxin (thioltransferase) activity in rat brain and liver mitochondria. Parkinsonism Relat. Disord. **8**(6): 395–400.
5. LUNDBERG, M., C. JOHANSSON, J. CHANDRA, *et al.* 2001. Cloning and expression of a novel human glutaredoxin (grx2) with mitochondrial and nuclear isoforms. J. Biol. Chem. **276**(28): 26269–26275.
6. WASHBURN, M.P. & W.W. WELLS. 1999. The catalytic mechanism of the glutathione-dependent dehydroascorbate reductase activity of thioltransferase (glutaredoxin). Biochemistry **38**(1): 268–274.
7. EHRHART, J. & G.D. ZEEVALK. 2001. Hydrogen peroxide removal and glutathione mixed disulfide formation during metabolic inhibition in mesencephalic cultures. J. Neurochem. **77:** 1496–1507.

Dopaminergic Neurons in Human Striatum and Neurogenesis in Adult Monkey Striatum

MARTINE COSSETTE, ANDRÉANNE BÉDARD, AND ANDRÉ PARENT

Centre de recherche Université Laval Robert-Giffard,
Beauport, Québec, Canada, G1J 2G3

KEYWORDS: basal ganglia; dopamine; Parkinson's disease; human brain; movement disorders; adult neurogenesis

INTRODUCTION

Dopaminergic neurons have been detected in the striatum (STR) of rats and monkeys, and their number was shown to increase in dopamine-denervated animals.[1-4] We also demonstrated the presence of such neurons in the human STR.[5] Because of its possible functional importance, we decided to characterize morphologically this unique striatal cell population in humans and investigate the possibility that new DA neurons are produced throughout adult life in the STR of monkeys.

METHODS

In a first set of experiments, quantitative stereological methods and immunofluorescence procedures were applied to postmortem tissues from 7 normal individuals (age range: 36–76 years; postmortem delay range: 3–30 hours). The chemical phenotype of the STR DA neurons was determined by using antibodies against dopamine-β-hydroxylase, dopamine transporter, neuronal nuclear protein (NeuN), and tyrosine hydroxylase (TH). In a second set of experiments, three adult male squirrel monkeys *(Saimiri sciureus)* were sacrificed 3 weeks following injections of bromodeoxyuridine (BrdU), a thymidine analogue; and their striata were examined for the presence of BrdU-labeled cells that express the neuronal marker NeuN. In both sets of experiments, a Zeiss LMS 510 confocal laser-scanning microscope served to image the fluorescence signals (see Ref. 6 for further technical details).

Address for correspondence: André Parent, Ph.D., Centre de recherche Université Laval Robert-Giffard, 2601, Chemin de la Canardière, Local F-6500, Beauport, Québec, Canada, G1J 2G3. Voice: 418-663-5747; fax: 418-663-8756.
andre.parent@anm.ulaval.ca

Ann. N.Y. Acad. Sci. 991: 346–349 (2003). © 2003 New York Academy of Sciences.

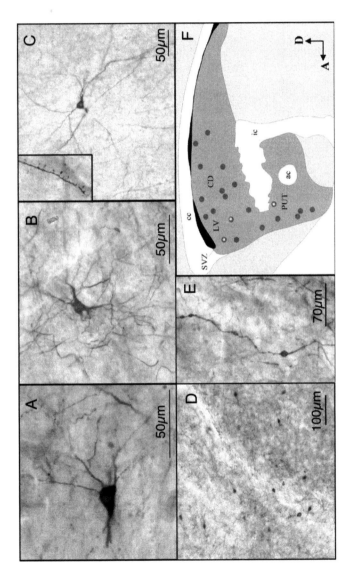

FIGURE 1. (**A–E**) Examples of DA neuronal profiles encountered in the human striatum. Medium (**A**) and small (**B**) TH+ neurons, together with a large multipolar TH+ neuron (**C**) whose dendrites are covered with spines, as shown at a higher magnification in the **inset.** (**D**) Low-power view of the ventral STR region that harbored numerous medium-sized TH+ neurons in two of the cases examined. (**E**) Example of thin and varicose TH+ fibers. Short segments of such fibers can easily be mistaken for small bipolar neurons. (**F**) Drawing of a sagittal section of monkey STR depicting the distribution and relative number of BrdU+ cells (*gray circles*) and BrdU+/NeuN+ cells (*gray circles with white core*), as seen 3 weeks after BrdU injection. ABBRE-VIATIONS: ac, anterior commissure; cc, corpus callosum; ic, internal capsule; LV, lateral ventricle; SVZ, subventricular zone.

RESULTS

Three types of DA neurons were encountered within the human STR. The most frequent ones had a round or oval perikarya of medium size (diameter: $20 \times 15–20$ μm) from which emerged 3–5 varicose aspiny dendrites (FIG. 1A). Neurons of the second type, which were about 50% less abundant than those of the first type, had a small cell body (diameter: $10 \times 10–15$ μm) with 3 or more varicose aspiny dendrites (FIG. 1B). Neurons of the third type, which represented less than 1% of the total population of STR DA neurons, had a large polygonal perikarya (diameter: 25–30 μm) with 4 or more dendrites endowed with spines (FIG. 1C). These 3 types of DA neurons were scattered throughout the entire extent of the caudate nucleus and putamen. However, in 2 of the 7 cases analyzed, a prominent cluster comprising 20–50 DA neurons per section occurred in the ventral STR, near the anterior commissure (FIG. 1D). Besides neurons, numerous TH-immunoreactive processes were present in the human STR (FIG. 1E). Short segments of these processes often displayed large swollen varicosities (diameter: 10–12 μm) and could thus easily be mistaken for small bipolar DA neurons. Such profiles were not taken into account in the present study because their varicosities lack NeuN immunoreactivity.

Various quantitative methods were used to evaluate the density of the STR DA neurons. The area of striatum was calculated with an image analysis system, and the neuronal densities were assessed by dividing the number of TH-positive neurons by the area of striatum surveyed. Because of the unequal size of our sample, factorial one-way ANOVA and Fisher's LSD methods were applied to compare the various density values. The Grubb's test was also used to look for the presence of outliers. The density of STR DA neurons varied significantly in the 7 individuals analyzed in the present study. The total number of DA neurons in the human STR ranged from 173 to 717, with a mean value estimated at 332 ± 199 neurons. However, this value is most likely an underestimate of the actual number of STR DA neurons, because only neuronal profiles that meet several stringent criteria were included in our sample. Furthermore, we did not include in the density measurements the ventral STR prolific zones that were encountered in 2 individuals and which could have raised the total number of STR DA neurons to about 3000.

Finally, numerous BrdU-labeled cells were visualized in the STR of monkeys injected with this thymidine analogue. Their number ranged from 5–50 per 40-μm-thick section. These BrdU+ cells were more abundant medially than laterally and displayed a rostrocaudal-decreasing gradient in caudate nucleus and putamen. Double immunofluorescence confocal studies have revealed that about 5–10% of the BrdU+ striatal cells expressed NeuN, a marker for mature neurons.

DISCUSSION

This study has allowed us to: (1) confirm the presence of DA neurons in the human STR; (2) characterize their morphological phenotype; (3) establish their topographical localization; and (4) estimate their number. Despite their relatively small number, these DA neurons could play an important role in the functional organization of the human STR in both health and disease. For example, they could compensate for the loss extrinsic DA innervation of the STR seen in Parkinson's disease by either upregulating their DA metabolic machinery or by increasing their number, as suggested by experimental studies in monkeys.[2] The absence of the aging pigment lipofuscin in the DA cells of the monkey STR has lead to the suggestion that proliferative progenitor cells might contribute to the increase in intrinsic STR DA cells seen in Parkinsonian monkeys.[2] This hypothesis is supported by the fact that new neurons are produced throughout adulthood in the STR of normal monkeys, as demonstrated here and elsewhere.[6] These findings raise the possibility of experimentally enhancing the recruitment of newborn DA neurons as a means to alleviate the symptoms of neurodegenerative diseases that affect the STR.

REFERENCES

1. DUBACH, M., *et al.* 1987. Primate neostriatal neurons containing tyrosine hydroxylase: immunohistochemical evidence. Neurosci. Lett. **75:** 205–210.
2. BETARBET, R., *et al.* 1997. Dopaminergic neurons intrinsic to the primate striatum. J. Neurosci. **17:** 6761–6768.
3. TASHIRO, Y., *et al.* 1989. Tyrosine hydroxylase-like immunoreactive neurons in the striatum of the rat. Neurosci. Lett. **97:** 6–10.
4. MEREDITH, G.E., *et al.* 1999. Immunocytochemical characterization of catecholaminergic neurons in the rat striatum following dopamine-depleting lesions. Eur. J. Neurosci. **11:** 3585–3596.
5. COSSETTE, M., *et al.* 1999. Extrastriatal dopaminergic innervation of human basal ganglia. Neurosci. Res. **34:** 51–54.
6. BÉDARD, A., *et al.* 2002. Proliferating cells can differentiate into neurons in the striatum of adult monkey. Neurosci. Lett. **328:** 213–216.

Secreted Factors from Primary Midbrain Glia Regulate Nurr1 Activity

Y. LUO[a] AND H. J. FEDEROFF[b]

[a]Department of Environmental Medicine and [b]Department of Neurology, Center for
Aging and Developmental Biology, University of Rochester School of Medicine,
Rochester, New York 14642, USA

KEYWORDS: dopamine; Nurr1; ligand; nuclear receptor; dopaminergic neurons; transcription factor

INTRODUCTION

Nurr1 is a member of the orphan nuclear receptor family. Previous studies have
demonstrated that Nurr1 is essential for the development of midbrain dopaminergic
(DA) neurons. However, the underlying mechanisms through which Nurr1 works are
still unknown. Overexpression of Nurr1 in neuronal progenitor cells is sufficient to
induce the dopaminergic phenotype only in the presence of secreted factors from
midbrain glia cells. Other studies also have demonstrated that the ligand binding domain of Nurr1 has the intrinsic capacity for transcriptional activation, depending on
cell type and mode of DNA binding. These data suggest that activity of Nurr1 might
be modulated by an unidentified coactivator and/or ligand in the developing and mature central nervous system.

In this study, we used different truncated forms of Nurr1 protein and a series of
reporter constructs to look at the regulation of Nurr1 by factors secreted by local glia
cells. Progenitor cells (C17.2) were transfected with full-length or truncated forms
of Nurr1 constructs and the reporter constructs. Cells were then incubated with either serum-free medium (SFM) or SFM combined with different percentages of conditioned medium (CM) from primary midbrain glia cells. The activity of Nurr1 was
assessed by the expression of reporter gene (lacZ or luciferase).

METHODS

Plasmids

Constructs containing full-length or truncated forms of Nurr1 are as shown in
FIGURES 1 and 2.

Address for correspondence: Howard J. Federoff, M.D., Ph.D., University of Rochester
School of Medicine, 601 Elmwood Ave., Rochester, NY 14642. Voice: 585-273-2190; fax: 585-
506-1957.

howard_federoff@urmc.rochester.edu

Ann. N.Y. Acad. Sci. 991: 350–353 (2003). © 2003 New York Academy of Sciences.

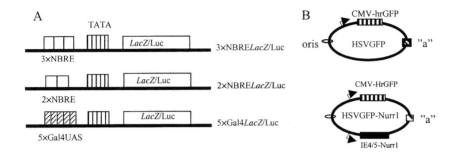

FIGURE 1. Nurr1 and NBRE reporter constructs. **(A)** The reporter constructs are composed of two or three copies of NBRE and Gal4UAS upstream of a minimal promoter and lacZ or Luciferase. **(B)** The herpes immediate early 4/5 promoter is used to drive expression of Nurr1, and the hrGFP is under the control of CMV promoter as a control.

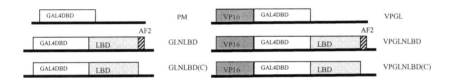

FIGURE 2. Nurr1 ligand binding domain constructs. Ligand binding domain of Nurr1 was fused to the Gal4 DNA binding domain. In NLBD C-terminal truncated form, NL-BD(C), the C-terminal transactivation domain (AF2 domain) is truncated. The VP16 activation domain (VP16AD) is fused to the N-terminus of the fusion constructs to examine the regulation of the NLBD on the activity of the N-terminus transactivation domain.

Primary Glia Culture and CM Collection

On embryonic day 18 (E18), embryos were removed from the uterus and placed into cold DMEM. Ventral mesencephalon was removed. Pooled tissue from 1–2 litters was minced into pieces of approximately 1 mm^3 and mechanically dissociated by triturating through Pasteur pipettes of decreasing bore size. Dissociated cells were plated into 60-mm dishes in 10% FBS DMEM. When confluent, cells were passaged into two T150 flasks and then allowed to reach confluence in about 3 days. Cells were washed three times with PBS and placed into SFM. After 3 days, CM was collected. Pooled CM was filter sterilized and stored at −80 °C until use.

Ultrafiltration of CM by YMT Membrane

CM was loaded onto Centriplus centrifugal filter devices containing various ultrafiltration membranes. The devices were centrifuged at 3000 × g at 4 °C for various times depending on the membrane type. The final volume of the concentrated fraction was less than 0.5 mL. The concentrated fraction was then diluted propor-

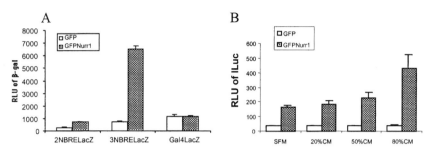

FIGURE 3. Nurr1 activity via NBRE is regulated by CM from midbrain glia. **(A)** Full-length Nurr1 induces the reporter gene expression in a NBRE-specific manner. Three copies of NBRE are more potent than two copies. Gal4UAS is not induced, demonstrating that the activation of NBRE is specific. **(B)** CM from midbrain glia cells enhances the activity of Nurr1 on 3NBRE constructs in a dose-dependent manner. GFP only was used as a control.

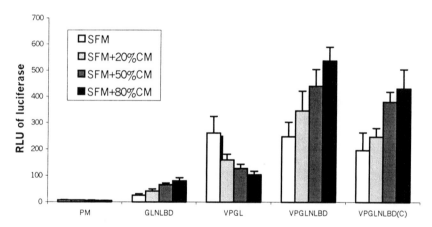

FIGURE 4. Conditioned medium regulates transcriptional activity through the ligand binding domain of Nurr1. Reporter gene expression after transfection of different constructs and treatment with CM is shown. The intrinsic AF2 activity of NLBD is demonstrated by the expression of reporter gene. Deletion of the AF2 core sequence completely abolished the activity in C17.2 cells (data not shown). The activity of NLBD was enhanced by CM in a dose-dependent manner. Moreover, although the NLBD(C) did not have transcriptional activity, it can regulate the VP16 AD activity in the presence of CM.

tionally into SFM and added to transfected cells. The filtratration fraction was also collected and tested.

RESULTS

Full-length Nurr1 protein activates reporter gene expression via a Nurr1-responsive element (NBRE), and CM from midbrain glia cells enhances the activity of Nurr1 in a dose-dependent manner (FIG. 3). Furthermore, the ligand binding domain

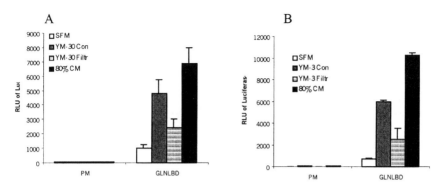

FIGURE 5. Concentrated and ultrafiltrated CM retained the enhancing activity for the Nurr1 ligand binding domain. C17.2 cells were cotransfected with the Gal4Luc reporter construct and GLNLBD. Conditioned medium was ultrafiltered through two types of YMT membrane (YM-3 retains molecules larger than 3KD, and YM-30 retains molecules larger than 30KD). The enhancing activity was effectively retained in concentrated fraction from both the YM30 **(A)** and YM-3 **(B)** membranes.

has an intrinsic transcriptional activity, which can be enhanced by the CM (FIG. 4). Our data demonstrate that a factor(s) in the CM from midbrain glia cells regulates the activity of Nurr1 through the ligand binding domain (LBD) and that the factor(s) can be concentrated by ultrafiltration (FIG. 5).

Development of Nurr1 Stable Cell Lines for the Identification of Downstream Targets

YU LUO,[a] LEIGH A. HENRICKSEN,[b] KATHLEEN A. MAGUIRE-ZEISS,[b]
AND HOWARD J. FEDEROFF[b]

[a]Department of Environmental Medicine and [b]Department of Neurology, Center for
Aging and Developmental Biology, University of Rochester School of Medicine,
Rochester, New York 14642, USA

KEYWORDS: dopamine; differential display; Nurr1; nuclear receptor; dopaminergic neurons; transcription factor

INTRODUCTION

Current evidence indicates that the transcription factor Nurr1 is critical for the development of midbrain dopaminergic (DA) neurons. First, transgenic mice lacking
Nurr1 function are devoid of DA neurons in the midbrain. Second, overexpression
of Nurr1, in combination with an unknown secretory factor from glia cells, is sufficient to induce the DA phenotype in neuronal progenitor cells (c17.2). However, the
cellular mechanism by which Nurr1 promotes the DA phenotype is still unknown.
Since Nurr1 is a transcription factor, we speculate that Nurr1 may exert its influence
on DA neurons by regulating the expression of a specific group of target genes. We
have developed cell lines with regulated Nurr1 expression and have begun to identify
potential downstream targets of Nurr1. The development of these cell lines will further our understanding of the role of Nurr1 in the development of DA neurons by
providing insight into the set(s) of genes regulated by Nurr1 function.

METHODS AND RESULTS

Autoreglated Bidirectional Expression Vector for Nurr1

Our laboratory has utilized an autoregulated bidirectional tetracycline-responsive
pBIG2i expression vector (FIG. 1) to establish stable expression of Nurr1 in the mesencephalic dopaminergic cell line MN9D. The bidirectional tetracycline-responsive
promoter is comprised of a $tetO_7$ element, a stronger CMV element that drives
cDNA expression, and a weak TK element to drive the transactivator (rtTA) expression. In addition, a selectable marker is added to allow for the production of stable

Address for correspondence: Howard J. Federoff, M.D., Ph.D., University of Rochester
School of Medicine, 601 Elmwood Ave., Rochester, NY 14642. Voice: 585-273-2190; fax: 585-
506-1957.
howard_federoff@urmc.rochester.edu

Ann. N.Y. Acad. Sci. 991: 354–358 (2003). © 2003 New York Academy of Sciences.

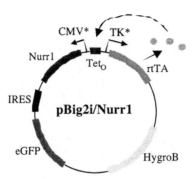

FIGURE 1. Schematic diagram of tetracycline-responsive vector pBig2I with Nurr1. (Adapted from Strathdee *et al.*[1])

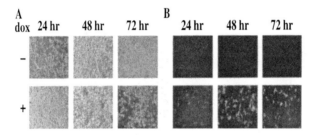

FIGURE 2. eGFP expression is induced following treatment with doxycycline in MN9D/Nurr1•IRES•eGFP cells. MN9D/Nurr1•IRES•eGFP cells were plated onto 24-well plates and induced with 2 µg/mL doxycycline for 24, 48, and 72 hours. Cells were plated at a density of 4×10^4 for 24- and 48-h time points and 1×10^4 for a 72-h time point. Following induction, cells were examined under phase contrast **(A)** and green fluorescence **(B)** to detect eGFP expression.

cell lines and an internal ribosome entry site in front of a codon-optimized enhanced green fluorescent protein coding region (human codon optimized eGFP), which allows for the monitoring of protein expression in live cells.

Production of Tetracycline-Responsive Autoregulated Stable MN9D

After establishing the appropriate concentration of hygromycin B for selection, MN9D cells were transfected with pBig2i containing either an eGFP or a Nurr1•IRES•eGFP insert. Following selection for 14 days, cells were isolated and expanded. Positive stable clones were detected by eGFP fluorescence after induction with doxycycline. Using both a cloning ring and the autoclone cell sorting method, we obtained a number of stable cell lines. The autoclone method produced pure clonal lines. FIGURE 2 demonstrates the effectiveness of this system for the regulated expression of eGFP and Nurr1 in MN9Ds. In the presence of doxycycline (Dox) eGFP expression is activated, while in the absence of Dox no eGFP fluorescence is observed.

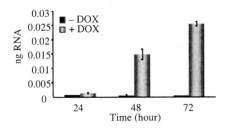

FIGURE 3. Nurr1 mRNA levels increase in a time-dependent manner following exposure to doxycycline. MN9D/Nurr1-eGFP cells were treated with Dox for 24, 48, or 72 hours. RNA was isolated, DNase I treated, and reverse transcribed. The amount of Nurr1 mRNA present was determined by qRT^2-PCR.

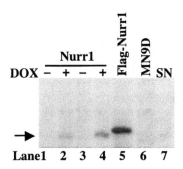

FIGURE 4. Following exposure to Dox, induction of Nurr1 is detected by Western blot analysis. Protein samples from two independent cell lines grown in the presence or absence of DOX were collected, separated by SDS-PAGE, and subjected to Western blot analysis. Nurr1 protein is detected only in Nurr1 stable cell lines following treatment with 2 μg/mL Dox (*arrow*; compare **lanes 1 and 3** to **lanes 2 and 4**). Positive controls include a BHK lysate containing Nurr1 fused to a Flag tag and transiently expressed **(lane 5)** and total protein from mouse substantia nigra (SN) **(lane 7)**. Nurr1 is not detected in the parental MN9D cell line **(lane 6)**.

Characterization of Nurr1 Stable Cell Lines

Nurr 1 mRNA expression was activated in this cell line after Dox treatment as determined by quantitative real-time PCR (qRT^2-PCR). The mRNA for Nurr1 increases approximately 15- to 25-fold after treatment with doxycycline for 48 hours (FIG. 3). As further confirmation, Nurr1 protein was induced as determined by Western blot analysis (FIG. 4). We have successfully used this approach to obtain multiple stable cell lines derived from MN9D cells.

Identification of Nurr1 Downstream Target Genes by Differential Display Analysis

Total RNA was extracted from MN9D Big2iNurr1 and Big2ieGFP cells with and without Dox (1 μg/mL) induction. Total RNA was subjected to differential display

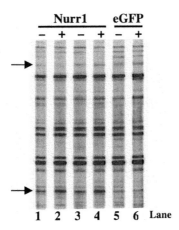

FIGURE 5. Differential display: treatment with DOX results in altered levels of selected mRNAs in stable Nurr1 cell lines. After 48-h incubation with 2 μg/mL Dox, mRNA was isolated and selectively amplified by PCR using primers designed for differential display in the presence of [^{33}P]dATP. Reaction products were separated on a 6% denaturing PAG and detected by phosphorimager. Shown is a representative gel. Transcripts that are either decreased or increased (*arrows*) are detected by comparing samples without **(lanes 1 and 3)** or with **(lanes 2 and 4)** Nurr1 expression (i.e., +/− Dox). These changes are absent in control lanes showing the parent expression vector containing only eGFP **(lanes 5 and 6)**. Typical changes range from 1.5- to 2-fold as quantitated by Imagequant (Molecular Dynamics).

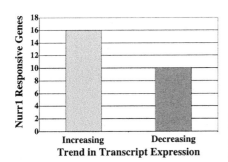

FIGURE 6. Summary of transcripts isolated by differential display. Bands identified by differential display with either an increase or decrease were excised and reamplified.

analysis according to the manufacturer (GenHunter; Nashville, TN). Following amplification, the samples were resolved on a denaturing PAGE and compared to each other. Transcripts more (or less) abundant were excised, reamplified, and isolated for further analysis and verification.

As shown in FIGURE 5, using one set of primers we visualize at least one differentially expressed gene following Nurr1 induction (arrows). This technique will allow for the identification and cloning of these differentially expressed genes. To date we have isolated 26 distinct transcripts (FIG. 6). As expected, comparison of these sequences with available databases results in both known genes and mRNAs of unknown function.

SUMMARY

We have employed the use of a vector containing a modified form of the tetracy-cline-inducible promoter system. There is minimal expression of Nurr1 in the "off" state. However, addition of doxycycline permits the expression of the reverse tetra-cycline transactivator (rtTA) gene and a Nurr1-IRES-eGFP transcriptional cassette from a bidirectional promoter. Thus, we are able to temporally follow downstream transcription events resulting from Nurr1 gain of function. We have established several Nurr1 clonal cell lines from the dopaminergic cell line MN9D. Currently, we are using differential display to identify changes in gene expression following the induc-tion of Nurr1 for 24, 48, and 72 hours. This approach detects genes whose expression is either increased or decreased following Nurr1 expression. We have detected tran-scripts with altered expresssion levels and are currently identifying the putative tar-get genes by sequencing.

REFERENCE

1. STRATHDEE, C.A., M.R. MCLEOD & J.R. HALL. 1999. Efficient control of tetracycline-responsive gene expression from an autoregulated bi-directional expression vector. Gene **229:** 21–29.

Index of Contributors

Alberí, L., 36–47
Ariano, M.A., 278–280
Arlotta, P., 229–236

Beal, M.F., 120–131
Bédard, A., 346–349
Benner, E.J., 319–321
Bernard, L.P., 342–345
Bezin, L., 307–310
Bhatt, L., 36–47
Biskup, T.M., 319–321
Boska, M.D., 319–321
Breidert, T., 214–228
Bremmer, S., 298–301
Brooks, D.J., 22–35
Brownell, A.-L., 281–283
Bubula, N., 339–341
Buchanan, T.M., 278–280
Burbach, J.P.H., 61–68
Burke, R.E., 69–79, 284–287

Carlson, K.A., 319–321
Casaceli, C., 315–318
Chen, I.Y., 281–283
Chen, L., 315–318
Chinopoulos, C., 111–119
Cho, J.W., 284–287
Choi, D.-K., 272–277
Chu, C.T., 288–290
Collier, T.J., 140–151
Conn, K., 330–332
Cossette, M., 346–349

Dawson, T.M., 80–92, 132–139
Dawson, V.L., 80–92, 132–139
DeLong, M.R., 199–213
Dervan, A.G., 291–294
Destache, C.J., 319–321
Doherty, S., 330–332
Duda, J.E., 295–297

Ehrhart, J., 342–345
Eisenhauer, P., 330–332

Fahn, S., 1–14
Farrer, M.J., 311–314
Federoff, H.J., ix, 152–166, 315–318, 350–353, 354–358
Fine, R., 330–332
Fisher, B., 298–301
Fiskum, G., 111–119

Gendelman, H.E., 319–321
Gherbassi, D., 36–47
Giasson, B.I., 295–297
Grissell, A.E., 278–280
Groc, L., 307–310
Gross, M., 339–341

Hamani, C., 15–21
Hardy, J., 167–170
Hartmann, A., 214–228
Hashimoto, M., 171–188
Hattori, N., 101–106
Heidenreich, K.A., 237–250
Heller, A., 339–341
Henricksen, L.A., 354–358
Hessefort, S., 339–341
Hirsch, E.C., 214–228
Hogg, E., 298–301
Hunot, S., 214–228
Hunter, T.J., 307–310

Imai, Y., 101–106
Ischiropoulos, H., 93–100

Jackson-Lewis, V., 272–277
Jakowec, M.W., 298–301
Jenkins, B.G., 281–283
Jiang, H., 307–310

Kadoya, C., 302–303
Kholodilov, N.G., 284–287
Kohbata, S., 302–303
Kress, G.J., 304–306

Lau, Y.-S., 291–294

Lee, V. M-Y., 107–110, 295–297
Levine, R.A., 307–310
Lim, K.L., 80–92
Lockhart, P.J., 311–314
Lozano, A.M., 15–21
Luo, Y., 350–353, 354–358

Macklis, J.D., 229–236
Magavi, S.S., 229–236
Maguire-Zeiss, K.A., 152–166, 354–358
Masliah, E., 171–188
Mayer-Pröschel, M., 251–271
McCarthy, M.K., 319–321
McGuire, S., 140–151
McNeill, T., 298–301
Meredith, G.E., 291–294
Meshul, C., 298–301
Michel, P.P., 214–228
Miller, R.M., 315–318
Mizuno, Y., 101–106
Mosley, R.L., 319–321

Nelson, J.A., 319–321
Nemechek, C., 319–321
Nixon, K., 298–301
Noble, M., 251–271

O'Farrell, C.A., 311–314

Parent, A., 346–349
Perlmann, T., 48–60
Petzinger, G.M., 298–301
Polster, B.M., 111–119
Power, J., 251–271
Przedborski, S., 189–198, 272–277

Reynolds, I.J., 304–306
Rockenstein, E., 171–188
Rousselet, E., 214–228

Schulz, J.D., 326–329
Seegal, 322–325
Sgadó, P., 36–47
Shaw, C.A., 326–329
Shimoji, M., 132–139
Simon, H.H., 36–47
Smidt, M.P., 61–68
Smith, J., 251–271
Smits, S., 61–68
Sortwell, C.E., 140–151
Starkov, A., 111–119
Steece-Collier, K., 140–151

Takahashi, R., 101–106
Teismann, P., 272–277
Tieu, K., 272–277
Totterdell, S., 291–294
Trojanowski, J.Q., 107–110, 295–297

Ullman, M.D., 330–332

Vila, M., 189–198, 272–277

Wallén, Å., 48–60
Wang, H., 132–139
Wang, X., 281–283
Wells, J., 330–332
West, A.B., 311–314
Wichmann, T., 199–213
Wilson, J.M.B., 326–329
Wissler, J.H., 333–338
Won, L., 339–341
Wu, D.C., 272–277

Yu, M., 281–283
Yu, S.-W., 132–139

Zeevalk, G.D., 342–345
Zelivyanskaya, M.L., 319–321
Zhu, J.-H., 288–290

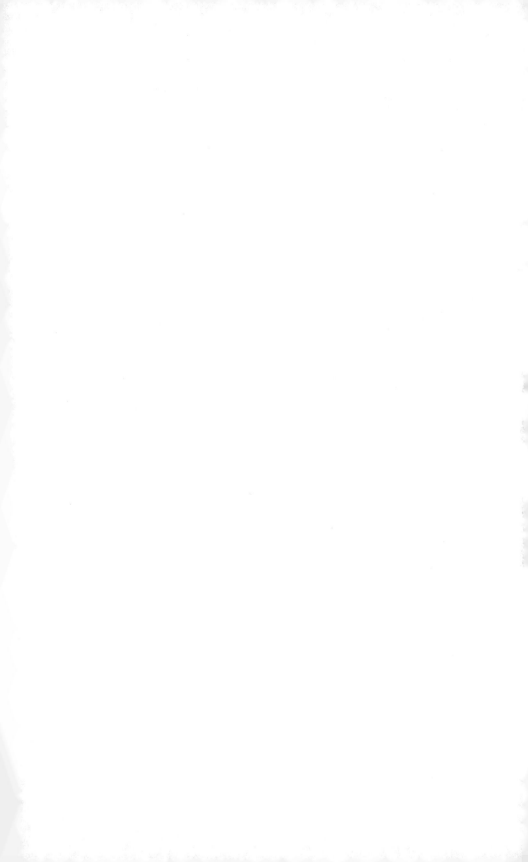

DATE DUE

New books— July 31, 2005